Cardiac Biomarkers

Cardiac Biomarkers
Expert Advice for Clinicians

Editor

Alan S Maisel MD

Professor of Medicine
Director, CCU and HF Program
Department of Medicine and Cardiology
VA Medical Center, University of California
San Diego, California, USA

JAYPEE BROTHERS MEDICAL PUBLISHERS (P) LTD.

New Delhi • Panama City • London

Jaypee Brothers Medical Publishers (P) Ltd.

Headquarters
Jaypee Brothers Medical Publishers (P) Ltd.
4838/24, Ansari Road, Daryaganj
New Delhi 110 002, India
Phone: +91-11-43574357
Fax: +91-11-43574314
Email: jaypee@jaypeebrothers.com

Overseas Offices

J.P. Medical Ltd.
83 Victoria Street London
SW1H 0HW (UK)
Phone: +44-2031708910
Fax: +02-03-0086180
Email: info@jpmedpub.com

Jaypee-Highlights Medical Publishers Inc.
City of Knowledge, Bld. 237, Clayton
Panama City, Panama
Phone: +507-317-0160
Fax: +507-301-0499
Email: cservice@jphmedical.com

Website: www.jaypeebrothers.com
Website: www.jaypeedigital.com

© 2012, Jaypee Brothers Medical Publishers

Inquiries for bulk sales may be solicited at: jaypee@jaypeebrothers.com

Editorial & Production : Shaila Prashar, Maheshweta Trivedi, Eti Dinesh, DC Gupta, Naren Aggarwal

Cardiac Biomarkers: Expert Advice for Clinicians / Ed. Alan S Maisel

First Edition: **2012**

ISBN 978-93-5025-564-3

Printed at: Sanat Printers, Kundli.

Dedicated to
my wife, Francine Fomon-Maisel
who has been a tremendous source of
support and love

Contents

Section 4: Biomarkers in Cardiorenal Desease

Section 5: Looking towards the Future

Contributors

EDITOR

Alan S Maisel MD
Professor of Medicine
Director, CCU and HF Program
Department of Medicine and Cardiology
VA Medical Center, University of California
San Diego, California, USA

CONTRIBUTING AUTHORS

Rudolf A de Boer MD PhD FESC
Department of Cardiology
University Medical Center Groningen
The Netherlands

Dinna N Cruz MD MPH
Director for Research
Department of Nephrology, Dialysis,
and Transplantation
San Bortolo Hospital
International Renal Research Institute
(IRRIV)
Vicenza, Italy

Lori B Daniels MD MAS FACC
Associate Professor of Medicine
Associate Director
Cardiac Care Unit
UCSD Division of Cardiology
Sulpizio Cardiovascular Center
San Diego, California, USA

Arrash Fard MD
Research Associate
VA San Diego Healthcare System
University of California
San Diego, California, USA

Gerasimos S Filippatos MD FACC
FCCP FESC
Department of Cardiology
Heart Failure Unit
Attikon University Hospital
Athens, Greece

Hanna Kim Gaggin MD MPH
Clinical Research Fellow
Graduate Medical Assistant
Division of Cardiology
Massachusetts General Hospital
Boston, Massachusetts, USA

Navaid Iqbal MD
Research Associate
VA San Diego Healthcare System
University of California
San Diego, California, USA

Allan S Jaffe MD
Professor of Medicine
Consultant in Cardiology and
Laboratory Medicine and Pathology
Chair, Core Clinical Laboratories
Services
Mayo Clinic and Medical School
Rochester, Minnesota, USA

James L Januzzi Jr MD FACC FESC
Associate Professor of Medicine
Harvard Medical School
Director, Cardiac Intensive Care Unit
Division of Cardiology
Massachusetts General Hospital
Boston, Massachusetts, USA

Manish Kaushik MD
Department of Nephrology, Dialysis
and Transplantation
San Bortolo Hospital
Vicenza, Italy
Department of Nephrology
Singapore General Hospital
Singapore

Payal Kohli MD
Fellow, Cardiovascular Division
Department of Medicine
Brigham & Women's Hospital
TIMI Study Group
Boston, Massachusetts, USA

Anna McDivit MD
Cardiology Fellow
Division of Cardiology
University of California
San Diego, California, USA

Ravindra L Mehta MBBS MD DM FACP
FRCP FASN
Professor of Clinical Medicine
Associate Chair for Clinical Research
Department of Medicine
Director of Clinical Nephrology and
Dialysis Programs
Division of Nephrology
Associate Director of the GCRC
UCSD Medical Center
University of California
San Diego, California, USA

Maxi Meissner PhD
Experimental Cardiology section
Department of Cardiology
University Medical Center Groningen
The Netherlands

Nils G Morgenthaler MD PhD MBA
Institut für Experimentelle
Endokrinologie
Charité Universitätsmedizin Berlin
Campus Virchow-Klinikum
Augustenburger
Berlin, Germany

David A Morrow MD MPH
Director, Levine Cardiac Unit
Cardiovascular Division
Brigham & Women's Hospital
Senior Investigator, TIMI Study Group
Associate Professor of Medicine
Harvard Medical School
Boston, Massachusetts, USA

John T Parissis MD
Associate Professor of Cardiology
Heart failure Unit
Attikon University Hospital
University of Athens
Athens, Greece

W Frank Peacock MD FACEP
Professor
Vice Chief, Emergency Medicine
Cleveland Clinic Foundation
Cleveland, Ohio, USA

Mark Richards MBChB MD PhD DSc FRACP
FRCP FRSNZ
Professor in Medicine
Director, Cardiovascular Research
Institute
University of Otago
Christchurch, New Zealand

Claudio Ronco MD
Director
Department of Nephrology, Dialysis,
and Transplantation
San Bortolo Hospital
International Renal Research Institute
(IRRIV)
Vicenza, Italy

Leo Slavin MD
Deparment of Cardiology
Southern California Permanente
Medical Group
San Marcos, California, USA

Adam Taleb MD
Post-Doctoral Fellow
Department of Medicine
Division of Cardiology
Vascular Medicine Program
University of California
San Diego, California, USA

Pam R Taub MD
Assistant Professor of Medicine
Board Certification in Internal Medicine
Board Certification in Nuclear
Cardiology
Cardiovascular Health - Women
University of California
San Diego, California, USA

Tertius Tuy
Duke-NUS Graduate Medical School
Singapore

Sotirios Tsimikas MD FACC FAHA FSCAI
Professor of Medicine
Director of Vascular Medicine
Department of Medicine
Division of Cardiology
Vascular Medicine Program
University of California
San Diego, California, USA

Dirk J van Veldhuisen MD PhD FESC FACC
Chairman and Professor of Cardiology
University Medical Center Groningen
The Netherlands

Alan HB Wu PhD DABCC
Professor of Laboratory Medicine
University of California
Section Chief, Clinical Chemistry, and
Toxicology
San Francisco General Hospital
San Francisco, California, USA

Yang Xue MD
Cardiology Fellow
UCSD Medical Center
University of California
San Diego, California, USA

Preface

Cardiac biomarkers have permeated our hospitals and research laboratories like no other time in the recent history. Thus, it is essential that healthcare practitioners have a clear understanding of this rapidly evolving field so that we can use them to better arm ourselves in the care of the patient. It is in this light that we present "Cardiac Biomarkers: Expert Advice for Clinicians."

We have divided this book in five sections. Section one deals with markers of cardiac risk. Here we give an overview of why this is such an important area covering some of the new exciting biomarkers. In specific, the oxidized phospholipids appear to play an ever-increasing role in detecting early cardiovascular risk.

In the section "Markers of cardiac ischemia," we tackle one of the most important and rapidly growing areas in medicine today—acute coronary syndrome. Understanding how the new "high-sensitive" troponins work is crucial to patient care, both for rapid diagnosis and effective triage. Besides exploring both the laboratory and the emergency department (ED) perspectives, we also offer insight on the potential new biomarkers for acute coronary ischemia that should add to the value of the new high-sensitivity troponins.

Natriuretic peptides (NPs) are firmly established as biomarkers for making the diagnosis of heart failure as well as ruling out heart failure in the patient presenting with shortness of breath. There are caveats to their use, such as renal failure, obesity, and the gray zone, and these are discussed as well as alogorithms for their use in the ED. NPs are extremely useful for risk stratification, and can help determine who should be admitted and potentially what treatment they should receive. Levels of NPs drop quickly as the volume overloaded patient is diuresed. Thus, using BNP levels should help one determine the optivolemic state and aid in discharge decisions. The lower the NP at discharge the less likely readmission will occur. The future for NPs will be discussed in terms of using these markers in the outpatient area. This will include as a monitor for decompensation as well as a way to guide outpatient therapy.

One of the most novel and relevant areas of biomarker translational work is in the setting of cardiorenal disease. The new definition of cardiorenal syndromes as well as the implications of these syndromes on medical management are discussed. Biomarkers of renal injury can be used to detect functional damage to the kidney up to two days before one sees the structural changes manifested by serum creatinine. These new biomarkers of early detection should allow us to target renal preventative therapy with more confidence as well as eventually target specific new treatments that will be developed. These treatments may include those that prevent renal toxicity from contrast media or nephrotoxic drugs. Additionally, renal injury markers might target a patient with sepsis for early dialysis, perhaps even before serum creatinine is elevated.

In the final section we take a look toward the future of biomarkers, with specific emphasis on a number of the most promising markers. Adrenomedullin appears to be perhaps the most robust biomarker of prognosis in patients with dsypnea and perhaps other diseases as well. Galectin-3, a marker of fibrosis, should allow us to target popoulations at risk for myocardial fibrosis and perhaps lead to the institution of early preventative treatment. ST-2 is a biomarker that transcends myocardial stretch and inflammation, and its future looks promising. Finally, copeptin, a pro-hormone surrogate for arginine vasopressin, may be a marker of early myocardial infarction as well as be a guide to heart failure treatemnt with a vasopressing antagonist.

Biomarkers are never stand-alone tests, but rather adjuncts to what the clinicians bring to the table with respect to their history-taking, physical examination, and other tests. There are always caveats and learning curves when using biomarkers. I believe in the following:

"Biomarkers will make a bad doctor worse and a good doctor better."

That is the purpose of this book. Make good doctors better.

Alan S Maisel
amaisel@ucsd.edu

Acknowledgments

I express my sincere gratitude to Steve Carter, Laboratory Manager for over twenty years who is instrumental for everything I accomplish.

I am thankful to the team at Jaypee Brothers Medical Publishers—Manoj Kumar, Sachin Dhawan, Shaila Prashar, Maheshweta Trivedi, Eti Dinesh, DC Gupta, and Naren Aggarwal—for their timely and consistent efforts to help complete this project.

Overview of Markers of Cardiac Risk

Lori B Daniels

INTRODUCTION

The past decade has seen an immense growth in the use of biomarkers in clinical care. Biomarkers are prevalent in numerous fields of medicine and are utilized in a wide variety of ways. These include screening for subclinical disease, diagnosis, risk stratification or prognosis, monitoring disease or titration of therapy, and determination of eligibility for specific therapies. Of all fields, cardiology is among the most prolific in its use of biomarkers, both novel and established, for the above applications. With an accelerating deluge of novel biomarkers emerging in the cardiovascular literature, it can be a daunting task to separate out the useful and promising ones from the rest. The chapter overviews some of the criteria for identifying valuable biomarkers of cardiac risk, and some of the emerging strategies and applications for these markers.

CRITERIA FOR A CLINICALLY USEFUL BIOMARKER

There are a large number of aspiring biomarkers, only a subset of which will rise through the ranks and be accepted into clinical care. As outlined by Morrow and de Lemos,[1] a clinically useful biomarker should meet several criteria. The first criteria relate to the measurability of the marker: the assay should be accurate and reproducible with good stability of the analyte, fast turnaround time, and a reasonable cost profile. Second, the biomarker should provide information that improves upon existing data and tests, as evidenced by multiple studies confirming an association between the marker and the outcome or disease, and with validated decision cut-points. Finally, use of the biomarker should in some way contribute to improved patient care. Of note, while an ideal biomarker was once thought to require both high sensitivity and high specificity, in most cases, it is perfectly acceptable to have one or the other (i.e., a high sensitivity troponin will have reduced specificity).

Uses of Biomarkers

Biomarkers may contribute to improved patient care in a number of different ways. Some biomarkers are useful for screening for subclinical disease (e.g., prostate specific antigen and prostate cancer), or for disease susceptibility (e.g., cholesterol levels and risk of coronary artery disease). Another application is in the diagnosis of overt disease as seen with cardiac troponin for diagnosing myocardial infarction, which is now incorporated into the "universal definition of myocardial infarction" and practice guidelines.[2] Biomarkers can be used for risk stratification and prognostication; for example, in the setting of heart failure or acute coronary syndrome, elevated levels of a number of markers have been associated with short- and long-term outcomes.[3-5] Another application is for monitoring and titration of therapy. Biomarkers can also assist clinicians with determining a patient's eligibility for specific therapies, for instance, by identifying a higher risk group, which may benefit from more aggressive treatments.[6] Often, one biomarker can fulfill several of these roles, for instance, natriuretic peptides, though initially heralded for their aid in diagnosing acute heart failure,[7] are also quite useful in risk stratification.[8] Additionally, they are gaining momentum in titration of outpatient therapy,[9] and have also been extensively evaluated for their ability to screen for subclinical cardiovascular disease.[10]

Evaluation of Markers

Recent guidelines described the appropriate evaluation of novel markers of cardiovascular risk, and outlined recommendations for the reporting of novel markers as well as the phases of evaluation, which each marker should be subject to.[11] This scientific statement emphasized that no single statistical measure can incorporate all important aspects of a marker's utility, and outlined the various assessments that should be considered. For any given study, these assessments include an estimate of the effect size and statistical significance of the marker alone, of the marker after adjustment for established risk factors, and of the marker added to a model with standard risk markers. In addition, the authors recommended describing the discrimination of the marker (the probability that the predicted risk, based on the marker, is higher for someone with disease than for someone without) by using both the improvement in the c-statistic (area under the receiver operator characteristic curve) for the novel marker when added to standard markers, as well as the integrated discrimination index. Finally, the statement suggested including measures of the marker's accuracy, including the observed versus expected event rates, and an assessment of how well the novel marker reclassifies individuals within established risk categories.

In evolving from a newly identified biomarker with uncharted potential, to an established marker with proven clinical benefit, a marker must complete several phases of evaluation.[11] Initially, proof of concept studies help identify potential novel markers by identifying a trend that shows different levels of the marker in individuals with a given outcome, compared to those without. The marker then must be prospectively validated in cohort studies, which show that it can predict the development of future outcomes, and that it adds incremental value to standard risk markers. Ultimately, a marker must have clinical utility and be cost-effective, and so studies are needed, which show that the marker changes not only treatment recommendations but also clinical outcomes in a meaningful and economical way.

CATEGORIES OF BIOMARKERS

Biomarkers of cardiovascular risk come in various forms, and can include hormones, enzymes, and other biologic proteins and substances. Most cardiovascular biomarkers fall into one of several categories (Table 1-1), though some markers can span several categories. For instance, growth differentiation factor-15 (GDF-15), a member of the transforming growth factor-β superfamily and originally identified in activated macrophages, is induced in the myocardium in response to ischemia, but is also potentially a marker of atherosclerosis, and to some degree, of more

Table 1-1	Categories of Biomarkers of Cardiovascular Risk[*]
Markers of myocardial strain, e.g., BNP, NT-proBNP, MR-proANP, osteoprotegerin, MR-proADM, copeptin	
Markers of myocardial cell damage, e.g., cardiac troponins (sensitive), creatine phosphokinase MB, myoglobin	
Markers of ischemia, e.g., ischemia modified albumin, heart-type fatty acid-binding protein, choline, MPO	
Markers of inflammation/vascular damage, e.g., CRP, IL-6, TNF-α, adiponectin, pentraxin 3	
Markers of extracellular matrix/remodeling/fibrosis, e.g., MMPs, tissue inhibitors of MMPs, collagen propeptides (pro-collagen 3), ST2, galectin-3	
Markers of atherosclerosis/unstable plaque, e.g., Lp(a), Lp-PLA$_2$, OxLDL, GDF-15, MPO, placental growth factor, PAPP-A, secretory phospholipase A$_2$, soluble fms-like tyrosine kinase 1, soluble ICAM 1, endothelin, osteopontin, NGAL	
Renal markers, e.g., cystatin C, creatinine, NGAL, urinary albumin:creatinine ratio, KIM-1, beta-trace protein	
Genetic markers, e.g., single nucleotide polymorphisms, structural variants	

[*]Categories are Not mutually exclusive.
BNP, B-type natriuretic peptide; CRP, C-reactive protein; GDF-15, growth differentiation factor-15; ICAM, intercellular adhesion molecule; IL-6, interleukin 6; KIM-1, kidney injury marker-1; Lp(a), lipoprotein (a); Lp-PLA$_2$, lipoprotein phospholipase A$_2$; MMPs, matrix metalloproteinases; MPO, myeloperoxidase; MR-proADM, mid-regional proadrenomedullin; MR-proANP, mid-regional proatrial natriuretic peptide; NGAL, neutrophil gelatinase associated lipocalin; NT-proBNP, N-terminal proBNP; OxLDL, oxidized low-density lipoprotein; PAPP-A, pregnancy-associated plasma protein A; TNF-α, tumor necrosis factor-α.

generalized myocardial stress. Thus, while the parsing of biomarkers into categories is somewhat contrived, it nonetheless provides an instructive framework.

Markers of Myocardial Injury

Myocardial injury occurs not only in the setting of acute coronary occlusion but also in several other well-documented situations.[12] Markers of myocardial injury include, most notably, the cardiac troponins. The expanding role played by sensitive cardiac troponins, as well as the ever-increasing number of studies validating their utility for risk prediction has led some to recently proclaim sensitive cardiac troponin testing to be an integral part of any cardiovascular risk assessment model.[13]

Markers of Myocardial Ischemia

It was previously believed that only irreversible damage to the cardiac myocyte would result in the release of cardiac troponins. Although this belief is no longer universally held, and the release of ever more sensitive cardiac troponin assays continues to challenge this view, the search for reliable markers of cardiac ischemia is ongoing. Thus far, even the most sensitive cardiac troponin assays cannot yet distinguish between unstable angina and noncardiac causes of chest pain, and many believe a marker of ischemia could help immensely with both risk stratification and with earlier diagnosis of acute coronary syndromes.[14]

Markers of Inflammation and Vascular Damage

Studies of markers of inflammation are prevalent throughout the cardiovascular literature because of the central role that inflammation is believed to play in the pathogenesis of both coronary artery disease and heart failure.[15] C-reactive protein (CRP) is an acute phase reactant synthesized by hepatocytes in response to a wide variety of inflammatory conditions.[16] While it is perhaps the most widely used of these in cardiology practice today, a good number of other markers within this category are emerging as well. Some of these newer biomarkers may be more specific to cardiac inflammation; whereas CRP is a nonspecific marker of inflammation, pentraxin 3, for example, is synthesized by cells that are directly involved in atherosclerosis, and seems to be triggered as a specific response to vascular damage (though it also plays a role in innate immunity).[17] As such, pentraxin 3 and other new, more specific markers may ultimately prove to be better indicators of the presence and progression of atherosclerosis, but for now, they lag significantly behind CRP in clinical studies and clinical experience.

Markers of Extracellular Matrix, Remodeling, and Fibrosis

Extracellular matrix turnover, ventricular remodeling, and myocardial fibrosis are central to the development of heart failure. Cardiac remodeling is linked to disease progression and to poor clinical outcomes in heart failure patients. Because of this, biomarkers reflecting these processes, including ST2 and galectin-3, have shown prognostic value in acute and chronic heart failure.[18,19] Since the biologic processes reflected by elevated levels of these markers are probably central to the development and progression of heart failure, these markers may also be important targets for therapy, or for identifying subsets of patients that are most likely to respond to intensified therapy.[20]

Markers of Atherosclerosis and Unstable Plaque

Categorizing a biomarker as either a marker of inflammation and vascular damage or a marker of atherosclerosis is somewhat arbitrary, given that inflammation and atherosclerosis go hand-in-hand. Nonetheless, several markers have shown clear associations with atherosclerosis, and some have the added property of being associated with destabilized atherosclerotic plaque, making them particularly attractive candidates for applications, such as early diagnosis of acute coronary syndrome. Myeloperoxidase (MPO), for instance, a protein produced by macrophages and polymorphonuclear neutrophils and released in the setting of inflammation, oxidizes lipids within low-density lipoprotein particles and promotes the formation of foam cells in atherosclerotic plaque. MPO is found at higher levels in ruptured, or culprit, plaques in patients with acute coronary syndrome, than in plaques from patients with stable coronary disease.[21,22] In fact, MPO may play a causal role in plaque rupture by degrading the collagen layer of atheroma.[23] Properties like these make MPO and other markers of atherosclerosis and plaque destabilization attractive candidates for evaluating susceptibility to and diagnosis of acute coronary syndromes.

Markers of Myocardial Strain

The natriuretic peptides, which include B-type natriuretic peptide (BNP) and the N-terminal fragment of its prohormone (NT-proBNP), as well as atrial natriuretic peptide (ANP) and the mid-regional fragment of the prohormone (MR-proANP), are currently the most widely used markers of myocardial strain or stress. In the setting of hemodynamic stress, such as ventricular wall dilation (especially of the left ventricle), hypertrophy, or increased cardiac wall tension, these prohormones are released and processed into biologically active natriuretic peptides, which can counteract the stress by inducing vasodilation, natriuresis, and diuresis.[24] Because of their profound ability to assist with diagnosis and prognosis across a wide variety of clinical settings, natriuretic peptides have, like the cardiac troponins, become an integral component of cardiovascular risk assessment. Nonetheless, several emerging markers of myocardial strain are gaining momentum as markers of cardiovascular risk in their own right, and several have been shown to add incremental information to the natriuretic peptides, implying that they are not merely identifying identical disease states.[25,26]

Markers of Renal Function/Injury

The close, interwoven relationship between cardiac disease and renal disease has been long appreciated with the two disease states sharing multiple risk factors, so it should come as no surprise that several markers of renal dysfunction also serve as markers of cardiovascular risk. One of the more recent additions is cystatin C, a protein secreted into the blood by almost all human cells. Cystatin C is a better marker of renal function than creatinine, and is also independent of age, sex, and lean muscle mass.[27] As a more accurate marker of renal function, cystatin C is also a stronger predictor of cardiovascular events than is creatinine or estimated glomerular filtration rate.[28-30] While the association of cystatin C with cardiovascular events is in part due to its improved estimation of renal function, cystatin C also reflects factors associated with cardiovascular disease even beyond its association with glomerular filtration rate.[31] Regardless of the reasons for the close association, markers of renal injury clearly have a leading role to play in cardiovascular risk assessment.

Genomic Markers

The burgeoning field of genomic medicine is leading to rapid advancements in the identification of potential cardiac risk markers, though their translation into the clinical realm is yet to be realized. For example, in a recent cohort study of over 19,000 women from the Women's Genome Health Study, a genetic risk score made up of 101 single nucleotide polymorphisms (SNPs) was constructed and compared to traditional cardiovascular risk factors for prediction of incident cardiovascular disease.[32] Disappointingly, the genetic risk score was unable to improve risk prediction models that used traditional cardiovascular risk factors. In fact, simply asking study participants about a family history of premature cardiovascular disease resulted in a highly significant improvement in risk prediction. As novel techniques are developed and more markers are identified, genomics may yet have a role to play in cardiovascular risk assessment.

EMERGING APPLICATIONS AND FUTURE APPROACHES

Serial Measurements

A recent trend in studies assessing cardiovascular risk is to evaluate the same biomarker at more than one point in time. Serial measurements of biomarkers, in theory, could improve risk assessment by providing a more dynamic view of risk, better reflecting change in subclinical or clinical disease. It might also be helpful for monitoring the response to therapeutic interventions. Because of intraindividual variability in biomarker measurements due to both day-to-day fluctuations and assay precision, assessment of serial measurements is not always straightforward; nonetheless, this approach has shown promise in several notable studies.[33-38]

Multimarker Approaches

Many attributes make biomarkers attractive candidates for use in cardiovascular risk assessment, including their ease of attainment, relatively low cost, and the links they provide to plausible pathophysiologic pathways. However, biomarkers also suffer from limitations. Biomarkers can have significant day-to-day intra-individual variability, as well as issues with assay precision and poor predictive values at the level of the individual patient.[39] Some of these limitations inherent in using an individual biomarker for risk stratification may potentially be overcome by a multimarker approach. Combining different biomarkers from distinct pathophysiologic pathways has the potential to improve risk stratification, and studies evaluating cardiovascular risk have begun to naturally evolve toward this approach. Thus far, the clinical studies using multiple biomarkers for cardiovascular risk assessment have shown mixed results.[40] Some studies using combinations of biomarkers for both prediction of the primary and secondary cardiovascular disease have found statistically significant albeit modest clinical improvements in prediction compared to a model with traditional risk factors (alone or with a single additional biomarker).[41-45] A few, though, have detailed substantially improved risk prediction with a multimarker approach.[5,46-52]

The two most obvious reasons for differing results in studies of multimarker panels are the choice of biomarkers comprising the panel, and the clinical scenario in which they are used. However, other reasons likely include the patient population targeted for risk assessment, the methods used to integrate results from the various markers, and the statistical metrics used to assess the results.[53] As methods and markers evolve and are optimized, multimarker panels are likely to assume a larger role in cardiovascular risk assessment.

Multimodal Approach

In addition to biomarkers, various other noninvasive methods for evaluating or screening for cardiovascular disease offer promise for improving cardiovascular risk assessment processes (Table 1-2). Noninvasive tests that measure endothelial cell function, coronary artery or other vascular calcification, carotid intimal thickening, hemodynamics, and exercise parameters, for example, are undergoing rapid improvements in methodology and are being validated in clinical studies. Combining various structural and functional markers, each representing different physiologic pathways (whether biomarkers [i.e., blood tests] or other measurements) in a "multimodal" approach is an extension of the concept of combining multiple biomarkers and could offer even further advances in risk assessment.

Table 1-2	Noninvasive Measures of Cardiovascular Risk	
Measures of subclinical atherosclerosis		**Measures of arterial stiffness**
Coronary artery calcification		Pulse wave velocity
Aortic calcification		Aortic augmentation index
Carotid intima-media thickness		**Exercise parameters**
Ankle-brachial index		Heart rate recovery
Measures of endothelial function		Exercise capacity
Flow-mediated vasodilation of brachial artery		

Putting It All Together

An approach to cardiovascular risk assessment that incorporates both biomarkers and noninvasive measures may ultimately prove to be the most useful in clinical practice, although the specific methods will necessarily vary based on the clinical situation. In the past, multimarker approaches were often deemed too complicated to make the jump from the literature to daily clinical practice. In today's world of smartphones, iPads, or tablet computers in the pocket of every white coat, even complicated risk assessment algorithms could potentially be fair game for daily use. Identifying the best markers to include and targeting the appropriate patient population to undergo testing will be the key to the success of any risk assessment approach.

For the moment, targeted marker assessment in selected individuals could certainly assist with screening, diagnosis, or prognostication, and might also point to new avenues for potential therapeutic targets. On the other hand, widespread and indiscriminate measurement of multiple biomarkers may not be warranted until further studies establishing cost-effectiveness and confirming improved clinical outcomes that result from an appropriate and specific response to the risk assessment results. Improved risk assessment is a worthy initial objective, but ultimately we await translation into improved prevention and treatment—a goal for which biomarkers will surely play an essential role.

REFERENCES

1. Morrow DA, de Lemos JA. Benchmarks for the assessment of novel cardiovascular biomarkers. *Circulation*. 2007;115:949-52.
2. Thygesen K, Alpert JS, White HD. Universal definition of myocardial infarction. *J Am Coll Cardiol*. 2007;50:2173-95.
3. Daniels LB, Maisel AS. Natriuretic peptides. *J Am Coll Cardiol*. 2007;50:2357-68.
4. Ohman EM, Armstrong PW, Christenson RH, Granger CB, Katus HA, Hamm CW, et al. Cardiac troponin T levels for risk stratification in acute myocardial ischemia. GUSTO IIA Investigators. *N Engl J Med*. 1996;335:1333-41.

5. Sabatine MS, Morrow DA, de Lemos JA, Gibson CM, Murphy SA, Rifai N, et al. Multimarker approach to risk stratification in non-ST elevation acute coronary syndromes: simultaneous assessment of troponin I, C-reactive protein, and B-type natriuretic peptide. *Circulation.* 2002;105:1760-3.

6. Morrow DA, Cannon CP, Rifai N, Frey MJ, Vicari R, Lakkis N, et al. Ability of minor elevations of troponins I and T to predict benefit from an early invasive strategy in patients with unstable angina and non-ST elevation myocardial infarction: results from a randomized trial. *JAMA.* 2001;286:2405-12.

7. Maisel AS, Krishnaswamy P, Nowak RM, McCord J, Hollander JE, Duc P, et al. Breathing not properly multinational study I. Rapid measurement of B-type natriuretic peptide in the emergency diagnosis of heart failure. *N Engl J Med.* 2002;347:161-7.

8. The hypertension detection and follow-up program: Hypertension detection and follow-up program cooperative group. *Prev Med.* 1976;5:207-15.

9. Maisel A, Mueller C, Adams K Jr, Anker SD, Aspromonte N, Cleland JG, et al. State of the art: using natriuretic peptide levels in clinical practice. *Eur J Heart Fail.* 2008;10:824-39.

10. Daniels LB. Natriuretic peptides and assessment of cardiovascular disease risk in asymptomatic persons. *Curr Cardiovasc Risk Rep.* 2010;4:120-7.

11. Hlatky MA, Greenland P, Arnett DK, Ballantyne CM, Criqui MH, Elkind MS, et al. Criteria for evaluation of novel markers of cardiovascular risk: a scientific statement from the American Heart Association. *Circulation.* 2009;119:2408-16.

12. Agewall S, Giannitsis E, Jernberg T, Katus H. Troponin elevation in coronary vs. non-coronary disease. *Eur Heart J.* 2011;32:404-11.

13. Apple FS. High-sensitivity cardiac troponin for screening large populations of healthy people: is there risk? *Clin Chem.* 2011;57:537-9.

14. Morrow DA, de Lemos JA, Sabatine MS, Antman EM. The search for a biomarker of cardiac ischemia. *Clin Chem.* 2003;49:537-9.

15. Anker SD, von Haehling S. Inflammatory mediators in chronic heart failure: an overview. *Heart.* 2004;90:464-70.

16. Castell JV, Gomez-Lechon MJ, David M, Fabra R, Trullenque R, Heinrich PC. Acute-phase response of human hepatocytes: regulation of acute-phase protein synthesis by interleukin-6. *Hepatology.* 1990;12:1179-86.

17. Mantovani A, Garlanda C, Bottazzi B, Peri G, Doni A, Martinez de la Torre Y, et al. The long pentraxin PTX3 in vascular pathology. *Vascul Pharmacol.* 2006;45:326-30.

18. de Boer RA, Voors AA, Muntendam P, van Gilst WH, van Veldhuisen DJ. Galectin-3: a novel mediator of heart failure development and progression. *Eur J Heart Fail.* 2009; 11:811-7.

19. Moore SA, Januzzi JL Jr. Found in translation soluble ST2 and heart disease. *J Am Coll Cardiol.* 2010;55:251-3.

20. Weir RA, Miller AM, Murphy GE, Clements S, Steedman T, Connell JM, et al. ST2: a potential novel mediator in left ventricular and infarct remodeling after acute myocardial infarction. *J Am Coll Cardiol.* 2010;55:243-50.

21. Buffon A, Biasucci LM, Liuzzo G, D'Onofrio G, Crea F, Maseri A. Widespread coronary inflammation in unstable angina. *N Engl J Med.* 2002;347:5-12.

22. Naruko T, Ueda M, Haze K, van der Wal AC, van der Loos CM, Itoh A, et al. Neutrophil infiltration of culprit lesions in acute coronary syndromes. *Circulation.* 2002;106:2894-2900.

23. Sugiyama S, Okada Y, Sukhova GK, Virmani R, Heinecke JW, Libby P. Macrophage myeloperoxidase regulation by granulocyte macrophage colony-stimulating factor in

human atherosclerosis and implications in acute coronary syndromes. *Am J Pathol.* 2001;158:879-91.

24. Nakao K, Ogawa Y, Suga S, Imura H. Molecular biology and biochemistry of the natriuretic peptide system. II: Natriuretic peptide receptors. *J Hypertens.* 1992;10:1111-4.

25. Januzzi JL Jr, Peacock WF, Maisel AS, Chae CU, Jesse RL, Baggish AL, et al. Measurement of the interleukin family member ST2 in patients with acute dyspnea: results from the PRIDE (Pro-Brain Natriuretic Peptide Investigation of Dyspnea in the Emergency Department) study. *J Am Coll Cardiol.* 2007;50:607-13.

26. Daniels LB, Clopton P, Laughlin GA, Maisel AS, Barrett-Connor E. Growth-differentiation factor-15 is a robust, independent predictor of 11-year mortality risk in community-dwelling older adults: the Rancho Bernardo study. *Circulation.* 2011;123:2101-10.

27. Herget-Rosenthal S, Trabold S, Pietruck F, Holtmann M, Philipp T, Kribben A. Cystatin C: efficacy as screening test for reduced glomerular filtration rate. *Am J Nephrol.* 2000; 20:97-102.

28. Shlipak MG, Sarnak MJ, Katz R, Fried LF, Seliger SL, Newman AB, et al. Cystatin C and the risk of death and cardiovascular events among elderly persons. *N Engl J Med.* 2005;352:2049-60.

29. Manzano-Fernandez S, Januzzi JL Jr, Boronat-Garcia M, Bonaque-Gonzalez JC, Truong QA, Pastor-Perez FJ, et al. Beta-trace protein and cystatin C as predictors of long-term outcomes in patients with acute heart failure. *J Am Coll Cardiol.* 2011;57:849-58.

30. Wu CK, Lin JW, Caffrey JL, Chang MH, Hwang JJ, Lin YS. Cystatin C and long-term mortality among subjects with normal creatinine-based estimated glomerular filtration rates: NHANES III (Third National Health and Nutrition Examination Survey). *J Am Coll Cardiol.* 2010;56:1930-6.

31. Mathisen UD, Melsom T, Ingebretsen OC, Jenssen T, Njolstad I, Solbu MD, et al. Estimated GFR associates with cardiovascular risk factors independently of measured GFR. *J Am Soc Nephrol.* 2011;22:927-37.

32. Paynter NP, Chasman DI, Pare G, Buring JE, Cook NR, Miletich JP, et al. Association between a literature-based genetic risk score and cardiovascular events in women. *JAMA.* 2010;303:631-7.

33. Anand IS, Fisher LD, Chiang YT, Latini R, Masson S, Maggioni AP, et al. Changes in brain natriuretic peptide and norepinephrine over time and mortality and morbidity in the Valsartan Heart Failure Trial (Val-HeFT). *Circulation.* 2003;107:1278-83.

34. Anand IS, Kempf T, Rector TS, Tapken H, Allhoff T, Jantzen F, et al. Serial measurement of growth-differentiation factor-15 in heart failure: relation to disease severity and prognosis in the Valsartan Heart Failure Trial. *Circulation.* 2010;122:1387-95.

35. Miller WL, Hartman KA, Burritt MF, Grill DE, Rodeheffer RJ, Burnett JC Jr, et al. Serial biomarker measurements in ambulatory patients with chronic heart failure: the importance of change over time. *Circulation.* 2007;116:249-57.

36. deFilippi CR, Christenson RH, Gottdiener JS, Kop WJ, Seliger SL. Dynamic cardiovascular risk assessment in elderly people. The role of repeated N-terminal pro-B-type natriuretic peptide testing. *J Am Coll Cardiol.* 2010;55:441-50.

37. deFilippi CR, de Lemos JA, Christenson RH, Gottdiener JS, Kop WJ, Zhan M, et al. Association of serial measures of cardiac troponin T using a sensitive assay with incident heart failure and cardiovascular mortality in older adults. *JAMA.* 2010;304:2494-2502.

38. Masson S, Latini R, Anand IS, Barlera S, Angelici L, Vago T, et al. Prognostic value of changes in N-terminal pro-brain natriuretic peptide in Val-HeFT (Valsartan Heart Failure Trial). *J Am Coll Cardiol.* 2008;52:997-1003.

39. Ware JH. The limitations of risk factors as prognostic tools. *N Engl J Med.* 2006;355: 2615-7.

40. Daniels LB. Multiple biomarker assessment in primary prevention of cardiovascular disease. *Curr Cardiovasc Risk Rep.* 2009;3:131-6.

41. Schnabel RB, Schulz A, Messow CM, Lubos E, Wild PS, Zeller T, et al. Multiple marker approach to risk stratification in patients with stable coronary artery disease. *Eur Heart J.* 2010;31:3024-31.

42. Wang TJ, Gona P, Larson MG, Tofler GH, Levy D, Newton-Cheh C, et al. Multiple biomarkers for the prediction of first major cardiovascular events and death. *N Engl J Med.* 2006;355:2631-9.

43. Melander O, Newton-Cheh C, Almgren P, Hedblad B, Berglund G, Engstrom G, et al. Novel and conventional biomarkers for prediction of incident cardiovascular events in the community. *JAMA.* 2009;302:49-57.

44. Kim HC, Greenland P, Rossouw JE, Manson JE, Cochrane BB, Lasser NL, et al. Multi-marker prediction of coronary heart disease risk: the women's health initiative. *J Am Coll Cardiol.* 2010;55:2080-91.

45. Olsen MH, Hansen TW, Christensen MK, Gustafsson F, Rasmussen S, Wachtell K, et al. N-terminal pro-brain natriuretic peptide, but not high sensitivity C-reactive protein, improves cardiovascular risk prediction in the general population. *Eur Heart J.* 2007;28: 1374-81.

46. Zethelius B, Berglund L, Sundstrom J, Ingelsson E, Basu S, Larsson A, et al. Use of multi-ple biomarkers to improve the prediction of death from cardiovascular causes. *N Engl J Med.* 2008;358:2107-16.

47. Blankenberg S, Zeller T, Saarela O, Havulinna AS, Kee F, Tunstall-Pedoe H, et al. Contribution of 30 biomarkers to 10-year cardiovascular risk estimation in 2 population cohorts: the MONICA, risk, genetics, archiving, and monograph (MORGAM) biomarker project. *Circulation.* 2010;121:2388-97.

48. Daniels LB, Laughlin GA, Clopton P, Maisel AS, Barrett-Connor E. Minimally elevated cardiac troponin T and elevated N-terminal pro-B-type natriuretic peptide predict mortality in older adults: results from the Rancho Bernardo Study. *J Am Coll Cardiol.* 2008;52:450-9.

49. Oemrawsingh RM, Lenderink T, Akkerhuis KM, Heeschen C, Baldus S, Fichtlscherer S, et al. Multimarker risk model containing troponin-T, interleukin 10, myeloperoxidase and placental growth factor predicts long-term cardiovascular risk after non-ST-segment elevation acute coronary syndrome. *Heart.* 2011;97:1061-6.

50. Pascual-Figal DA, Manzano-Fernandez S, Boronat M, Casas T, Garrido IP, Bonaque JC, et al. Soluble ST2, high-sensitivity troponin T- and N-terminal pro-B-type natriuretic peptide: complementary role for risk stratification in acutely decompensated heart failure. *Eur J Heart Fail.* 2011.

51. Velagaleti RS, Gona P, Larson MG, Wang TJ, Levy D, Benjamin EJ, et al. Multimarker approach for the prediction of heart failure incidence in the community. *Circulation.* 2010;122:1700-6.

52. Nozaki T, Sugiyama S, Koga H, Sugamura K, Ohba K, Matsuzawa Y, et al. Significance of a multiple biomarkers strategy including endothelial dysfunction to improve risk stratification for cardiovascular events in patients at high risk for coronary heart disease. *J Am Coll Cardiol.* 2009;54:601-8.

53. Daniels LB, Maisel AS. Multiple marker approach to risk stratification in patients with stable coronary artery disease: to have or have not. *Eur Heart J.* 2010;31:2980-3.

The OxPL/apoB Assay: A Predictor of Cardiovascular Disease and Events[*]

Adam Taleb, Sotirios Tsimikas

INTRODUCTION

Oxidative stress is considered to be a key mechanism for the initiation and progression of atherosclerosis and the development of cardiovascular disease (CVD).[1,2] Excessive oxidative stress occurs in response to many underlying cardiovascular risk factors, such as hypercholesterolemia, hypertension, diabetes mellitus, and underlying genetic predisposition. Oxidative stress and subsequent oxidation of low-density lipoprotein (OxLDL) is created through the reaction of reactive oxygen species, such as superoxide anion, and hydrogen peroxide and peroxynitrite. These oxidative species are generated during cellular metabolic pathways by lipoxygenases, myeloperoxidase, nitric oxide synthase, NADPH oxidase, xanthine oxidase, and other oxidases, with polyunsaturated fatty acids, lipoproteins, and amino acids, causing their modification to proinflammatory and atherogenic particles. One LDL particle is composed of approximately 600 molecules of free cholesterol (FC), 1,600 molecules of cholesteryl esters (CE), 700 molecules of phospholipids (PL), and 185 molecules of triglycerides (TG). The polyunsaturated acyl chains of CE, PL, and TG are vulnerable to oxidation, as is the sterol of FC and CE. LDL contains one molecule of apolipoprotein B-100, made of 4,536 amino acid residues, with many exposed lysines, which can be directly oxidized or modified by lipid oxidation products.[3] Due to its molecular composition, LDL is particularly susceptible to oxidation and OxLDL is considered among the strongest proinflammatory components of vulnerable plaques.[4]

Oxidation of low-density lipoprotein leads to the generation of a variety of oxidation specific epitopes (OSE), such as the oxidized phospholipid (OxPL) and malondialdehyde (MDA) epitopes on LDL. Oxidation of LDL is thought to occur primarily in the vessel wall rather than in plasma, which is strongly enriched in antioxidants. These OSE are biologically active and upregulate adhesion molecules to attract monocytes into the vessel wall, mediate proinflammatory responses in cytokines and upregulation of proinflammatory genes, promote macrophage

---

[*]This chapter was adapted from Taleb A, Witztum JL, **Tsimikas S**. Oxidized phospholipids on apolipoprotein B-100 (OxPL/apoB) containing lipoproteins: A biomarker predicting cardiovascular disease and cardiovascular events. *Biomarkers in Medicine* 2011;In press.

retention and apoptosis,[5,6] and are cytotoxic. These OSE are pro-atherogenic by enhancing the unregulated uptake of OxLDL in macrophages through specific pathways generating activated macrophage foam cells (Figure 2-1). Accumulation of foam cells leads to fatty streak formation. Foam cell necrosis and/or apoptosis and continued accumulation of oxidized lipids in the extracellular space eventually lead to atheroma formation.

OSE are also potent immunogens and lead to activation of T-cells and B-cells, resulting in the generation of autoantibodies to specific epitopes, which have been described in both humans and animals.[7-9] In mice, natural antibodies, secreted from OxLDL-specific B-1 cell lines, bind to OSE, block uptake of OxLDL by macrophages,

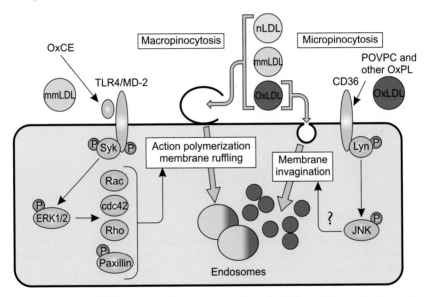

Figure 2-1 Oxidized lipid moieties induce lipoprotein accumulation in macrophages. Macrophage lipoprotein uptake mechanisms can be separated into: (i) macropinocytosis, when actin polymerization and extensive membrane ruffling result in the ruffles closing into large endosomes and capture of large volumes of extracellular material, including all classes of native and oxidized LDL present in the vicinity of the cell; and (ii) micropinocytosis, when ligand-receptor binding leads to membrane invagination and nearly stoichiometric internalization of the ligand or the lipoprotein carrying this ligand. mmLDL and polyoxygenated oxidized cholesterol esters (OxCEs) induce Syk recruitment to TLR4, Syk, and TLR4 phosphorylation and subsequent ERK½-dependent activation of small GTPases Rac, cdc42, and Rho and phosphorylation of paxillin, leading to actin reorganization and membrane ruffling. Resulting macropinocytosis promotes foam cell formation.[71] Binding of OxLDL or OxPL to CD36 initiates Lyn-dependent phosphorylation of JNK, which is essential for CD36-mediated OxLDL uptake, although the mechanism linking JNK with the membrane dynamics is unclear.[72] The TLR4- and CD36-mediated uptake mechanisms are only examples; there are numerous other PRRs involved in oxidation-specific epitope-stimulated lipoprotein internalization by macrophages. *From* Miller YI, Choi SH, Wiesner P, Fang L, Harkewicz R, Hartvigsen K, et al. Oxidation-specific epitopes are danger-associated molecular patterns recognized by pattern recognition receptors of innate immunity. *Circ Res.* 2011;108:235-48.

recognize apoptotic cells, and are deposited in atherosclerotic lesions, suggesting a role of the innate immunity system in protecting hosts against these pro-inflammatory antigens (Figure 2-2).

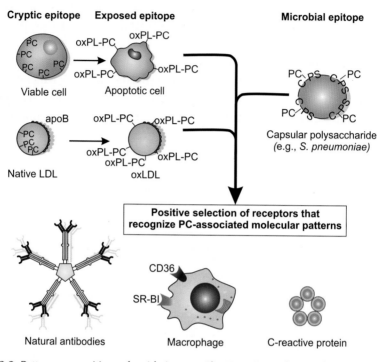

Figure 2-2 Pattern recognition of oxidation-specific DAMPs and microbial PAMPs. Using the example of the PC epitope, in this illustration, we demonstrate our hypothesis of the emergence and positive selection of multiple PRRs that recognize common epitopes, shared by modified self and microbial pathogens. According to this hypothesis, oxidation of plasma membrane phospholipids in apoptotic cells alters the conformation of the PC head group, yielding an exposed epitope, accessible to recognition by macrophage scavenger receptors, natural antibodies, and pentraxins, such as CRP. These PRRs were selected to clear apoptotic cells from developing or regenerating tissues. Recognition by the same receptors of the PC epitope of capsular polysaccharide in Gram-positive bacteria (e.g., *S. pneumoniae*) strengthened positive selection of these PRRs and probably helped select additional strong proinflammatory components to PRR-dependent responses. (Note the PC on the bacteria is not part of a phospholipid.) Finally, oxidized lipoproteins, prevalent in experimental animals and humans as a result of enhanced oxidative stress, dyslipidemia and impact of environmental factors, bear OxPLs with the PC epitope exposed in an analogous manner to that of apoptotic cells. This leads to OxLDL recognition by PRRs and initiation of innate immune responses. The balance between proinflammatory responses of cellular PRRs and atheroprotective roles of natural antibodies plays an important role in the development of atherosclerosis. There are likely many more oxidation-specific epitopes that represent such DAMPs and corresponding PRRs that represent respective innate responses. DAMPs, danger-associated molecular patterns; PAMPs, pathogen-associated molecular patterns; PRRs, pattern recognition receptors; PC, phosphocholine. *From* Miller YI, Choi SH, Wiesner P, Fang L, Harkewicz R, Hartvigsen K, et al. Oxidation-specific epitopes are danger-associated molecular patterns recognized by pattern recognition receptors of innate immunity. *Circ Res.* 2011;108:235-48.

OxPL play an important role in atherosclerosis and accumulate in human and mouse lesions. Specific OxPL have been identified as major regulators of many cell types present in the vessel wall, including endothelial cells, smooth muscle cells, macrophages, dendritic cells, and platelets.[10,11] Furthermore, several receptors and signaling pathways associated with OxPL action have been identified and shown to be upregulated in human lesions.[11,12] OxPL mediate plaque destabilization, being present in higher quantities (70-fold) in plaque than plasma.[4,13] OxPL are key components of OxLDL, apoptotic cells and atherosclerotic lesions, and are important contributors to early events in atherogenesis by activating proinflammatory genes, leading to inflammatory cascades in the vessel wall.[10,11] The complex interplay of oxidized lipids, inflammatory processes, endothelial dysfunction, platelet activation, and thrombosis ultimately leads to plaque progression and/or disruption. Immune mechanisms and inflammatory cells play a central role throughout all these events, resulting in atherosclerotic lesions having many features of a chronic inflammatory disease.[1,14]

We have cloned a series of immunodominant IgM antibodies (Abs) binding to OxLDL from apoE$^{-/-}$ mice.[9,15,16] E06 is a well-characterized murine monoclonal antibody (mAb) that binds to the phosphocholine (PC) headgroup of oxidized but not native phospholipids.[17] E06 is encoded by non-mutated germline genes and is 100% identical in the variable region to the T15 natural Ab, which provides the optimal protection to mice against lethal infection with *S. pneumoniae*.[18] E06/T15 binds to PC exposed on OxPLs on Cu-oxidized LDL, as well as OxPL present on apoptotic cells, but also to PC coupled to techoic/lipotechoic acid on the cell wall of bacteria, such as *S. pneumoniae*. Indeed, E06 recognizes OxPL on an equimolar basis when simply present as a PC salt or as PC on OxPL such as POVPC [1-palmitoyl-2-(5-oxovaleroyl)-sn-glycero-3-phosphocholine] attached to a variety of different peptides, as well as PC on OxPL covalently linked (via its *sn-2* oxidized side chain) to a variety of synthetic peptides irrespective of amino acid sequence.[17] E06 inhibits OxLDL uptake by macrophages, preventing recognition by scavenger receptors, and inhibits a number of other proinflammatory properties of OxPL generated via acute lung injury and infections.[19,20] E06 also exhibits other important biological functions, such as inhibition of uptake of apoptotic cells by macrophages *in vitro*,[16,21-23] but promotes complement-mediated enhanced clearance of apoptotic cells *in vivo*.[24] Interestingly, pneumococcal vaccination of cholesterol-fed LDLR$^{-/-}$ mice increased the T15/E06 titers and, most strikingly, reduced the progression of atherosclerosis.[25,26] Overall, these data suggest that PC-based OxPL represents a pathogen-associated molecular pattern and that effector molecules, such as IgM natural Abs (i.e., antibody E06/T15), scavenger receptors (e.g., CD36 and SR-B1), and CRP of the innate immune system evolved to bind and potentially neutralize them.[27]

OxPL/apoB METHODOLOGY

Using E06, we have developed a chemiluminescent ELISA to detect OxPL on human apolipoprotein B-100 (OxPL/apoB) containing lipoprotein particles in plasma. This well-validated assay has been previously described in detail.[28-31] The assay is performed by plating overnight murine monoclonal antibody MB47 (50 µL at 5 µg/mL),[32,33] which captures a saturating amount of apoB-100 on all apoB-containing lipoproteins from plasma. After washing, the plates are coated with 1% bovine serum albumin in tris (hydroxymethyl) aminomethane–buffered saline. Plasma (50 µL of 1:50 dilution) is added and allowed to incubate for 75 minutes. This initial step is designed so that each well captures a constant, saturating amount of apoB-100 from plasma (1–2 mg/mL, significantly less than plasma levels of apoB in humans), and, therefore, normalizes the OxPL measure to an equal fraction of each patient's apoB-100 levels. Thus, by definition, it is independent of apoB and LDL-C levels. Biotinylated E06 (1 µg/mL) is added and allowed to incubate for 1 hour. Alkaline phosphatase Neutravidin (1:40,000 dilution) is added for 1 hour. LumiPhos (25 µL) is added for 75 minutes to detect OxPL per apoB particle (e.g., to yield OxPL/apoB ratio). The apoB in the denominator is not the plasma level of each patient's apoB, but the amount captured on the microtiter well plate. Because an equal amount of apoB-100 is captured in each well from each subject, the denominator is 1 and thus, the actual read out is the amount of OxPL as detected by E06. This is detected by chemiluminescent technique and reported in relative light units (RLU) in 100 ms (Figure 2-3).

In an early version of this assay prior to 2006, parallel plates were used to document that the wells captured equal amounts of apoB by first capturing apoB with MB47 and then adding the biotinylated murine monoclonal antibody MB24 to quantitate the amount of captured apoB, which detects a separate apoB epitope.

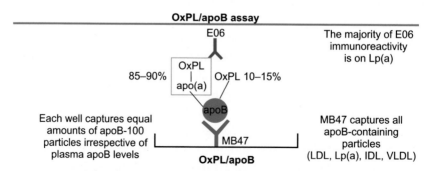

Figure 2-3 Schematic representation of the OxPL/apoB assay. Microtiter well plates are coated with the murine antibody MB47 and plasma added to bind apolipoprotein B-100 particles. OxPL on apoB-100 are then detected with biotinylated murine monoclonal antibody E06.

Dividing the RLU from the E06 assay with the RLU from the MB24 assay results in a true OxPL/apoB ratio. Subsequently, we showed that the correlation between OxPL/apoB RLU vs OxPL/apoB ratio was r = 0.99 in more than 1,500 samples.[31] Therefore, this additional step is not performed routinely in current human studies and the data are presented as OxPL/apoB in RLU, measured as the E06 binding only. The OxPL/apoB assay is highly specific to the number of OxPL epitopes on individual apoB-100 particles, but does not measure the total amount of OxPL in plasma. Table 2-1 displays the various studies performed with this assay.

RELATIONSHIP OF OxPL/apoB AND Lp(a): Lp(a) AS A PREFERENTIAL CARRIER OF E06-DETECTABLE OxPL

Several early clinical studies documented, unexpectedly, that OxPL/apoB correlated strongly with Lp(a),[30,34,35] and not with LDL as expected.[29] Lp(a), which is secreted from the liver, is an independent, causal, genetic risk factor for cardiovascular death and myocardial infarction, and this risk is continuous and linear with increasing Lp(a) levels.[36-43] A physiological role of Lp(a) and the underlying mechanisms through which it contributes to CVD are still unknown. However, we have shown that Lp(a) preferentially binds OxPL, compared to other lipoproteins[44] and have proposed that a unique physiological role of Lp(a) may be to bind and transport proinflammatory OxPL in plasma. This would suggest that a sufficient and low level of Lp(a) is beneficial. Indeed, a J-shaped curve relates Lp(a) levels to CVD,[45,46] suggesting that a small amount of Lp(a) (2–7 mg/dL) is associated with reduced CVD risk, but higher levels with increased risk (> 25 mg/dL). The OxPL content may also explain this pathophysiological role.[29] When present at high plasma concentrations, Lp(a) would be more atherogenic than native LDL, as it binds with increased affinity to arterial intimal proteoglycans[47] resulting in increased intimal concentration of LDL along with associated proinflammatory OxPL. This hypothesis is now supported by several levels of evidence, including: (i) the correlation of OxPL/apoB and Lp(a) in multiple clinical studies;[28,45,48] (ii) the presence of OxPL- Lp(a) detected by immunoprecipitation and ultracentrifugation experiments demonstrating that ~85% of E06 reactivity (i.e., OxPL) coimmunoprecipitated with Lp(a);[44] (iii) *in vitro* transfer studies showing that OxPL from OxLDL are preferentially transferred to Lp(a) compared to LDL in a time/temperature dependent fashion;[44] (iv) extraction of purified human Lp(a) with organic solvents followed by LC/MS/MS studies showing that 30–70% of OxPL, both E06-detectable and E06-non-detectable, are extractable; (v) lack of evidence of oxidation of Lp(a) itself, such as the presence of MDA epitopes;[44] (vi) large clinical studies showing CVD event prediction by elevated baseline levels of OxPL/apoB, particularly those with small isoforms;[31,44,45,48-50] and (vii) accentuation of CVD risk and event prediction by OxPL/apoB with either lipoprotein-associated phospholipase A$_2$ (Lp-PLA$_2$) or secretory-PLA$_2$ (sPLA$_2$), suggesting an additive effect of substrate (OxPL) and enzyme activity of phospholipases.[45,48]

Table 2-1 Clinical Studies Examining the Role of OxPL/apoB in Cardiovascular Disease

Study	Year	Study name	Patient population	Number of patients/samples	Outcome change in OxPL/apoB levels
Wu et al.[66]	1999		Borderline hypertension (BHT)	146/146	Increased in BHT and may reflect early vascular changes
Penny et al.[67]	2001	UCSD regression study	Hypercholesterolemic patients undergoing quantitative angiography before/after lipid lowering therapy	29/54	Related significantly to the severity of endothelial dysfunction and was the single most powerful independent risk factor
Tsimikas et al.[30]	2003	ACS	Acute coronary syndromes, acute MI, unstable angina, stable CAD	66/272	Increase after acute MI
Tsimikas et al.[34]	2004	Toronto PCI	Patients with stable angina pectoris undergoing PCI	141/1269	Increase immediately after PCI and return to baseline after 6 hours
Segev et al.[68]	2005				No relationship to restenosis
Tsimikas et al.[35]	2004	MIRACL	Impact of atorvastatin in ACS	2341/4682	Increase 9.6% with atorvastatin 80 mg/day
Fraley et al.[69]	2009				Baseline levels varied according to specific CVD risk factors and were largely independent of inflammatory biomarkers
Silaste et al.[59]	2004		Healthy young women	37/74	Increase 19–27% with low-fat, high vegetable diet
Tsimikas et al.[49]	2005	MAYO	Coronary angiography	504/504	Strong and graded association with presence and extent of CAD

Continued

Continued

Study	Year	Study name	Patient population	Number of patients/samples	Outcome change in OxPL/apoB levels
Tsimikas et al.[31]	2006	BRUNECK	Random sample of population (40–79 years old males and females)	765/1436	Predict presence and progression of carotid and femoral atherosclerosis
Kiechl et al.[45]	2007				Predict 10-year CVD event rates independently of traditional risk factors, hsCRP, and FRS
Rodenburg et al.[58]	2006		Children with familial hypercholesterolemia and unaffected siblings	256/512	Increase 29% with Step II AHA diet; increase 49% with pravastatin 40 mg/day
Bossola et al.[70]	2007		End-stage renal failure patients undergoing chronic hemodialysis	52/104	Reduced in end-stage renal failure patients following hemodialysis
Ky et al.[57]	2008	PROXI	Hypercholesterolemic patients were randomized to different type and dose of statin	120/240	Increased 26% with pravastatin 40 mg/day and 20% with atorvastatin 80 mg/day
Choi et al.[63]	2008	REVERSAL	Patients with CAD who underwent coronary IVUS and assigned to statin therapy	214/428	Increased 48% with atorvastatin 80 mg/day and 39% with pravastatin 40 mg/day
Tsimikas et al.[50]	2009	Dallas Heart Study	Multiethnic, probability-based sample of the Dallas county population	3481/3481	Vary according to race/ethnicity, are independent of cardiovascular risk factors and are inversely associated with apo(a) isoform size

Continued

Continued

Study	Year	Study name	Patient population	Number of patients/samples	Outcome change in OxPL/apoB levels
Tsimikas et al.[48]	2010	EPIC–Norfolk study	45–79 years old healthy males and females followed for 6 years	2160/2160	The highest tertiles are associated with higher risk of CAD events
Budoff et al.[61]	2009	Garlic study	Asymptomatic patients with CAD treated with aged garlic extract plus supplement followed with coronary artery calcium scan (CAC)	60/120	Increase with aged garlic extract predicts lack of CAC progression
Ahmadi et al.[60]	2010				Increase with aged garlic extract correlates with improvement in vascular function
Arai et al.[54]	2010	I4399M SNP	Carriers and noncarriers of I4399M single nucleotide LPA polymorphism	174/174	Elevated in carriers than in noncarriers, while patients with small apolipoprotein(a) isoforms had the highest OxPL/apoB levels
Faghihnia et al.[62]	2010	CHORI	Healthy subjects consuming a high-fat low-carbohydrate (HFLC) diet and a LFHC diet	63/126	OxPL/apoB and OxPL/apo(a) are increased by a LFHC diet
Total: 21				10609/15782	

In the Dallas Heart Study, OxPL/apoB levels were measured in 3,481 subjects (1,831 Black, 1,047 White, and 603 Hispanic) and correlated with age, gender, cardiovascular risk factors, Lp(a) and apolipoprotein(a) isoforms. Significant differences in OxPL/apoB levels were noted among racial subgroups, with Blacks having the highest levels, compared to Whites and Hispanics (p < 0.001 for each comparison, figure 2-4). OxPL/apoB levels generally did not correlate with age, gender, or cardiovascular risk factors. In the overall cohort, OxPL/apoB levels

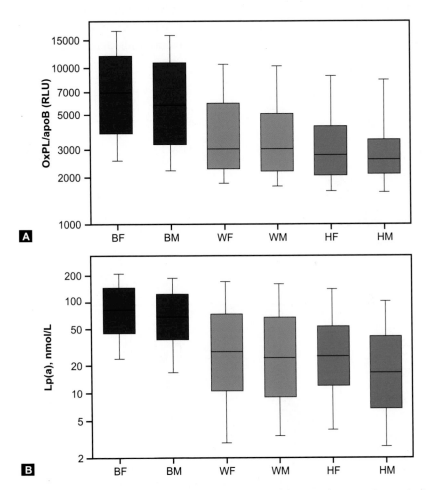

Figure 2-4 Levels of **A,** OxPL/apoB. **B,** Lp(a), categorized by racial group. Boxes indicate medians, 25th and 75th percentile, whiskers indicate 10th and 90th percentile. Differences among racial groups are all significant (p < 0.001). BF, Black females; BM, Black males; WF, White females; WM, White males; HF, Hispanic females; HM, Hispanic males. *From* Tsimikas S, Clopton P, Brilakis ES, Marcovina SM, Khera A, Miller ER, et al. Relationship of oxidized phospholipids on apolipoprotein B-100 particles to race/ethnicity, apolipoprotein(a) isoform size, and cardiovascular risk factors: results from the Dallas Heart Study. *Circulation.* 2009;119:1711-9.

strongly correlated with Lp(a) (r = 0.85, p < 0.001), with the shape of the relationship demonstrating a "reverse L" shape for log-transformed values (Figure 2-5). The highest correlation was present in Blacks, followed by Whites and Hispanics, and was dependent on apo(a) isoform size, and became progressively weaker with larger isoforms. The size of the major apolipoprotein(a) isoform (number of kringle type-IV repeats) was negatively associated with OxPL/apoB (r = –0.49, p < 0.001) and Lp(a) (r = –0.61, p < 0.001), irrespective of racial group. After adjusting for apolipoprotein(a) isoform size, the relationship between OxPL/apoB and Lp(a) remained significant (r = 0.67, p < 0.001, table 2-2). The association of OxPL with small apolipoprotein(a) isoforms, where a similar relationship is present among all racial subgroups despite

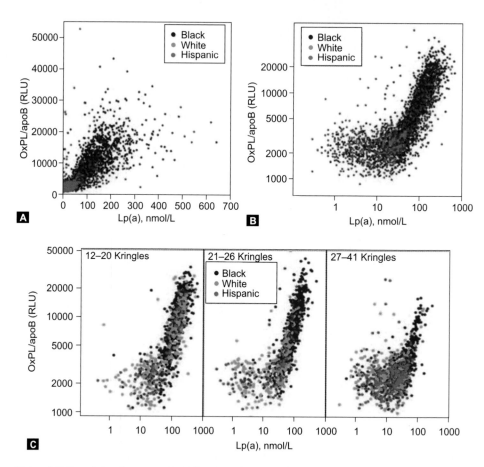

Figure 2-5 Correlation between OxPL/apoB and Lp(a) in the Dallas Heart Study. **A,** Relationship plotted on a geometric scale. **B,** Relationship plotted on a logarithmic scale. **C,** Relationship in the entire cohort according to apo(a) isoform sizes. *From* Tsimikas S, Clopton P, Brilakis ES, Marcovina SM, Khera A, Miller ER, et al. Relationship of oxidized phospholipids on apolipoprotein B-100 particles to race/ethnicity, apolipoprotein(a) isoform size, and cardiovascular risk factors: results from the Dallas Heart Study. *Circulation.* 2009;119:1711-9.

Table 2-2	Spearman Correlation (r-values) between Lp(a) and OxPL/apoB by Race and Sex						
Correlation	*All*	*BF*	*BM*	*WF*	*WM*	*HF*	*HM*
Lp(a) vs OxPL/apoB	0.84[*]	0.87[*]	0.87[*]	0.72[*]	0.68[*]	0.69[*]	0.53[*]
Correlation between major apolipoprotein(a) allele and OxPL/apoB by race-sex							
apolipoprotein(a) vs OxPL/apoB	−0.50[*]	−0.47[*]	−0.48[*]	−0.46[*]	−0.46[*]	−0.50[*]	−0.32[*]
Correlation between Lp(a) and OxPL/apoB by race-sex stratified by # of apolipoprotein(a) isoforms in the major allele							
12–20	0.85[*]	0.81[*]	0.84[*]	0.84[*]	0.85[*]	0.85[*]	0.80[*]
21–26	0.88[*]	0.86[*]	0.85[*]	0.74[*]	0.62[*]	0.80[*]	0.69[*]
27–41	0.47[*]	0.67[*]	0.71[*]	0.16[†]	0.13[†]	0.38[*]	0.25[*]

[*]$p < 0.001$; [†]$p < 0.05$.
BF, Black females; BM, Black males; WF, White females; WM, White males; HF, Hispanic females; HM, Hispanic males.
From Tsimikas S, Clopton P, Brilakis ES, Marcovina SM, Khera A, Miller ER, et al. Relationship of oxidized phospholipids on apolipoprotein B-100 particles to race/ethnicity, apolipoprotein(a) isoform size, and cardiovascular risk factors: results from the Dallas Heart Study. *Circulation.* 2009;119:1711-9.

differences in plasma Lp(a) levels, may be a key determinant of cardiovascular risk. In summary, this suggests that the OxPL/apoB levels reflect the most atherogenic Lp(a) particles, irrespective of race, and may allow clinical selection of risk profiles above and beyond measuring Lp(a) levels, as recently shown in the EPIC-Norfolk study.[48]

RELATIONSHIP OF OxPL/apoB AND CARDIOVASCULAR DISEASE

Association with Acute Coronary Syndromes and Percutaneous Coronary Intervention

Acute coronary syndromes (ACS) are associated with increased oxidative stress.[51-53] In two studies, it was demonstrated that acute increases occur in OxPL/apoB in patients following ACS[30] or during uncomplicated percutaneous coronary intervention (PCI),[34] suggesting generation and/or release of oxidized lipids into the circulation from atherosclerotic lesions. In a prospective study in patients with ACS,[30] it was demonstrated that OxPL/apoB levels rise rapidly by approximately 54% after an acute myocardial infarction and then tend to decrease toward baseline levels over the next seven months (Figure 2-6). In comparison, no significant changes were noted in patients with stable CAD, patients with normal coronary angiograms and a control group of healthy subjects followed for the same period of time. Further supporting this finding, a follow-up study demonstrated that OxPL/apoB and Lp(a) levels also acutely increased [by 36% (P < 0.0001) (Figure 2-7) and 64% (P < 0.0001), respectively] immediately following PCI.[34] Interestingly, the OxPL/apoB levels returned to baseline by 6 hours and precipitation experiments showed that immediately after PCI, approximately 50% of OxPLs were present on Lp(a) whereas

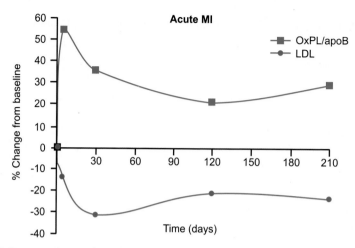

Figure 2-6 Percent change from baseline in OxPL/apoB measured by antibody E06. The p values at the 30-, 120-, and 210-day labels represent differences between groups at each time point. Changes in LDL-C are given for comparison. *From* Tsimikas S, Bergmark C, Beyer RW, Patel R, Pattison J, Miller E, et al. Temporal increases in plasma markers of oxidized low-density lipoprotein strongly reflect the presence of acute coronary syndromes. *J Am Coll Cardiol.* 2003;41:360-70, with permission.

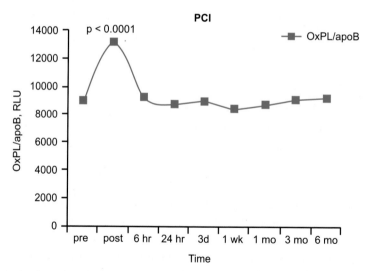

Figure 2-7 Absolute changes in relative light units (RLU) in OxPL/apoB after PCI. *P < 0.001 compared with other time points. *Modified from* Tsimikas S, Lau HK, Han KR, Shortal B, Miller ER, Segev A, et al. Percutaneous coronary intervention results in acute increases in oxidized phospholipids and lipoprotein(a): short-term and long-term immunologic responses to oxidized low-density lipoprotein. *Circulation.* 2004;109:3164-70.

the other 50% were present on non-Lp(a) apoB-100 particles. By 6 hours after PCI, however, more than 90% of OxPL were again present on Lp(a), suggesting that, when present, Lp(a) preferentially binds and transports mobilized OxPL.[44]

Association with Coronary Artery Disease

The relationship of OxPL/apoB to coronary artery disease (CAD) was shown in 504 patients immediately before undergoing clinically indicated coronary angiography.[49] OxPL/apoB levels were strongly and independently correlated with the presence and extent of angiographically documented CAD, particularly in patients 60 years of age or younger. A graded increase in levels was associated with more advanced disease, defined by > 50% diameter stenosis and measured as 1-, 2-, or 3-vessel CAD. In patients less than 60 years of age, compared with the lowest quartile, patients in the highest quartile of OxPL/apoB had odds ratios (OR) for CAD of 3.12 (P = 0.004), a relationship that was markedly accentuated in the setting of hyperlipidemia [OR 16.8] (Table 2-3). In the entire cohort, OxPL/apoB levels were independently associated with obstructive CAD for all clinical and lipid measures except one,

Table 2-3	Relationship of OxPL/apoB with CAD According to the Presence or Absence of Hypercholesterolemia (HC)				
Patient Group	Oxidized Phospholipid: Apo B-100 ratio				P value
	No HC		HC		
	% with CAD	OR (95% CI)	% with CAD	OR (95% CI)	
All patients					
Quartile I	29	1.00	67	4.93 (2.31–10.5)	
Quartile II	44	1.92 (0.91–4.06)	56	3.10 (1.54–6.25)	
Quartile III	38	1.47 (0.68–3.19)	64	4.36 (2.16–8.79)	
Quartile IV	39	1.54 (0.70–3.40)	77	8.13 (3.88–17.1)	< 0.001
Age ≤ 60 yr					
Quartile I	14	1.00	61	9.33 (2.64–33.0)	
Quartile II	27	2.21 (0.61–7.97)	37	3.53 (1.03–12.0)	
Quartile III	28	2.33 (0.64–8.45)	57	8.00 (2.51–25.5)	
Quartile IV	43	4.59 (1.39–15.1)	74	16.8 (5.11–55.2)	< 0.001
Age > 60 yr					
Quartile I	45	1.00	71	3.00 (1.10–8.18)	
Quartile II	61	1.85 (0.67–5.15)	68	2.57 (1.01–6.54)	
Quartile III	48	1.11 (0.39–3.14)	71	2.90 (1.11–7.58)	
Quartile IV	31	0.55 (0.15–1.92)	80	4.95 (1.76–13.9)	0.003

For the OxPL/apoB ratio, quartiles I through IV correspond to the following values: < 0.047, 0.047–0.089, > 0.089–0.294, and > 0.294, respectively. The P values indicate whether any two of the eight groups (defined by quartile and hypercholesterolemia status) have significantly different proportions of subjects with CAD.

OR, odds ratio; CI, confidence interval.

From Tsimikas S, Brilakis ES, Miller ER, McConnell JP, Lennon RJ, Kornman KS, et al. Oxidized phospholipids, Lp(a) lipoprotein, and coronary artery disease. N Engl J Med. 2005;353:46-57, with permission.

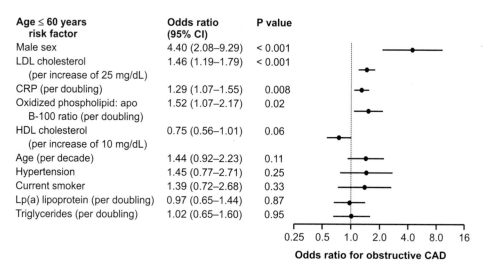

Age ≤ 60 years risk factor	Odds ratio (95% CI)	P value
Male sex	4.40 (2.08–9.29)	< 0.001
LDL cholesterol (per increase of 25 mg/dL)	1.46 (1.19–1.79)	< 0.001
CRP (per doubling)	1.29 (1.07–1.55)	0.008
Oxidized phospholipid: apo B-100 ratio (per doubling)	1.52 (1.07–2.17)	0.02
HDL cholesterol (per increase of 10 mg/dL)	0.75 (0.56–1.01)	0.06
Age (per decade)	1.44 (0.92–2.23)	0.11
Hypertension	1.45 (0.77–2.71)	0.25
Current smoker	1.39 (0.72–2.68)	0.33
Lp(a) lipoprotein (per doubling)	0.97 (0.65–1.44)	0.87
Triglycerides (per doubling)	1.02 (0.65–1.60)	0.95

Odds ratio for obstructive CAD

Figure 2-8 Odds Ratios for obstructive CAD associated with selected risk factors among patients 60 years of age or younger from the multivariable analysis. Risk factors are shown in descending order of significance. In this analysis, Lp(a) lipoprotein was forced into the model with the oxidized phospholipid:apo B-100 ratio. CI, confidence interval; LDL, low-density lipoprotein; CRP, C-reactive protein, oxidized phospholipid:apo B-100 ratio: the ratio of oxidized phospholipid content per particle of apolipoprotein B-100; HDL, high-density lipoprotein. *From* Tsimikas S, Brilakis ES, Miller ER, McConnell JP, Lennon RJ, Kornman KS, et al. Oxidized phospholipids, Lp(a) lipoprotein, and coronary artery disease. *N Engl J Med.* 2005;353:46-57, with permission.

Lp(a), suggesting a common biologic influence on CAD risk. However, in patients aged 60 years or less, OxPL/apoB remained an independent predictor of CAD, even with Lp(a) in the model (Figure 2-8). These observations support the hypothesis that much of the risk attributable to Lp(a) levels can be explained by the binding of OxPL by Lp(a) lipoprotein, but that in younger patients, an additional risk associated with OxPL may be present, perhaps through proinflammatory pathways independent of Lp(a).

Relationship to Peripheral Artery Disease

The utility of OxPL/apoB in predicting the presence and progression of carotid and femoral atherosclerosis was evaluated in the Bruneck study, a large prospective population-based survey of 40- to 79-year-old men and women initiated in 1990.[31] Serial plasma levels of OxPL/apoB were acquired in 765 and 671 subjects in 1995 and 2000, respectively. The cohort was evaluated for baseline cardiovascular events and also followed for progression of atherosclerosis with serial measurement of femoral and carotid intima-media thickness (IMT) and atherosclerosis. OxPL/apoB levels were strongly and significantly associated with the presence, extent, and

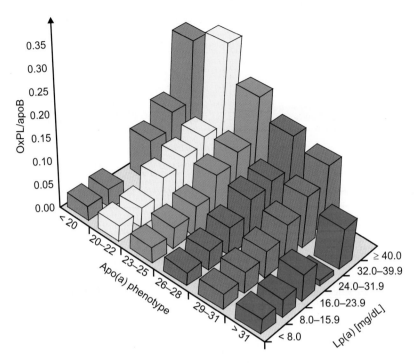

Figure 2-9 Three-dimensional plot of OxPL/apoB levels according to Lp(a) mass and apolipoprotein (a) [Apo(a)] phenotypes expressed as the number of kringle IV-type 2 repeats. The OxPL/apoB levels presented are geometric means (taken as the antilog of the mean of log-transformed OxPL/apoB values). *From* Tsimikas S, Kiechl S, Willeit J, Mayr M, Miller ER, Kronenberg F, et al. Oxidized phospholipids predict the presence and progression of carotid and femoral atherosclerosis and symptomatic cardiovascular disease: five-year prospective results from the Bruneck study. *J Am Coll Cardiol*. 2006;47:2219-28, with permission.

development (1995–2000) of carotid and femoral atherosclerosis and predicted the presence of symptomatic cardiovascular disease. The highest tertile of OxPL/apoB was associated with a higher odds ratio for the presence (in 1995) and development (1995–2000) of carotid and femoral atherosclerosis (Figure 2-9), compared with the lowest tertile. Both OxPL/apoB and Lp(a) levels showed similar associations with atherosclerosis severity and progression, suggesting a common biological influence on atherogenesis. This study, also, showed for the first time that the association of OxPL/apoB and Lp(a) was strongest in those subjects with the highest Lp(a) concentration but smallest apo(a) isoforms, suggesting that OxPL/apoB levels may be related to the number of K-IV2 repeats (Figure 2-10).

Prediction of Cardiovascular Events

The Bruneck study[31,45] was the first prospective epidemiological study to demonstrate the prognostic utility of OxPL/apoB levels in predicting future death, myocardial

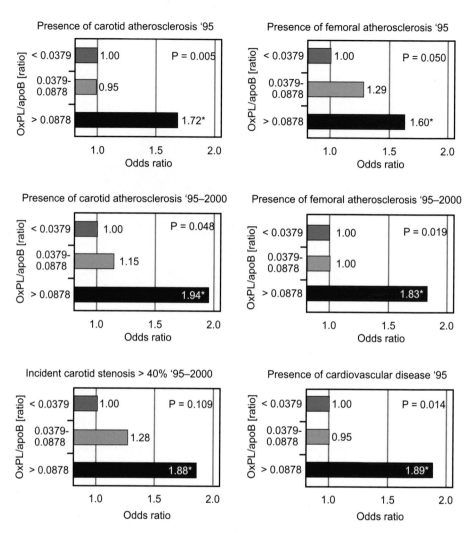

Figure 2-10 Multivariate analysis showing the association of oxidized phospholipids (OxPL)/apolipoprotein B-100 particle (apoB) tertile groups with presence and progression of carotid and femoral artery atherosclerosis and with cardiovascular disease. *p < 0.05 for the comparison between the first tertile group (reference category) and the third tertile group. The p values presented in the figures are the overall p values for the three tertiles (test for trend). *From* Tsimikas S, Kiechl S, Willeit J, Mayr M, Miller ER, Kronenberg F, et al. Oxidized phospholipids predict the presence and progression of carotid and femoral atherosclerosis and symptomatic cardiovascular disease: five-year prospective results from the Bruneck study. *J Am Coll Cardiol.* 2006;47:2219-28, with permission.

infarction, stroke, and TIA and revascularization. OxPL/apoB levels measured at baseline in an unselected population derived from the general community predicted the development of cardiovascular events over a 10-year prospective follow-up period. In multivariable analysis, which included traditional risk factors,

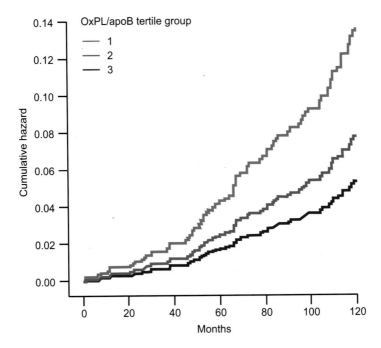

Figure 2-11 Cumulative hazard curves of incident CVD from 1995 to 2005 for tertiles of OxPL/apoB In the Bruneck Study. *From* Kiechl S, Willeit J, Mayr M, Viehweider B, Oberhollenzer M, Kronenberg F, et al. Oxidized phospholipids, lipoprotein(a), lipoprotein-associated phospholipase A_2 activity, and 10-year cardiovascular outcomes: prospective results from the Bruneck study. *Arterioscler Thromb Vasc Biol.* 2007;27:1788-95.

hsCRP, and lipoprotein-associated phospholipase A_2 (Lp-PLA$_2$) activity, subjects in the highest tertile of OxPL/apoB had a significantly higher risk of cardiovascular events than those in the lowest tertile (hazard ratio[95% CI] 2.4[1.3–4.3], P = 0.004) (Figure 2-11). These results were confirmed in the prospective case-control study nested in the EPIC (European Prospective Investigation of Cancer)-Norfolk cohort of 45- to 79-year-old apparently healthy men and women followed for 6 years.[48] Cases consisted of participants in whom fatal or nonfatal CAD developed, matched by sex, age, and enrollment time with controls without CAD. Baseline levels of OxPL/apoB and Lp(a) were measured in 763 cases and 1,397 controls. After adjusting for age, smoking, diabetes, low- and high-density lipoprotein cholesterol, and systolic blood pressure, the highest tertiles of OxPL/apoB were associated with a significantly higher risk of CAD events (odds ratios: 1.67; p < 0.001) compared with the lowest tertiles (Table 2-4).

Furthermore, OxPL/apoB levels provided additional predictive value to the Framingham Risk Score (FRS). By measuring OxPL/apoB in each tertile of FRS, the predicted risk can be either increased or decreased depending on the tertiles of OxPL/apoB. This would allow fine tuning of risk prediction and more accurate

Table 2-4	Odds Ratios (95% CI) for CAD for Tertiles of OxPL/apoB in the EPIC-Norfolk Study			
OxPL/apoB	Tertile 1 < 1,150 RLUs	Tertile 2 1,150–2,249 RLUs	Tertile 3 > 2,249 RLUs	p trend linearity
Entire cohort				
Unadjusted	1.00	1.21 (0.97–1.52)	1.61 (1.29–2.01)	< 0.001
Adjusted model 1*	1.00	1.32 (1.04–1.68)	1.67 (1.32–2.12)	< 0.001
Adjusted model 2**	1.00	1.27 (1.01–1.60)	1.66 (1.32–2.09)	< 0.001
Men				
Unadjusted	1.00	1.31 (0.99–1.75)	1.59 (1.20–2.11)	0.001
Adjusted model 1*	1.00	1.43 (1.05–1.94)	1.65 (1.21–2.24)	0.001
Adjusted model 2**	1.00	1.42 (1.06–1.92)	1.70 (1.26–2.29)	< 0.001
Women				
Unadjusted	1.00	0.96 (0.67–1.39)	1.60 (1.12–2.28)	0.009
Adjusted model 1*	1.00	1.05 (0.70–1.56)	1.67 (1.14–2.44)	0.007
Adjusted model 2**	1.00	0.97 (0.67–1.41)	1.58 (1.10–2.26)	0.01

*Model 1 matched for sex, age, and enrollment time and adjusted for diabetes, smoking, systolic blood pressure, and LDL and HDL cholesterol.
**Model 2 matched for sex, age, and enrollment time, and adjusted for Framingham Risk Score.
From Tsimikas S, Mallat Z, Talmud PJ, Kastelein JJ, Wareham NJ, Sandhu MS, et al. Oxidation-specific biomarkers, lipoprotein(a), and risk of fatal and nonfatal coronary events. J Am Coll Cardiol. 2010;56:946-55, with permission.

assessment of treatment options. For example, in the Bruneck Study, the graded increase in CVD risk across OxPL/apoB tertile groups was evident in the low-risk, moderate-risk, and high-risk groups as defined by the FRS (Figure 2-12A).[45] This result was validated in the EPIC-Norfolk study (Figure 2-12B).[48] Finally, OxPL/apoB values are independent of metabolic syndrome parameters.[48]

Receiver-operator Characteristic c-index Values

To assess the predictive value of the utility of these biomarkers above the FRS, receiver-operator characteristic unconditional c-indexes were generated.[48] The c-index for the FRS was 0.584 (95% CI: 0.558–0.609), a relatively low value that reflects the fact that age and sex were already accounted for as part of the matching design. Adding individual biomarkers to the FRS shows that the c-index increased from 0.584 (95% CI: 0.558–0.609) to 0.618 (95% CI: 0.593–0.642), in progressing order of myeloperoxidase mass, Lp-PLA$_2$ activity, OxPL/apoB, hsCRP, Lp(a), secretory phospholipase A$_2$ (sPLA$_2$) mass, and sPLA$_2$ activity. Adding biomarkers to FRS until all biomarkers were present in the model progressively increased the c-index from 0.584 (95% CI: (0.558–0.609) to 0.651 (95% CI: 0.627–0.675) (Table 2-5).

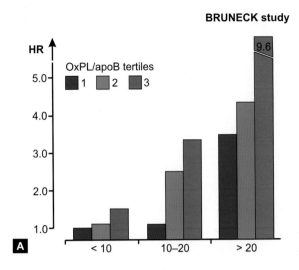

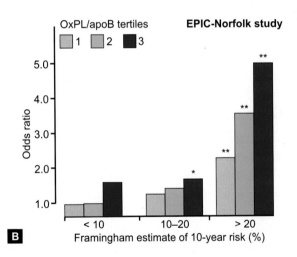

Figure 2-12 A, Relationship between tertile groups of OxPL/apoB ratio (< 0.0379, 0.0379–0.0878, > 0.0878; A) and CVD risk within each Framingham Risk Score Group. Framingham Risk Score was calculated as low risk (<10% risk of events over 10 years), moderate risk (10–20%), and high risk (> 20%). *From* Kiechl S, Willeit J, Mayr M, Viehweider B, Oberhollenzer M, Kronenberg F, et al. Oxidized phospholipids, lipoprotein(a), lipoprotein-associated phospholipase A$_2$ activity, and 10-year cardiovascular outcomes: prospective results from the Bruneck study. *Arterioscler Thromb Vasc Biol.* 2007;27:1788-95. **B,** Relationship between tertile groups of OxPL/apoB RLU (< 1,150, 1,151–2,249, and > 2,249 RLUs) and future CAD risk within each Framingham Risk Score group. *p < 0.05 and **p < 0.001 for comparison of each tertile of the respective biomarkers with the lowest tertile in the low Framingham Risk Score category of each biomarker. *From* Tsimikas S, Mallat Z, Talmud PJ, Kastelein JJ, Wareham NJ, Sandhu MS, et al. Oxidation-specific biomarkers, lipoprotein(a), and risk of fatal and nonfatal coronary events. *J Am Coll Cardiol.* 2010;56:946-55.

Table 2-5	c-index Values for Receiver Operating Curves in the EPIC-Norfolk Study
FRS	0.584 (0.558–0.609)
FRS, MPO	0.586 (0.561–0.612)
FRS, Lp-PLA$_2$	0.587 (0.562–0.613)
FRS, OxPL/apoB	0.597 (0.572–0.623)
FRS, hsCRP	0.605 (0.580–0.630)
FRS, Lp(a)	0.607 (0.582–0.632)
FRS, sPLA$_2$ mass	0.609 (0.584–0.634)
FRS, sPLA$_2$ activity	0.618 (0.593–0.642)
FRS, MPO, Lp-PLA$_2$	0.590 (0.565–0.616)
FRS, MPO, Lp-PLA$_2$, OxPL/apoB	0.603 (0.578–0.628)
FRS, MPO, Lp-PLA$_2$, OxPL/apoB, hsCRP	0.614 (0.590–0.639)
FRS, MPO, Lp-PLA$_2$, OxPL/apoB, hsCRP, Lp(a)	0.625 (0.600–0.649)
FRS, MPO, Lp-PLA$_2$, OxPL/apoB, hsCRP, Lp(a), sPLA$_2$ mass	0.635 (0.610–0.659)
FRS, MPO, Lp-PLA$_2$, OxPL/apoB, hsCRP, Lp(a), sPLA$_2$ mass, sPLA$_2$ activity	0.651 (0.627–0.675)

FRS, Framingham Risk Score; MPO, myeloperoxidase.
From Tsimikas S, Mallat Z, Talmud PJ, Kastelein JJ, Wareham NJ, Sandhu MS, et al. Oxidation-specific biomarkers, lipoprotein(a), and risk of fatal and nonfatal coronary events. *J Am Coll Cardiol.* 2010;56: 946-55, with permission.

Relationship of OxPL/apoB to Lp(a), Lp-PLA$_2$ and sPLA$_2$

In prior studies, we had shown that OxPL/apoB reflect the biological activity of small apo(a) isoforms associated with high Lp(a) levels.[45,50] Furthermore, the OxPL/apoB assay represents OxPL bound by Lp(a) (approximately 85–90%) and non-Lp(a) apoB (10–15%), on average.[44] This relationship is not constant and depends on the underlying LPA genetics, where small isoforms are associated with high OxPL/apoB and high correlations with Lp(a),[50,54] but large isoforms with low Lp(a) levels (i.e., < 25 mg/dL) with weak to absent correlations.[50] To assess whether adding Lp(a) levels to OxPL/apoB enhances predictive value for CVD events, we performed a 3 × 3 tertile analysis in evaluating relationship to CAD events in EPIC-Norfolk. This demonstrated that the relationship of OxPL/apoB and Lp(a) to fatal and nonfatal CAD was accentuated in the highest tertiles of both biomarkers (OR: 1.77, 95% CI: 1.31-2.37), suggesting that they can provide independent and additive information for risk prediction (Figure 2-13).[48]

Lp-PLA$_2$ and sPLA$_2$ are enzymes that react with OxPLs and cleave the oxidized fatty acid side chain at the sn2 position of OxPL to generate lysophosphatidylcholine and an oxidized free fatty acid. Both of these biomarkers have been associated with the prediction of higher cardiovascular events when elevated and are targets of ongoing therapeutic trials to inhibit their activities.[55] Because OxPL and phospholipases

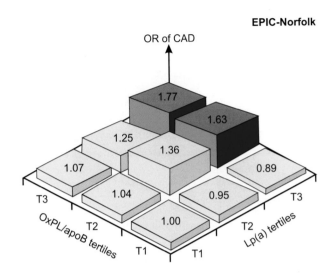

Figure 2-13 Odds Ratios for fatal and nonfatal CAD based on tertiles of OxPL/apoB and Lp(a). The tertile cutoffs for OxPL/apoB are < 1,150, 1,151–2,249, and > 2,249 RLUs and < 7.25, 7.25–11.69, and > 11.69 mg/dL for Lp(a). *From* Tsimikas S, Mallat Z, Talmud PJ, Kastelein JJ, Wareham NJ, Sandhu MS, et al. Oxidation-specific biomarkers, lipoprotein(a), and risk of fatal and nonfatal coronary events. *J Am Coll Cardiol.* 2010;56:946-55, with permission.

may share similar pathophysiology, we evaluated whether the combination of these biomarkers provides enhanced predictive value. In the Bruneck Study, the strength of the association between OxPL/apoB and CVD risk significantly increased with increasing Lp-PLA$_2$ activity (P = 0.018 for interaction) (Figure 2-14A). Similarly, the odds ratio of CAD events associated with the highest tertiles of OxPL/apoB was significantly potentiated (approximately doubled) by the highest tertiles of sPLA$_2$ activity and mass (Figure 2-14B). In clinical risk prediction, using combinations of these biomarkers may allow stronger predictive value for ascertaining CVD risk.

Change in OxPL/apoB and Therapeutic Interventions

Originally, we developed the OxPL/apoB measure as an indicator of minimally oxidized LDL in plasma that might reflect the overall content of circulating OxLDL. We surmised that the OxPL/apoB ratio would increase during hypercholesterolemia and atherosclerosis progression and decrease during atherosclerosis regression. Counterintuitively, we have found the opposite, in both animals[56] and humans.[35,57-63] As demonstrated in Tsimikas et al.,[64] in New Zealand White rabbits and cynomolgus monkey models of atherosclerosis, which do not have Lp(a) or their Lp(a) does not bind OxPL and/or has E06 immunoreactivity, respectively, the OxPL/apoB ratio increased 50–100% in plasma in the setting of lesion regression, concomitant with reduced presence of OxPL in atherosclerotic lesions (Figure 2-15). Note that the

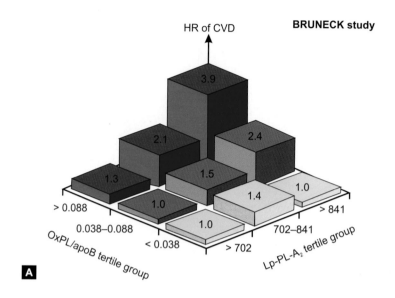

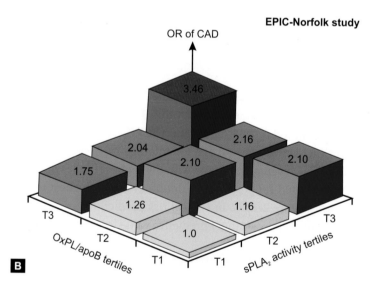

Figure 2-14 A, Relationship between OxPL/apoB (A) tertile groups and CVD risk according to tertiles of Lp-PLA$_2$ activity. *From* Kiechl S, Willeit J, Mayr M, Viehweider B, Oberhollenzer M, Kronenberg F, et al. Oxidized phospholipids, lipoprotein(a), lipoprotein-associated phospholipase A$_2$ activity, and 10-year cardiovascular outcomes: prospective results from the Bruneck study. *Arterioscler Thromb Vasc Biol.* 2007;27:1788-95. **B,** Odds ratios for CAD based on tertiles of OxPL/apoB and sPLA$_2$ activity. The tertile cutoffs for OxPL/apoB are < 1,150 relative light units (RLUs), 1,151–2,249 RLUs, and > 2,249 RLUs, and for sPLA$_2$ activity levels < 4.05, 4.05–4.83, and > 4.83 nmol/min/mL. *From* Tsimikas S, Mallat Z, Talmud PJ, Kastelein JJ, Wareham NJ, Sandhu MS, et al. Oxidation-specific biomarkers, lipoprotein(a), and risk of fatal and nonfatal coronary events. *J Am Coll Cardiol.* 2010;56: 946-55, with permission.

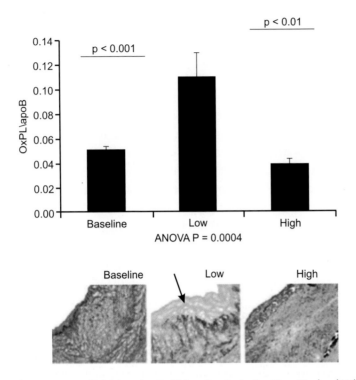

Figure 2-15 The upper panel depicts the OxPL/apoB ratio in the New Zealand White (NZW) rabbit study in the baseline (n = 15), low-cholesterol (N = 10), and high-cholesterol (N = 5) groups. The lower panel depicts immunochemistry of NZW aortas with antibody E06 staining (brown color pattern) for OxPL in the baseline, low-cholesterol, and high-cholesterol diet groups. The arrow represents lack of OxPL at the luminal surface in a representative rabbit with preexisting atherosclerosis that was subsequently switched to a low-cholesterol diet. Note that the OxPL staining in the middle panel has disappeared from the luminal surface, while the OxPL/apoB level goes up in plasma, suggesting a flux of OxPL from the vessel wall to the circulation during dietary induced regression. *From* Tsimikas S, Aikawa M, Miller FJ Jr, Miller ER, Torzewski M, Lentz SR, et al. Increased plasma oxidized phospholipid:apolipoprotein B-100 ratio with concomitant depletion of oxidized phospholipids from atherosclerotic lesions after dietary lipid-lowering: a potential biomarker of early atherosclerosis regression. *Arterioscler Thromb Vasc Biol.* 2007;27:175-81.

oxidized phospholipid staining in the middle panel of figure 2-15 has disappeared from the luminal surface, while the OxPL/apoB level goes up in plasma, suggesting a flux of OxPL from the vessel wall to the circulation during dietary induced regression. This observation suggests that efflux of OxPL from arterial lesions into plasma occurs preferentially early during atherosclerosis regression, even more extensively than depletion of apoB-100 or physical plaque regression. These data suggest that changes in the OxPL/apoB ratio may reflect early atherosclerosis regression. Similarly, in human studies with low fat diets,[57,59] aged garlic supplementation[60,61] and statin therapy,[35,57,58,63] (Table 2-1) significant increases in OxPL/apoB have been noted shortly after the initiation of the intervention. Although the etiology of these changes are not fully defined, the data are consistent across studies and are associated with treatments considered to be of clinical benefit. For example, in the MIRACL trial, an increase in OxPL/apoB and Lp(a) was observed at 16 weeks after initiation of atorvastatin therapy, consistent with a decreased recurrence of clinical events, while no such change was observed in the placebo arm. Similarly, an increase in OxPL/apoB, and Lp(a) in response to aged garlic supplements was associated with less progression of coronary artery calcium and improvement in vascular function.[60,61] Based on the animal data, one may postulate a flux of OxPL, from sites of vessel injury or inflammation to the circulation, where they are bound to apoB lipoproteins. In humans, the OxPL preferentially bind to Lp(a), but we have also noted an increase in the Lp(a) levels as well, suggesting that perhaps there is some signaling mechanism leading to increased Lp(a) levels in these settings. These findings are consistent with our suggestion noted above that a "physiological" role of Lp(a) may be to bind and transport cellular sources of OxPL, such as from apoptotic cells or during normal cellular metabolism where OxPL may be generated. Whether these increases in OxPL/apoB found in the settings of low fat diets, statin therapy, or other potentially beneficial interventions are biomarkers of enhanced efflux from the artery of OxPL, and hence a surrogate of regression, remains to be established. The apparent paradox is that OxPL/apoB remain a strongly independent predictor of CVD in prospective studies, yet here we find they are increased, at least in the short-term, in settings of effective therapy. We suggest that a resolution of this paradox may be that with continued therapy, the initial efflux into plasma of OxPL will return to baseline, and the elevated OxPL/apoB will revert to basal levels, or even lower, consistent with reduced risk caused by the intervention. These ideas are currently being tested by extended analyses of adequately powered prospective intervention trials. If confirmed, an early rise in OxPL/apoB might then be used as a useful surrogate biomarker of a beneficial intervention. Such biomarkers are urgently needed.

CONCLUSION AND FUTURE DIRECTIONS

Oxidized phospholipids are strongly implicated in several aspects of cardiovascular disease. The OxPL/apoB assay provides diagnostic information in strongly reflecting the presence and progression of cardiovascular disease and prognostic information for predicting future cardiovascular events. It independently complements established risk factors in risk prediction, is independent of the metabolic syndrome and optimizes the predictive value of the FRS. Importantly, from a pathophysiological perspective, OxPL/apoB appears to most closely reflect the biological activity of the most atherogenic Lp(a) particles that are associated with both high Lp(a) levels and small apo(a) isoforms. Since apo(a) isoforms are laborious and expensive to measure, OxPL/apoB levels may accurately reflect the CVD risk of these atherogenic lipoproteins. With Lp(a) now being established as an independent, genetic risk factor for CVD, it may become a target of therapy in future studies. In fact, the antisense oligonucleotide mipomersen and a more specific antisense oligonucleotide targeted to KIV-2 repeats of apo(a) have recently been shown to reduce plasma levels of Lp(a)/apo(a), and their associated OxPL, by 75–86% in Lp(a)-transgenic mice,[64,65] setting the stage for future clinical development.

Currently, the OxPL/apoB assay is a research tool but the large clinical database already established suggests that with standardization of the methodology, it will be a useful biomarker that can be used clinically for risk stratification. Future research will focus on the early (and possibly late) changes in OxPL/apoB that occur with therapeutic interventions and whether therapeutic decisions can be guided by assessing these changes in response to the intervention. Finally, since OxPL are implicated in a variety of disorders that have oxidative stress as a key component, such as Alzheimer's disease, multiple sclerosis, non-alcoholic steatohepatitis, rheumatologic diseases, such as lupus and rheumatoid arthritis, infectious disease, and cancer, it would be of interest to assess whether OxPL/apoB and related oxidative biomarkers are associated with and predict noncardiovascular outcomes in patients with these disorders.

Disclosure

Dr. Tsimikas is named as co-inventor of patents and patent applications owned by the University of California for the clinical use of oxidation-specific antibodies. Dr. Tsimikas is a consultant to Quest and ISIS, Inc. and has received investigator-initiated research funding from Merck, Inc. and Pfizer, Inc.

REFERENCES

1. Glass CK, Witztum JL. Atherosclerosis. the road ahead. *Cell.* 2001;104:503-16.
2. Navab M, Reddy ST, Van Lenten BJ, Fogelman AM. HDL and cardiovascular disease: atherogenic and atheroprotective mechanisms. *Nat Rev Cardiol.* 2011;advance online publication.
3. Steinberg D, Parthasarathy S, Carew TE, Khoo JC, Witztum JL. Beyond cholesterol. Modifications of low-density lipoprotein that increase its atherogenicity. *N Engl J Med.* 1989;320:915-24.
4. Nishi K, Itabe H, Uno M, Kitazato KT, Horiguchi H, Shinno K, et al. Oxidized LDL in carotid plaques and plasma associates with plaque instability. *Arterioscler Thromb Vasc Biol.* 2002;22:1649-54.
5. Seimon TA, Nadolski MJ, Liao X, Magallon J, Nguyen M, Feric NT, et al. Atherogenic lipids and lipoproteins trigger CD36-TLR2-dependent apoptosis in macrophages undergoing endoplasmic reticulum stress. *Cell Metab.* 2010;12:467-82.
6. Tabas I, Ron D. Integrating the mechanisms of apoptosis induced by endoplasmic reticulum stress. *Nat Cell Biol.* 2011;13:184-90.

7. Salonen JT, Yla-Herttuala S, Yamamoto R, Butler S, Korpela H, Salonen R, et al. Autoantibody against oxidised LDL and progression of carotid atherosclerosis. *Lancet.* 1992;339:883-7.

8. Palinski W, Rosenfeld ME, Yla-Herttuala S, Gurtner GC, Socher SS, Butler SW, et al. Low density lipoprotein undergoes oxidative modification in vivo. *Proc Natl Acad Sci U S A.* 1989;86:1372-6.

9. Palinski W, Ord VA, Plump AS, Breslow JL, Steinberg D, Witztum JL. ApoE-deficient mice are a model of lipoprotein oxidation in atherogenesis. Demonstration of oxidation-specific epitopes in lesions and high titers of autoantibodies to malondialdehyde-lysine in serum. *Arterioscler Thromb.* 1994;14:605-16.

10. Berliner JA, Leitinger N, Tsimikas S. The role of oxidized phospholipids in atherosclerosis. *J Lipid Res.* 2009;50 Suppl:S207-12. Epub 2008 Dec 4.

11. Bochkov VN, Oskolkova OV, Birukov KG, Levonen AL, Binder CJ, Stockl J. Generation and biological activities of oxidized phospholipids. *Antioxid Redox Signal.* 2010;12: 1009-59.

12. Greenberg ME, Li XM, Gugiu BG, Gu X, Qin J, Salomon RG, et al. The Lipid Whisker Model of the Structure of Oxidized Cell Membranes. *J Biol Chem.* 2008;283:2385-96.

13. Van Dijk RA, Shaw PX, Kolodgie F, et al. Differential Expression of Oxidation-Specific Epitopes and Lipoprotein (a) Reflect the Presence of Progressive and Ruptured Plaques in Human Coronary Arteries. Submited 2010.

14. Libby P. Inflammation in atherosclerosis. *Nature.* 2002;420:868-874.

15. Horkko S, Bird DA, Miller E, Itabe H, Leitinger N, Subbanagounder G, et al. Monoclonal autoantibodies specific for oxidized phospholipids or oxidized phospholipid-protein adducts inhibit macrophage uptake of oxidized low-density lipoproteins. *J Clin Invest.* 1999;103:117-28.

16. Shaw PX, Horkko S, Chang MK, Curtiss LK, Palinski W, Silverman GJ, et al. Natural antibodies with the T15 idiotype may act in atherosclerosis, apoptotic clearance, and protective immunity. *J Clin Invest.* 2000;105:1731-40.

17. Friedman P, Horkko S, Steinberg D, Witztum JL, Dennis EA. Correlation of antiphospholipid antibody recognition with the structure of synthetic oxidized phospholipids. Importance of Schiff base formation and aldol condensation. *J Biol Chem.* 2002;277: 7010-20.

18. Briles DE, Forman C, Hudak S, Claflin JL. Anti-phosphorylcholine antibodies of the T15 idiotype are optimally protective against Streptococcus pneumoniae. *J Exp Med.* 1982;156:1177-85.

19. Imai Y, Kuba K, Neely GG, Yaghubian-Malhami R, Perkmann T, van Loo G, et al. Identification of oxidative stress and Toll-like receptor 4 signaling as a key pathway of acute lung injury. *Cell.* 2008;133:235-49.

20. Cruz D, Watson AD, Miller CS, Montoya D, Ochoa MT, Sieling PA, et al. Host-derived oxidized phospholipids and HDL regulate innate immunity in human leprosy. *J Clin Invest.* 2008;118:2917-28.

21. Boullier A, Li Y, Quehenberger O, Palinski W, Tabas I, Witztum JL, et al. Minimally oxidized LDL offsets the apoptotic effects of extensively oxidized LDL and free cholesterol in macrophages. *Arterioscler Thromb Vasc Biol.* 2006;26:1169-76.

22. Chang MK, Bergmark C, Laurila A, Hörkkö S, Han KH, Friedman P, et al. Monoclonal antibodies against oxidized low-density lipoprotein bind to apoptotic cells and inhibit their phagocytosis by elicited macrophages: evidence that oxidation-specific epitopes mediate macrophage recognition. *Proc Natl Acad Sci U S A.* 1999;96:6353-8.

23. Chang MK, Binder CJ, Miller YI, Subbanagounder G, Silverman GJ, Berliner JA, et al. Apoptotic cells with oxidation-specific epitopes are immunogenic and proinflammatory. *J Exp Med.* 2004;200:1359-70.

24. Ogden CA, Kowalewski R, Peng Y, Montenegro V, Elkon KB. IGM is required for efficient complement mediated phagocytosis of apoptotic cells in vivo. *Autoimmunity.* 2005;38:259-64.

25. Binder CJ, Horkko S, Dewan A, et al. Pneumococcal vaccination decreases atherosclerotic lesion formation: molecular mimicry between Streptococcus pneumoniae and oxidized LDL. *Nat Med.* 2003;9:736-43.

26. Hartvigsen K, Chou MY, Hansen LF, Shaw PX, Tsimikas S, Binder CJ, et al. The role of innate immunity in atherogenesis. *J Lipid Res.* 2009;50 Suppl:S388-93. Epub 2008 Dec 22.

27. Miller YI, Choi SH, Wiesner P, Fang L, Harkewicz R, Hartvigsen K, et al. Oxidation-specific epitopes are danger-associated molecular patterns recognized by pattern recognition receptors of innate immunity. *Circ Res.* 2011;108:235-48.

28. Fraley AE, Tsimikas S. Clinical applications of circulating oxidized low-density lipoprotein biomarkers in cardiovascular disease. *Curr Opin Lipidol.* 2006;17:502-9.

29. Tsimikas S, Witztum JL. The role of oxidized phospholipids in mediating lipoprotein(a) atherogenicity. *Curr Opin Lipidol.* 2008;19:369-77.

30. Tsimikas S, Bergmark C, Beyer RW, Patel R, Pattison J, Miller E, et al. Temporal increases in plasma markers of oxidized low-density lipoprotein strongly reflect the presence of acute coronary syndromes. *J Am Coll Cardiol.* 2003;41:360-70.

31. Tsimikas S, Kiechl S, Willeit J, Mayr M, Miller ER, Kronenberg F, et al. Oxidized phospholipids predict the presence and progression of carotid and femoral atherosclerosis and symptomatic cardiovascular disease: five-year prospective results from the Bruneck study. *J Am Coll Cardiol.* 2006;47:2219-28.

32. Young SG, Smith RS, Hogle DM, Curtiss LK, Witztum JL. Two new monoclonal antibody-based enzyme-linked assays of apolipoprotein B. *Clin Chem.* 1986;32:1484-90.

33. Young SG, Witztum JL, Casal DC, Curtiss LK, Bernstein S. Conservation of the low density lipoprotein receptor-binding domain of apoprotein B. Demonstration by a new monoclonal antibody, MB47. *Arteriosclerosis.* 1986;6:178-88.

34. Tsimikas S, Lau HK, Han KR, Shortal B, Miller ER, Segev A, et al. Percutaneous coronary intervention results in acute increases in oxidized phospholipids and lipoprotein(a): short-term and long-term immunologic responses to oxidized low-density lipoprotein. *Circulation.* 2004;109:3164-70.

35. Tsimikas S, Witztum JL, Miller ER, Sasiela WJ, Szarek M, Olsson AG, et al. High-dose atorvastatin reduces total plasma levels of oxidized phospholipids and immune complexes present on apolipoprotein B-100 in patients with acute coronary syndromes in the MIRACL trial. *Circulation.* 2004;110:1406-12.

36. Rhoads GG, Dahlen G, Berg K, Morton NE, Dannenberg AL. Lp(a) lipoprotein as a risk factor for myocardial infarction. *JAMA.* 1986;256:2540-44.

37. Seed M, Hoppichler F, Reaveley D, McCarthy S, Thompson GR, Boerwinkle E, et al. Relation of serum lipoprotein(a) concentration and apolipoprotein(a) phenotype to coronary heart disease in patients with familial hypercholesterolemia. *N Engl J Med.* 1990;322:1494-99.

38. Dangas G, Ambrose JA, D'Agate DJ, Shao JH, Chockalingham S, Levine D, et al. Correlation of serum lipoprotein(a) with the angiographic and clinical presentation of coronary artery disease. *J Am Coll Cardiol.* 1999;83:583-5.

39. Danesh J, Collins R, Peto R. Lipoprotein(a) and coronary heart disease. Meta-analysis of prospective studies. *Circulation.* 2000;102:1082-5.

40. Marcovina SM, Koschinsky ML, Albers JJ, Skarlatos S. Report of the National Heart, Lung, and Blood Institute Workshop on Lipoprotein(a) and Cardiovascular Disease: recent advances and future directions. *Clin Chem.* 2003;49:1785-96.

41. Bennet A, Di Angelantonio E, Erqou S, Eiriksdottir G, Sigurdsson G, Woodward M, et al. Lipoprotein(a) levels and risk of future coronary heart disease: Large-scale prospective data. *Arch Intern Med.* 2008;168:598-608.

42. Berglund L, Anuurad E. Role of Lipoprotein(a) in Cardiovascular Disease: Current and Future Perspectives. *J Am Coll Cardiol.* 2008;52:132-4.

43. Kamstrup PR, Benn M, Tybjaerg-Hansen A, Nordestgaard BG. Extreme lipoprotein(a) levels and risk of myocardial infarction in the general population: the Copenhagen City Heart Study. *Circulation.* 2008;117:176-84.

44. Bergmark C, Dewan A, Orsoni A, Merki E, Miller ER, Shin MJ, et al. A novel function of lipoprotein [a] as a preferential carrier of oxidized phospholipids in human plasma. *J Lipid Res.* 2008;49:2230-9.

45. Kiechl S, Willeit J, Mayr M, Viehweider B, Oberhollenzer M, Kronenberg F, et al. Oxidized phospholipids, lipoprotein(a), lipoprotein-associated phospholipase A_2 activity, and 10-year cardiovascular outcomes: prospective results from the Bruneck study. *Arterioscler Thromb Vasc Biol.* 2007;27:1788-95.

46. Berg K, Dahlen G, Christophersen B, Cook T, Kjekshus J, Pedersen T. Lp(a) lipoprotein level predicts survival and major coronary events in the Scandinavian Simvastatin Survival Study. *Clin Genet.* 1997;52:254-61.

47. Pillarisetti S, Paka L, Obunike JC, Berglund L, Goldberg IJ. Subendothelial retention of lipoprotein (a). Evidence that reduced heparan sulfate promotes lipoprotein binding to subendothelial matrix. *J Clin Invest.* 1997;100:867-74.

48. Tsimikas S, Mallat Z, Talmud PJ, Kastelein JJ, Wareham NJ, Sandhu MS, et al. Oxidation-specific biomarkers, lipoprotein(a), and risk of fatal and nonfatal coronary events. *J Am Coll Cardiol.* 2010;56:946-55.

49. Tsimikas S, Brilakis ES, Miller ER, McConnell JP, Lennon RJ, Kornman KS, et al. Oxidized phospholipids, Lp(a) lipoprotein, and coronary artery disease. *N Engl J Med.* 2005;353:46-57.

50. Tsimikas S, Clopton P, Brilakis ES, Marcovina SM, Khera A, Miller ER, et al. Relationship of oxidized phospholipids on apolipoprotein B-100 particles to race/ethnicity, apolipoprotein(a) isoform size, and cardiovascular risk factors: results from the Dallas Heart Study. *Circulation.* 2009;119:1711-9.

51. Ehara S, Ueda M, Naruko T, Haze K, Itoh A, Otsuka M, et al. Elevated levels of oxidized low density lipoprotein show a positive relationship with the severity of acute coronary syndromes. *Circulation.* 2001;103:1955-60.

52. Holvoet P, Lee DH, Steffes M, Gross M, Jacobs DR Jr. Association between circulating oxidized low-density lipoprotein and incidence of the metabolic syndrome. *JAMA.* 2008;299:2287-93.

53. Holvoet P, Vanhaecke J, Janssens S, van de Werf F, Collen D. Oxidized LDL and malondialdehyde-modified LDL in patients with acute coronary syndromes and stable coronary artery disease. *Circulation.* 1998;98:1487-94.

54. Arai K, Luke MM, Koschinsky ML, Miller ER, Pullinger CR, Witztum JL, et al. The I4399M variant of apolipoprotein(a) is associated with increased oxidized phospholipids on apolipoprotein B-100 particles. *Atherosclerosis.* 2010;209:498-503.

55. Mallat Z, Lambeau G, Tedgui A. Lipoprotein-associated and secreted phospholipases A in cardiovascular disease: roles as biological effectors and biomarkers. *Circulation.* 2010;122:2183-200.

56. Tsimikas S, Aikawa M, Miller FJ Jr, Miller ER, Torzewski M, Lentz SR, et al. Increased plasma oxidized phospholipid:apolipoprotein B-100 ratio with concomitant depletion of oxidized phospholipids from atherosclerotic lesions after dietary lipid-lowering: a potential biomarker of early atherosclerosis regression. *Arterioscler Thromb Vasc Biol.* 2007;27:175-81.

57. Ky B, Burke A, Tsimikas S, Wolfe ML, Tadesse MG, Szapary PO, et al. The influence of pravastatin and atorvastatin on markers of oxidative stress in hypercholesterolemic humans. *J Am Coll Cardiol.* 2008;51:1653-62.

58. Rodenburg J, Vissers MN, Wiegman A, Miller ER, Ridker PM, Witztum JL, et al. Oxidized low-density lipoprotein in children with familial hypercholesterolemia and unaffected siblings: effect of pravastatin. *J Am Coll Cardiol.* 2006;47:1803-10.

59. Silaste ML, Rantala M, Alfthan G, Aro A, Witztum JL, Kesäniemi YA, et al. Changes in dietary fat intake alter plasma levels of oxidized low-density lipoprotein and lipoprotein(a). *Arterioscler Thromb Vasc Biol.* 2004;24:498-503.

60. Ahmadi N, Tsimikas S, Hajsadeghi F, Saeed A, Nabavi V, Bevinal MA, et al. Relation of oxidative biomarkers, vascular dysfunction, and progression of coronary artery calcium. *Am J Cardiol.* 2010;105:459-66.

61. Budoff MJ, Ahmadi N, Gul KM, Liu ST, Flores FR, Tiano J, et al. Aged garlic extract supplemented with B vitamins, folic acid and L-arginine retards the progression of subclinical atherosclerosis: a randomized clinical trial. *Prev Med.* 2009;49:101-7.

62. Faghihnia N, Tsimikas S, Miller ER, Witztum JL, Krauss RM. Changes in lipoprotein(a), oxidized phospholipids, and LDL subclasses with a low-fat high-carbohydrate diet. *J Lipid Res.* 2010;51:3324-30.

63. Choi SH, Chae A, Miller E, Messig M, Ntanios F, DeMaria AN, et al. Relationship between biomarkers of oxidized low-density lipoprotein, statin therapy, quantitative coronary angiography, and atheroma: volume observations from the REVERSAL (Reversal of Atherosclerosis with Aggressive Lipid Lowering) study. *J Am Coll Cardiol.* 2008;52:24-32.

64. Merki E, Graham MJ, Mullick AE, Miller ER, Crooke RM, Pitas RE, et al. Antisense oligonucleotide directed to human apolipoprotein B-100 reduces lipoprotein(a) levels and oxidized phospholipids on human apolipoprotein B-100 particles in lipoprotein(a) transgenic mice. *Circulation.* 2008;118:743-53.

65. Merki E, Graham M, Taleb A, Leibundgut G, Yang X, Miller ER, et al. Antisense Oligonucleotide Lowers Plasma Levels of Apolipoprotein (a) and Lipoprotein (a) in Transgenic Mice. *J Am Coll Cardiol.* 2011;57:1611-21.

66. Wu R, de Faire U, Lemne C, Witztum JL, Frostegard J. Autoantibodies to OxLDL are decreased in individuals with borderline hypertension. *Hypertension.* 1999;33:53-9.

67. Penny WF, Ben-Yehuda O, Kuroe K, Long J, Bond A, Bhargava V, et al. Improvement of coronary artery endothelial dysfunction with lipid-lowering therapy: heterogeneity of segmental response and correlation with plasma-oxidized low density lipoprotein. *J Am Coll Cardiol.* 2001;37:766-74.

68. Segev A, Strauss BH, Witztum JL, Lau HK, Tsimikas S. Relationship of a comprehensive panel of plasma oxidized low-density lipoprotein markers to angiographic restenosis in patients undergoing percutaneous coronary intervention for stable angina. *Am Heart J.* 2005;150:1007-14.

69. Fraley AE, Schwartz GG, Olsson AG, Kinlay S, Szarek M, Rifai N, et al. Relationship of oxidized phospholipids and biomarkers of oxidized low-density lipoprotein with cardiovascular risk factors, inflammatory biomarkers, and effect of statin therapy in patients with acute coronary syndromes: Results from the MIRACL (Myocardial

Ischemia Reduction With Aggressive Cholesterol Lowering) trial. *J Am Coll Cardiol.* 2009;53:2186-96.

70. Bossola M, Tazza L, Merki E, Giungi S, Luciani G, Miller ER, et al. Oxidized low-density lipoprotein biomarkers in patients with end-stage renal failure: Acute effects of hemodialysis. *Blood Purif.* 2007;25:457-65.

71. Choi SH, Harkewicz R, Lee JH, Boullier A, Almazan F, Li AC, et al. Lipoprotein accumulation in macrophages via toll-like receptor-4-dependent fluid phase uptake. *Circ Res.* 2009;104:1355-63.

72. Rahaman SO, Lennon DJ, Febbraio M, Podrez EA, Hazen SL, Silverstein RL. A CD36-dependent signaling cascade is necessary for macrophage foam cell formation. *Cell Metab.* 2006;4:211-21.

Diagnosis and Risk Stratification of Acute Coronary Syndrome

Tertius Tuy, W Frank Peacock

INTRODUCTION

Cardiovascular disease accounts for over 800,000 deaths a year and is the number one killer in America, averaging 1 in every 2.9 deaths.[1] Approximately half of these deaths will be attributed to coronary heart disease. In the US, over the course of one year there will be in excess of 785,000 new cases of coronary heart disease and 470,000 recurrent heart attacks.[1]

The most frequent complaint in patients presenting with coronary heart disease is chest pain. However, as many of a third of the patients will not suffer any chest pain, instead they will present with nonspecific symptoms, such as weakness, dizziness, shortness of breath, or altered mental status.[2] In fact, chest pain by itself may be a nonspecific presentation. While emergency departments (ED) nationwide receive over 5.8 million cases of chest pain a year,[3] only one-third of these patients will ultimately be diagnosed with acute coronary syndrome (ACS).[4,5]

ACS may be defined as a sudden occlusion to the coronary arteries (e.g., plaque rupture, embolus, etc.) that causes reversible or irreversible cardiac ischemia. ACS patients may be further divided into those with unstable angina or MI. Timely assessment of ACS allows for early reperfusion therapy, salvation of viable myocardium, and overall minimization of morbidity and mortality. Unless there is a high index of suspicion, nonspecific signs and symptoms in ACS often pose a challenge to both triage nurses and clinicians. Patients suffering from MI without chest pain have lower rates of aggressive therapy and therefore have higher rates of adverse outcomes.[2] Currently, the misdiagnosis rate for both acute myocardial infarction (AMI) and unstable angina (UA) is approximately 2-3%.[6-8] Failure to diagnose ACS can have fatal consequences for the patient and legal ramification for the clinician. In patients with UA and AMI, the 30-day mortality in those erroneously diagnosed and discharged was 70–90% greater than those hospitalized.[9] With such serious implications, a strategy of risk stratification and diagnostic protocols, which include electrocardiography, cardiac biomarker, or imaging modalities, is highly desirable.

CLINICAL EXAMINATION

History

In the ED, the second most common presenting chief complaint is chest pain (CP). With an extensive list of potential causes (Table 3-1), arriving at a diagnosis can be a challenging process. Although ACS is not the most frequent cause of CP, it is one of the most important diagnoses to exclude. In assessing for ACS, the clinical examination provides minimal information and is often nondiagnostic. Risk factors for ACS include advanced age, male gender, and a history of diabetes, prior MI, previous episodes of angina, and tobacco use.[10] Yet, neither their presence clinches the diagnosis of ACS, nor does their absence eliminate its possibility.

Consideration of historical factors in the diagnosis of ACS is controversial. Some analyses have shown that pain described as pressure, exacerbated by exertion, or radiated to the arms or shoulders were indicative of MI (Both LR+ and CI > 1).[11] Other have found that with the exception of right arm radiation (LR = 3.24; CI: 1.57–6.88), the nature, site, and radiation of the chest pain were not predictive, since the confidence intervals for both the positive and negative likelihood ratio (LR) spanned unity.[12] Regardless, the diagnostic benefits are curbed by the poor sensitivity of these symptoms (< 50%).[13] Furthermore, advancing age can render a history almost ineffective. The Internet Tracking Registry for Acute Coronary Syndromes (i*trACS),

Table 3-1 Differentials for Chest Pain	
Cardiovascular	**Gastrointestinal**
Ischemic	Gastroesophageal reflux disease
Stable angina	Esophageal spasm
Variant angina	Esophagitis
Unstable angina	Biliary colic
Myocardial infarction	Cholecystitis
Heart failure	Pancreatitis
Nonischemic	Peptic ulcer disease
Aortic dissection	Mediastinitis
Myocarditis	**Musculoskeletal**
Pericarditis	Costochondritis
Heart failure	Chest wall muscle strain
Pulmonary hypertension	
	Psychogenic
Pulmonary	Depression
Pneumonia	Anxiety
Pneumothorax	Hypochondriasis
Pulmonary embolus	

a multi-center registry of over 17,000 patients, found that except for the presence of left arm pain (p = 0.006), a history of typical chest pain was not helpful in the diagnosis for patients older than 75 years of age who suffered from ACS.[14]

In real life, the clinical picture is usually more ambiguous as patients can present with atypical chest pain (e.g., chest pain described as pleuritic or sharp, worsened by positional change or palpation, not exacerbated by exertion, or unresponsive to nitroglycerin).[11] Although generally indicative of noncardiac etiologies, atypical CP is ultimately nonspecific. One retrospective study showed that 23% of atypical chest pains had significant stenosis (> 50%) on cardiac CT.[15] Therefore, a minimal work-up for ACS is warranted even for atypical chest pain, and will reduce mortality and morbidity associated with an ACS misdiagnosis.[16]

In the most challenging presentations, chest pain may be completely absent. For these patients, a high index of suspicion is required. The Global Registry of Acute Coronary Events (GRACE) was a multinational, prospective, observational study involving over 20,000 ACS patients. In GRACE, 8.4% of the ACS patients had no symptoms of CP, which led to a tenfold higher chance of being misdiagnosed (23.8 vs 2.4%), compared to those with typical chest pain.[17] The consequences of misdiagnosis were grave, as those with atypical presentations had delayed revascularization, were likely to forgo needed intervention, had an increased morbidity (higher complications like heart failure, cardiogenic shock, arrhythmia, and renal failure) and elevated mortality (13.0 vs 4.3%, p < 0.001).[17] Instead of CP, these patients were more likely to complain of breathlessness (41.5–49.3%), diaphoresis (26.2–27.8%), nausea and vomiting (24.3–25.8%), syncope or presyncope (19.1–21.4%), palpitations (4.8%), or jaw pain (6.1%).[17-20] Factors that are associated with atypical presentations are advanced age, gender,[18,21] diabetes,[5,17,21,22] hypertension, and history of heart failure (Figure 3-1).[17] Moreover, an analysis of the Worcester Heart Attack Study investigated the effects of both age group and gender on the likelihood of atypical presentation in ACS. For women less than 65 or greater than 75 years of age, the incidence of ACS with CP was less than that of men; however, between 65 and 75 years of age, women with ACS had similar incidence of CP.[23]

Physical Examination

The physical examination is often of little use in the diagnosis of ACS, unless there are complications (e.g., cardiac failure, arrhythmia, acute valvular dysfunction, shock, etc.). Alternatively, patients may exhibit no signs at all. The greatest value of the physical examination is the finding of an alternative diagnosis, e.g., unifocal rales secondary to pneumonia. Unilateral limb swelling, acute dyspnea, and chest pain may indicate pulmonary embolus; orthopnea and jugular venous distension may indicate heart failure; rales with hypotension may suggest cardiogenic shock, or a pain exacerbated by palpation or movement may indicate a muscular skeletal

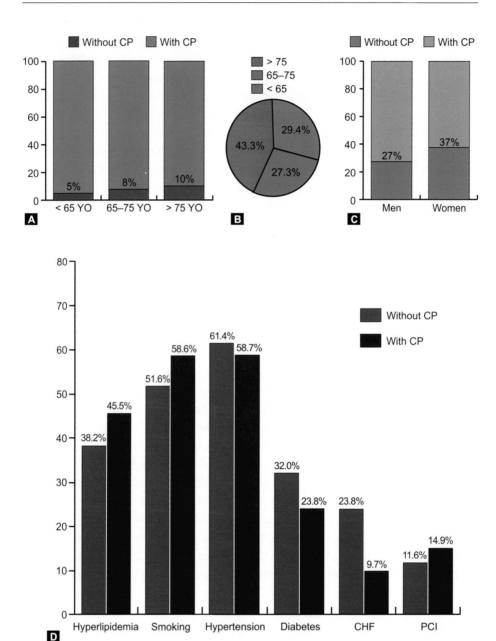

Figure 3-1 A, Atypical presentation of ACS with advancing age. **B,** Breakdown of atypical presentation in ACS by age group. **C,** Atypical presentation of ACS according to gender. **D,** Effects of cardiovascular risk factors on atypical presentation of ACS. ACS, acute coronary syndrome; CHF, congestive heart failure; PCI, percutaneous coronary intervention. *Data from* Brieger D, Eagle KA, Goodman SG, Steg PG, Budaj A, White K, et al. Acute coronary syndromes without chest pain, an underdiagnosed and undertreated high-risk group: insights from the Global Registry of Acute Coronary Events. *Chest.* 2004;126:461-9.

etiology. However, even when signs of alternative diagnoses are present, the possibility of ACS cannot be entirely ruled out. Thus, even for patients whose likely diagnosis is non-ACS CP, at a minimum, ECG and baseline cardiac biomarkers should be considered.

Electrocardiogram (ECG)

The ECG is instrumental in the work-up of ACS, as it can give an indication of presence of ischemia, infarction, and their respective location. It is a quick bedside evaluation which can detect coronary artery occlusion within minutes of its onset. Patients presenting to the ED with chest discomfort or anginal equivalent should have an initial ECG within the first 10 minutes of arrival and possibly 15–30 minutes thereafter, if symptoms persist or change, to assess for ischemic development.[24] The typical ECG progression of a ST-elevation myocardial infarction (STEMI) initially develops an increase in amplitude of T wave, followed by ST-elevation, T-wave inversion and Q-wave evolution. However, these signs are not specific to infarction and their differential diagnoses should be considered (Table 3-2).[25] Depending on the criteria used, ST-elevation on a 12 lead ECG has a sensitivity of 45–68% for MI and specificity of 81–98%.[26]

A normal or nondiagnostic ECG does not preclude the possibility of ACS, since ST-elevation may be entirely absent (e.g., non-ST-elevated myocardial infarction or UA). Likewise, depending on the timing, the physicians may misinterpret a normalizing ST-segment, which can occur 12 hours after the onset of CP and gradually continues to normalize over the following two weeks. Furthermore,

Table 3-2 Differentials for ECG Changes	
Increased T-wave amplitude	**Q-waves**
Hyperkalemia	Left ventricular hypertrophy
Benign early repolarization	False lead poling
Left ventricular hypertrophy	Left bundle branch block
Acute myocardial infarction	Pre-excitation in Wolf Parkinson White syndrome
ST-elevation	Hypertrophic obstructive cardiomyopathy
Acute myocardial infarction	
Left ventricular hypertrophy	**T-wave inversion**
Left or right bundle branch block	Stroke
Left ventricular aneurysm	Long QTc
Nonspecific intraventricular conduction defect	Pacemaker
Benign early repolarization	
Pericarditis	

location of the infarct may erroneously be negative. With standard ECG, a left circumflex artery occlusion may remain hidden or have a nondiagnostic ECG pattern in 32%[27] of patients and a right-sided ECG may improve the diagnostic accuracy.[24] In the Acute Cardiac Ischemia Time-Insensitive Predictive Instrument (ACI-TIPI) trial, a multicenter prospective study with over 10,000 patients, among 681 MI patients evaluated with ECG, 19.5% had a normal or nondiagnostic initial ECG while 33.3% of confirmed UA had a normal or nondiagnostic ECG.[9] MI patients having a nondiagnostic ECG were more likely to be misdiagnosed and erroneously discharged (1.3 vs 9.0%, p = 0.001).[9] A postmortem analysis of 100 MI death cases showed that for those with undiagnosed MI, ECG was suggestive or diagnostic in 25.5%, nonspecific in 31.9%, and normal or insufficient in 42.5%.[28] To reduce misdiagnosis, implementing a strategy of serial ECGs has improved the detection of ACS. In fact, one study demonstrated that serial ECG was able to correctly identify 16.2% more AMI patients than a single initial ECG.[29] Nevertheless, when the ECG does not show obvious ischemia, cardiac biomarkers are necessary to determine the diagnosis.

CARDIAC BIOMARKERS

Cardiac biomarkers have long been implemented in the diagnosis of ACS especially to diagnose non-STEMI (NSTEMI). While many different markers have been utilized, the current standard is for the use of cardiac specific troponin, either I or T. If troponin is unavailable, the MB fraction of creatinine kinase may be utilized. The use of other markers is generally discouraged by many professional society guidelines. With a suspicion of myocardial ischemia, MI can be diagnosed by having a rise and fall of cardiac markers over the 99th percentile of the upper reference limit.[30] The detection of myocardial necrosis markers is highly dependent on the amount cardiac necrosis and its timing (Figure 3-2).[31]

On initial assessment the sensitivities of biomarkers for MI do not reach 100%, despite having high specificities. The accepted cardiac biomarkers, when assayed within 3 hours of MI symptoms, have low sensitivities (< 65%) and may be falsely negative.[32,33] As time progresses, the sensitivities of the biomarkers improve variably (Figure 3-3).[33] To improve sensitivities, cardiac biomarkers are assayed serially and in combination to one another. Currently, creatine kinase, CK-MB, myoglobin, and troponin, are used nationwide in EDs for the evaluation of ACS.

Creatine Kinase

Creatine kinase (CK) is a cytosolic enzyme that catalyzes the phosphorylation of creatinine. It is found primarily in skeletal muscle, cardiac muscle, and the brain. Total CK has been used as a marker of acute myocardial injury; however, with a sensitivity of 37% and specificity of 87%, it is no longer used as a primary marker

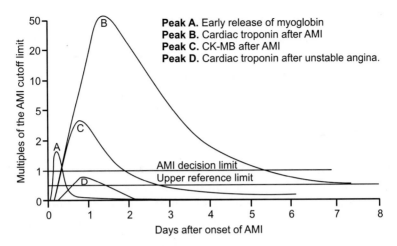

Figure 3-2 Timing of detection of various biomarkers following acute myocardial infarction. Data are plotted on a relative scale, where 1.0 is set at the AMI cutoff concentration. AMI, acute myocardial infarction; CAD, coronary artery disease; CKMB, creatine kinase MB fraction. *From* Wu AH, Apple FS, Gibler WB, Jesse RL, Warshaw MM, Valdes R Jr. National Academy of Clinical Biochemistry Standards of Laboratory Practice: recommendations for the use of cardiac markers in coronary artery diseases. *Clin Chem.* 1999;45:1104-21, with permission.

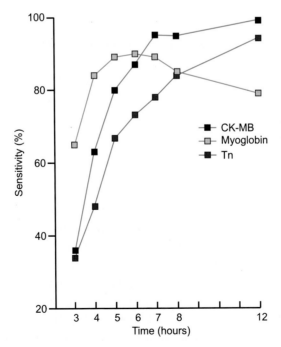

Figure 3-3 Sensitivities of cardiac biomarkers over a 12-hour time course. *Data from* de Winter RJ, Koster RW, Sturk A, Chen D, Harakal C, Addonizio VP, et al. Value of myoglobin, troponin T, and CK-MB$_{mass}$ in ruling out an acute myocardial infarction in the emergency room. *Circulation.* 1995;92:3401-7.

of cardiac necrosis.[34] Typically, it is elevated above the reference range of normal within 3–8 hours, and peaks around 24 hours[32] after myocardial infarction. Yet, in the context of acute CP, total CK specificity remains modest, since even skeletal muscle microtrauma can cause a 40-fold rise in CK (IM injections, strenuous muscular activity, etc.).[35] With the need for a more cardiac specific assay, the CK-MB assay was developed.

CK-MB

CK has three dimeric isoenzyme forms: CK-MM, CK-BB, and CK-MB. In the ED, a rising CK-MB has been associated with the clinical diagnosis of MI (p = 0.04) but not UA.[36] Following an AMI, circulating CK-MB typically rises within 3–4 hours and peaks around 12–24 hours. However, CK-MB may not be diagnostic until eight to twelve hours after onset of symptoms.[37] CK-MB is found predominantly in the heart, accounting for up to 30% of CK activity there, yet it can also be found in small level in skeletal muscle, intestines, uterus, prostate, and diaphragm (1–3%).[38,39] Thus, a rise in circulating CK-MB is not entirely specific to myocardial damage and could be caused by large amounts of skeletal muscle disease (i.e., rhabdomyolysis, muscular degeneration, abnormal muscle regeneration, etc.). Regardless, with acute non-traumatic chest pain, CK-MB is useful in the diagnosis of ACS. Most recently, the CK-MB enzyme assay has been replaced by the $CK-MB_{mass}$ assay, which provides better sensitivity and negative predictive value (NPV). In a meta-analysis by Balk et al. on patients with chest pain, the initial CK-MB (threshold range 5–8 ng/mL) had a sensitivity of 42% and the specificity of 97% for AMI.[34] Further, overall serial measurements raised sensitivity to 79%, while specificity remained about the same at 96%.[34] With its shorter half-life, CK-MB is able to detect reinfarction, if the troponin levels are elevated and serial CK-MB shows a rising trend then reinfarction should be considered.[40]

Myoglobin

Myoglobin is an oxygen-binding cytoplasmic protein located within cardiac and skeletal myocytes. After an MI, the intracellular myoglobin within the cardio-myocytes is rapidly released at rates faster than those of CK-MB and troponins. Following its release, the serum myoglobin concentration becomes abnormal in about one hour, double the normal levels within 2 hours, peaks at 4 hours, and within 8–12 hours returns to baseline, as it is rapidly cleared by the kidneys. This rapid rise and fall makes myoglobin useful in excluding the diagnosis of AMI within 6 hours of presentations.[32] Balk et al. demonstrated that diagnosis of AMI with myoglobin (threshold range of 70–110 ng/mL) produced a 49% sensitivity and a 91% specificity in patients with a normal chest X-ray and no suspicion of trauma, renal failure, or skeletal muscle damage.[34] However, due to myoglobin's abundance in both skeletal and cardiac muscle,[37] its specificity is highly dependent on the pretest probability, diagnostic threshold, and the timing at which it was measured. Some studies have quoted the specificity of myoglobin anywhere between 21 and 43%.[41,42] With 1–2 hour serial measurements, sensitivity improved to 89% and specificity decreased to 87%.[34] Thus, serial measurements give myoglobin the potential for rapid rule-out of MI.

Cardiac Troponin

Cardiac troponin (cTn) is a structural component of cardiomyocytes, found at small quantities in the cytoplasm and large quantities in the thin filaments. Among its three subunits (C, I, and T), the I and T subunits are highly specific to cardiac cells. The I and T subunits have the same diagnostic capabilities in regards to sensitivity, specificity, NPV, and positive predictive value (PPV). They have replaced CK-MB as the gold standard for detecting ischemic myocardial event and remote infarction. The American College of Cardiology/American Heart Association (ACC/AHA) 2007 guidelines suggest that, when available, cardiac-specific troponin is the preferred marker in the detection of cardiac injury. Upon cardiomyocyte destruction and myofibril degradation, troponin is released to circulate in the blood. After 3–6 hours from the ischemic event, the cytosolic pool of troponin is first detectable in the blood-stream. This leads to an initially poor sensitivity within the first 3 hours. Troponin peaks at 12 hours post-MI, and remains elevated for 10–14 days afterward, the result of continued proteolysis of the myocardial contractile apparatus.[43,44] Balk et al. showed that when diagnosing AMI, initial troponin I and T (threshold range 0.1–0.6 ng/mL) had poor sensitivity (39%), but adequate specificity (93%).[34] Moreover, serial measurements of cTn raised the sensitivity by nearly 2.5-fold, resulting in a sensitivity of 90–100% and a specificity of 83–96%.[34] However, regardless of the high serial sensitivity with the current diagnostic thresholds, detection of reinfarction is sometimes challenging because of cTn's long half-life.

High Sensitivity Troponin (hs-Tn)

Troponin assays are evolving to improve sensitivity early after MI. Newer and improved analysis methods allow for lowered limits of detection and thus decrease the 99th percentile cutoff of normal while maintaining a coefficient of variation of 10%.[45] Reichlin et al. showed that high sensitivity assays improved diagnosis of AMI over standard troponin assays at presentations (hs-Tn AUC 0.95 vs standard AUC 0.90) and at 3 hours from the onset of chest pain (hs-Tn 0.92 vs standard 0.76).[46] One study by Januzzi showed that a precommercial hs-TnT had a 99th percentile of healthy population cutoff of 13 pg/mL. This new hs-Tn threshold is highly predictive of ACS (OR 9.0 CI: 3.9–20.9, p < 0.001), detecting 27% more ACS cases compared to normal troponins (p = 0.001).[47] A study by Melanson et al. investigated NSTEMI patients who initially had negative troponin levels. These patients had troponin

Table 3-3	Etiologies of Troponin Elevation without Overt Cardiac Ischemia
Arrhythmia	Myocarditis (Coxsackievirus, Parvovirus B19, Kawasaki disease, sarcoidosis, etc.)
Endocarditis	
Cardiac surgery (ablation, biopsy, percutaneous coronary intervention, etc.)	Snake venom exposure
	Valvular disease (especially aortic)
Cardiomyopathy (hypertrophic obstructive cardiomyopathy, Takotsubo syndrome, etc.)	Vasculopathy
	Acute neurological disease (cerebrovascular accident, subarachnoid hemorrhage, etc.)
Cardioversion	Carbon monoxide poisoning
Congestive heart failure	Critically ill patients (respiratory failure, GI bleeds, sepsis, large burns, etc.)
Coronary vasospasm	
Drug toxicity (adriamycin, 5 FU, and herceptin)	Hypothyroidism
	Inflammatory diseases
Hypertensive emergencies and hypotension	Postoperative noncardiac surgery
Infiltrative diseases (amyloidosis, hemachromatosis, sarcoidosis, scleroderma, etc.)	Pulmonary embolism
	Pulmonary hypertension (severe)
Intracardiac device induced (pacing, ICD firings, etc.)	Renal failure
	Vital exhaustion
Myocardial trauma	

assessed at 0 hour (initial measurement), 6–9 hours, and 12–24 hours. The hs-TnI was positive for AMI in the initial measurement for 61.2% of the patients. In fact, hs-TnI diagnosed AMI before conventional Tn in 64.1% of the patients, and AMI was diagnosed an average of 564 minutes earlier.[48] Hs-Tn is slowly gaining use because of its improved ability to diagnose and detect infarcts of minimal size.[40] However, with higher sensitivity, there is a diminished specificity, thus increasing the rate of non-ACS troponin elevations (Table 3-3). Therefore, when interpreting hs-Tn levels it is crucial to understand the clinical likelihood of ACS.

APPLYING MARKERS: WHAT THE GUIDELINES RECOMMEND

The American College of Emergency Physicians (ACEP) advocates several biomarker recommendations, stratified by the strength of data, for evaluating ED patients with CP.[49] Level A recommendations have the largest amount of supporting literature, while level B recommendations have less certain but still supporting literature. The only level A recommendation advises that non-MI ACS (i.e., unstable angina) cannot be rule out by biomarkers. Below are three level B recommended strategies, which may be used to exclude NSTEMI.

1. If onset of anginal symptoms occurs 8–12 hours prior to ED presentation, a one time negative troponin and CK-MB$_{mass}$.

2. If onset of anginal symptoms occurs less than 8 hours prior to ED presentation, a negative serial measurements of myoglobin with CK-MB$_{mass}$, or serial measurements troponin at baseline and 90 minutes.
3. If onset of anginal symptoms occurs less than 8 hours prior to ED presentation, a negative 2-hour delta CK-MB$_{mass}$ with a 2-hour delta troponin.

The European Society of Cardiology (ESC) differs from ACEP in their biomarker recommendations.[50] They indicate that for patients presenting within 12 hours of onset of last chest pain episode, a single negative troponin on presentation cannot preclude NSTEMI, since patients' troponin levels may be initially negative and subsequently rise within the following hours. Furthermore, a repeated marker measurement is indicated at 6–12 hours after presentation or last episode of chest pain, to rule out myocardial damage. However, if the initial troponin measurement is taken after 12 hours or more from the last occurrence of chest pain, a single negative troponin measurement is sufficient to rule out NSTEMI. Lastly, since myoglobin is neither specific nor sensitive in detection of myocardial injury, the ESC recommends troponin as the biomarker of choice.

Multimarker Approach

A multi-marker approach has been extensively investigated for rapid rule-out of MI patients who present to the ED within 6 hours of symptom onset. By combining serial measures of early and late markers of cardiac necrosis, the multimarker approach can raise sensitivity to as high as 95%.[24] The use of 90-minute serial myoglobin in conjunction with serial troponin or CK-MB has been proven effective in ruling out MI.[51] Yet, positive results are inadequate to confirm the diagnosis of an MI as this approach lacks specificity. Physicians should carefully consider when implementing therapy based on the positive results.

Lastly, there are a multitude of biomarkers in the pipeline being investigated for their role in diagnosis, rule-out, and risk stratification of ACS (Table 3-4).[44,52-54] However, their utility is as yet unclear and supersedes the scope of this article.

Risk Stratification

Several models of risk stratifications have been developed to manage patients better. They include the thrombolysis in myocardial infarction (TIMI), GRACE, and platelet glycoprotein IIb/IIIa in unstable angina using integrilin therapy (PURSUIT) risk scores. In both the TIMI and GRACE risk score, troponin has a role in stratification. Patients with elevated troponins are at risk for future ischemic events. Suspected ACS patients with positive cTn and normal CK-MB had higher rate of MI within 30 days of initial presentation compared to those with normal cTn and CK-MB.[55-57]

Table 3-4	List of Emerging Biomarkers in ACS	
Endothelial activation	**Ischemia**	
ET1/CTproET1	Ischemic modified albumin	
Adrenomedullin	Heart-type fatty-acid-binding protein	
Plaque rupture, inflammation, and atherothrombosis	Glycogen phosphorylase-BB	
CRP/hsCRP	**Cardiac stress**	
Serum amyloid A	BNP/NT-proBNP	
Pregnancy-associated plasma protein A	MR-ProANP	
Placental growth factor	GDF-15	
Myeloperoxidase	ST-2	
Matrix metalloproteinase	**Miscellaneous**	
Lectin-like oxidized LDL receptor 1 (LOX-1)	Cystatin C	
Choline	Copeptin	
Soluble CD40L		
P-selectin		
Soluble fibrin		

Natriuretic peptides (NPs) are cardiac proteins released in response to volumetric and pressure stress on the heart. Although they are commonly used for the evaluation of heart failure in dyspneic patients, they have been suggested as a potential biomarker of ACS. NPs may be found elevated within hours of MI symptoms.[58] Yet, NPs have low specificity and sensitivity for ACS, which leads to a limited diagnostic utility, if used alone.[59] ACS patients may only have a modest elevation of NPs or none at all, depending on the timing and severity of ischemia. Additionally, elevated NPs indicate cardiac stress, but do not necessarily indicate its etiology.

Perhaps of greater utility is NPs ability to prognosticate. The Treat Angina with Aggrastat and Determine Cost of Therapy with Invasive or Conservative Strategy—Thrombolysis in Myocardial Infarction (TACTICS-TIMI) trial showed that elevated B-type natriuretic peptide (BNP) was a significant predictor of MI and death within 10 months of AMI.[60] On admission > 80 pg/mL BNP was associated with sevenfold higher mortality.[59] Likewise, when the cleavage product of the precursor to BNP (NT-proBNP) was measured within 3 hours of ACS symptoms, a NT-proBNP > 107 ng/L was also associated with a threefold risk of death compared to those with lower levels.[61] For these reasons, according to ACC/AHA guidelines for unstable angina/NSTEMI, NP measurement for risk stratification in ACS[24] should be taken into consideration. This compares to the National Association of Clinical Biochemistry guidelines, which suggest that therapeutic benefits of NP levels are uncertain.[38]

AFTER THE RULE-OUT

Myocardial infarction can be excluded by the absence of any detectable marker changes during serial sampling. However, the exclusion of MI does not complete the evaluation in patients with potential unstable angina, which by definition has no marker evidence of necrosis. In patients with suspected unstable angina, further testing is required. Functional and diagnostic testing includes exercise treadmill testing (ETT), stress myocardial perfusion imaging (MPI), or stress echocardiography. Also, when patients are symptomatic, some institutions are implementing rest MPI or echocardiography. If provocative testing is negative, patients may be discharged with an outpatient follow-up evaluation. However, when provocative testing is positive, further inhospital evaluation (e.g., coronary angiography) is required.

The current ACC/AHA guidelines for stress testing and management of NSTEMI/ unstable angina recommend ETT without imaging should be performed as the initial test in low to intermediate risk patients with ischemic symptoms, if they can exercise.[62] Pharmacological stress testing with imaging is an alternative for patients unable to walk and exercise.

Determination of which diagnostic test to perform is dependent on the ability of the patient to exercise and the physician's stress ECG interpretation skills. Other factors that influence the diagnostic test strategy are the standard institutional practices, the expertise in each test technique, and the availability of each modality (both physical and temporal). For most chest pain centers, ETT is first line test used for diagnostic testing of CAD and inducible ischemia. Yet, there are certain clinical circumstances in which stress MPI and echocardiography may be used as an alternative.

MPI uses a radioactive tracer injection (e.g., technetium-99m based isotope) to visualize ischemic and infarcted myocardium. It requires 30–60 minutes incubation but results can be delayed for up to 2–4 hours depending on the availability of the facility and technicians. It has a high sensitivity for infarct at 92% but falters at specificity of 63–71%.[63] The limitation of perfusion scanning is that it is unable to differentiate old from new infarct. Additionally, it detects relative hypoperfusion, so severe multivessel disease can have falsely normal results.

Pharmacologic stress testing with MPI or echocardiography is indicated for patients with exercise intolerance (e.g., physical limitations, pulmonary disease, or peripheral arterial disease, etc.). When performing pharmacologic stress testing, vasodilator (dipyridamole or adenosine) or dobutamine are used to induce cardiac stress. Since adenosine and dipyridamole are highly effective in diagnosis and risk stratification they are the agents of choice. Dobutamine is an alternative used only when vasodilators are contraindicated (e.g., bronchospastic disease). It is relatively understudied, has an increased number of side effects, and has a decreased effectiveness in producing coronary flow heterogeneity compared to vasodilators.[64] Compared to exercise stress, pharmacologic stress testing has equivalent sensitivities and specificities for diagnosing CAD.[65] Yet, patients undergoing pharmacologic stress MPI have a higher incidence of cardiac death than those with exercise stress MPI, regardless of whether the images were normal or not.[66] It should be noted that the increased risk is a reflection of a more severe patient population who were unable to perform exercise stress testing because of comorbidity, and not an indicator a reduction of prognostic accuracy of pharmacological stress testing.

Rest MPI, another risk stratification technique, uses the patients' rest symptoms as the "stress." During or shortly after anginal symptoms in the ED, an isotopic tracer is injected to visualize the heart. Old infarctions as well as acute ischemia and infarction show up as perfusion defects. Since a normal perfusion scan is associated with very low clinical risks, patients may be discharged home and managed with outpatient stress MPI looking for underlying CAD.

For patients able to exercise with baseline ECG abnormalities, stress echocardiography is an equally viable method for risk stratification. Stress echocardiography is performed using standard echocardiography equipment and thus it is noninvasive, inflicts no radiation exposure, and its results are made available immediately. Furthermore, echocardiography produces functional and structural information, therefore giving insight into both ischemic and nonischemic etiologies (e.g., valvular heart disease, cardiomyopathy, etc.).[67]

FUTURE

Coronary CT angiography (CTA) produces high resolution images of the coronary arteries, allowing for visualization of vessel blockage or abnormalities. Resolution of CTA is improved by slowing heart rate ~60 bpm with β-blockade, prospective and retrospective ECG gated analysis, and breath holding maneuver. CTA is able to classify patients into categories of patients free of CAD, having non-obstructive disease, or identifying the cohort with significant stenosis. Furthermore, CTA can differentiate calcified and non-calcified stenosis. With these abilities it has been used in the work-up of acute chest pain. A study by Goldstein et al. showed that CTA was able to immediately excluded 75% of their CP cases, which reduced both diagnosis time (3.4 hours vs 15.0 hours, p < 0.001) and overall costs ($1,586 vs $1,872, p < 0.001).[68] A large prospective trial, rule-out myocardial infarction using computer assisted tomography (ROMICAT), demonstrated that CTA detected coronary plaque and significant stenosis with a sensitivity of 100% and 77% for ACS, respectively, and a NPV of 100 and 98%, respectively. However, the specificity and PPV of coronary plaque (54% and 17%) and of significant stenosis for ACS (87% and 35%) was low, since these did not necessarily lead to ACS.[69] CTA is now being applied to visualize the pulmonary vasculature and aortic arch, which helps rule out other important causes of CP like pulmonary embolus and aortic dissection.

Coronary artery calcium (CAC) scoring identifies calcified plaques within the coronary arteries. In patients with CP and a calcium score of zero, < 1% had cardiac chest pain; while 97% of cardiac chest pain patients had evidence of calcification on CT. At a CAC cutoff score of 36, the sensitivity for ACS was 90%; specificity was 85%; PPV was 44%; and NPV was 99%.[70] Although calcium scoring had an adequate diagnostic accuracy in evaluation of CP in ED (0.88 AUC ROC), unlike CTA it is unable to detect uncalcified plaques on its own.[71]

SUMMARY

The work-up for ACS is a rapidly evolving field, which has led to the advancement of timely and noninvasive methods. Although cardiac imaging provides a quick visualization of coronary anatomy, cardiac biomarkers still remain the mainstay in the diagnosis of NSTEMI. Biomarkers technology has developed methods to improve sensitivity; meanwhile newer biomarkers are being discovered that address the full range of ACS pathology (i.e., ischemia, necrosis, inflammation, etc.). Ultimately, both cardiac biomarkers and imaging have aided in the diagnosis and risk stratification ACS, reduced unneeded stay, and minimized overall costs.

REFERENCES

1. loyd-Jones D, Adams RJ, Brown TM, Carnethon M, Dai S, De Simone G, et al. Executive summary: heart disease and stroke statistics—2010 update: a report from the American Heart Association. *Circulation.* 2010;121:948-54.
2. Canto JG, Shlipak MG, Rogers WJ, Malmgren JA, Frederick PD, Lambrew CT, et al. Prevalence, clinical characteristics, and mortality among patients with myocardial infarction presenting without chest pain. *JAMA.* 2000;283:3223-9.
3. Nawar EW, Niska RW, Xu J. National Hospital Ambulatory Medical Care Survey: 2005 emergency department summary. *Adv Data.* 2007;1-32.
4. Storrow AB, Gibler WB. Chest Pain Centers: Diagnosis of Acute Coronary Syndromes. *Ann Emerg Med.* 2000;35:449-61.
5. Coronado BE, Pope JH, Griffith JL, Beshansky JR, Selker HP. Clinical features, triage, and outcome of patients presenting to the ED with suspected acute coronary syndromes but without pain: a multicenter study. *Am J Emerg Med.* 2004;22:568-74.
6. McCarthy BD, Beshansky JR, D'Agostino RB, Selker HP. Missed diagnoses of acute myocardial infarction in the emergency department: results from a multicenter study. *Ann Emerg Med.* 1993;22:579-82.
7. Schiff GD, Hasan O, Kim S, Abrams R, Cosby K, Lambert BL, et al. Diagnostic Error in Medicine: Analysis of 583 Physician-Reported Errors. *Arch Intern Med.* 2009;169:1881-7.
8. Fesmire FM, Hughes AD, Fody EP, Jackson AP, Fesmire CE, Gilbert MA, et al. The Erlanger chest pain evaluation protocol: a one-year experience with serial 12-lead ECG monitoring, two-hour delta serum marker measurements, and selective nuclear stress testing to identify and exclude acute coronary syndromes. *Ann Emerg Med.* 2002;40: 584-94.

9. Pope JH, Aufderheide TP, Ruthazer R, Woolard RH, Feldman JA, Beshansky JR, et al. Missed diagnoses of acute cardiac ischemia in the emergency department. *N Engl J Med.* 2000;342:1163-70.

10. Pope JH, Ruthazer R, Beshansky JR, Griffith JL, Selker HP. Clinical Features of Emergency Department Patients Presenting with Symptoms Suggestive of Acute Cardiac Ischemia: A Multicenter Study. *J Thromb Thrombolysis.* 1998;6:63-74.

11. Swap CJ, Nagurney JT. Value and Limitations of Chest Pain History in the Evaluation of Patients With Suspected Acute Coronary Syndromes. *JAMA.* 2005;294:2623-29.

12. Goodacre S, Pett P, Arnold J, Chawla A, Hollingsworth J, Roe D, et al. Clinical diagnosis of acute coronary syndrome in patients with chest pain and a normal or non-diagnostic electrocardiogram. *Emerg Med J.* 2009;26:866-70.

13. Hwang SY, Park EH, Shin ES, Jeong MH. Comparison of factors associated with atypical symptoms in younger and older patients with acute coronary syndromes. *J Korean Med Sci.* 2009;24:789-94.

14. Han JH, Lindsell CJ, Hornung RW, Lewis T, Storrow AB, Hoekstra JW, et al. The elder patient with suspected acute coronary syndromes in the emergency department. *Acad Emerg Med.* 2007;14:732-9.

15. Bonello L, Armero S, Jacquier A, Com O, Sarran A, Sbragia P, et al. Non-invasive coronary angiography for patients with acute atypical chest pain discharged after negative screening including maximal negative treadmill stress test. A prospective study. *Int J Cardiol.* 2009;134:140-3.

16. El-Menyar A, Zubaid M, Sulaiman K, AlMahmeed W, Singh R, Alsheikh-Ali AA, et al. Atypical presentation of acute coronary syndrome: a significant independent predictor of in-hospital mortality. *J Cardiol.* 2011;57:165-71.

17. Brieger D, Eagle KA, Goodman SG, Steg PG, Budaj A, White K, et al. Acute coronary syndromes without chest pain, an underdiagnosed and undertreated high-risk group: insights from the Global Registry of Acute Coronary Events. *Chest.* 2004;126:461-9.

18. Canto JG, Goldberg RJ, Hand MM, Bonow RO, Sopko G, Pepine CJ, et al. Symptom presentation of women with acute coronary syndromes: myth vs reality. *Arch Intern Med.* 2007;167:2405-13.

19. Dey S, Flather MD, Devlin G, Brieger D, Gurfinkel EP, Steg PG, et al. Sex-related diffe-rences in the presentation, treatment and outcomes among patients with acute coronary syndromes: the Global Registry of Acute Coronary Events. *Heart.* 2009;95:20-6.

20. Peterson ED, Alexander KP. Learning to suspect the unexpected: Evaluating women with cardiac syndromes. *Am Heart J.* 1998;136:186-8.

21. Stephen SA, Darney BG, Rosenfeld AG. Symptoms of acute coronary syndrome in women with diabetes: An integrative review of the literature. *Heart Lung.* 2008;37:179-89.

22. DeVon HA, Penckofer SM, Zerwic JJ. Symptoms of unstable angina in patients with and without diabetes. *Res Nurs Health.* 2005;28:136-43.

23. Milner KA, Vaccarino V, Arnold AL, Funk M, Goldberg RJ. Gender and age differences in chief complaints of acute myocardial infarction (Worcester Heart Attack Study). *Am J Cardiol.* 2004;93:606-8.

24. ACC/AHA 2007 Guidelines for the Management of Patients With Unstable Angina/Non-ST-Elevation Myocardial Infarction: Executive Summary: A Report of the American College of Cardiology/American Heart Association Task Force on Practice Guidelines (Writing Committee to Revise the 2002 Guidelines for the Management of Patients With Unstable Angina/Non-ST-Elevation Myocardial Infarction): Developed in Collaboration with the American College of Emergency Physicians, the Society for Cardiovascular Angiography and Interventions, and the Society of Thoracic Surgeons: Endorsed by the

American Association of Cardiovascular and Pulmonary Rehabilitation and the Society for Academic Emergency Medicine. *Circulation.* 2007;116:803-77.

25. Nable JV, Brady W. The evolution of electrocardiographic changes in ST-segment elevation myocardial infarction. *Am J Emerg Med.* 2009;27:734-46.

26. Menown IB, Mackenzie G, Adgey AA. Optimizing the initial 12-lead electrocardiographic diagnosis of acute myocardial infarction. *Eur Heart J.* 2000;21:275-83.

27. Berry C, Zalewski A, Kovach R, Savage M, Goldberg S. Surface electrocardiogram in the detection of transmural myocardial ischemia during coronary artery occlusion. *Am J Cardiol.* 1989;63:21-6.

28. Zarling EJ, Sexton H, Milnor P Jr. Failure to diagnose acute myocardial infarction. The clinicopathologic experience at a large community hospital. *JAMA.* 1983;250:1177-81.

29. Fesmire FM, Percy RF, Bardoner JB, Wharton DR, Calhoun FB, Usefulness of automated serial 12-lead ECG monitoring during the initial emergency department evaluation of patients with chest pain. *Ann Emerg Med.* 1998;31:3-11.

30. Thygesen K, Alpert JS, White HD, Jaffe AS, Apple FS, Galvani M, et al. Universal Definition of Myocardial Infarction. *Circulation.* 2007;116:2634-53.

31. Wu AH, Apple FS, Gibler WB, Jesse RL, Warshaw MM, Valdes R Jr. National Academy of Clinical Biochemistry Standards of Laboratory Practice: recommendations for the use of cardiac markers in coronary artery diseases. *Clin Chem.* 1999;45:1104-21.

32. Hudson MP, Christenson RH, Newby LK, Kaplan AL, Ohman EM. Cardiac markers: point of care testing. *Clin Chim Acta.* 1999;284:223-37.

33. de Winter RJ, Koster RW, Sturk A, Chen D, Harakal C, Addonizio VP, et al. Value of Myoglobin, Troponin T, and CK-MBmass in Ruling Out an Acute Myocardial Infarction in the Emergency Room. *Circulation.* 1995;92:3401-7.

34. Balk EM, Ioannidis JPA, Salem D, Chew PW, Lau J. Accuracy of biomarkers to diagnose acute cardiac ischemia in the emergency department: a meta-analysis. *Ann Emerg Med.* 2001;37:478-94.

35. Lott J, Stang J. Serum enzymes and isoenzymes in the diagnosis and differential diagnosis of myocardial ischemia and necrosis. *Clin Chem.* 1980;26:1241-50.

36. Hedges JR, Gibler WB, Young GP, Hoekstra JW, Slovis C, Aghababian R, et al. Multicenter study of creatine kinase-MB use: effect on chest pain clinical decision making. *Acad Emerg Med.* 1996;3:7-15.

37. Christenson RH, Newby LK, Ohman EM. Cardiac markers in the assessment of acute coronary syndromes. *Md Med J.* 1997;18-24.

38. NACB WRITING GROUP MEMBERS, Morrow DA, Cannon CP, Jesse RL, Newby LK, Ravkilde J, Storrow AB, et al. National Academy of Clinical Biochemistry Laboratory Medicine Practice Guidelines: Clinical characteristics and utilization of biochemical markers in acute coronary syndromes. *Circulation.* 2007;115:e356-75.

39. Apple FS. Tissue specificity of cardiac troponin I, cardiac troponin T and creatine kinase-MB. *Clin Chim Acta.* 1999;284:151-9.

40. Alpert JS, Thygesen K, Antman E, Bassand JP. Myocardial infarction redefined—a consensus document of The Joint European Society of Cardiology/American College of Cardiology committee for the redefinition of myocardial infarction. *J Am Coll Cardiol.* 2000;36:959-69.

41. Davis CP, Barrett K, Torre P, Wacasey K. Serial myoglobin levels for patients with possible myocardial infarction. *Acad Emerg Med.* 1996;3:590-7.

42. Bhayana V, Cohoe S, Pellar TG, Jablonsky G, Henderson AR. Combination (multiple) testing for myocardial infarction using myoglobin, creatine kinase-2 (mass), and troponin T. *Clin Biochem.* 1994;27:395-406.

43. Hamm CW. Acute coronary syndromes. The diagnostic role of troponins. *Thromb Res.* 2001;103:S63-9.

44. Chan D, Ng L. Biomarkers in acute myocardial infarction. *BMC Med.* 2010;8:34.

45. Morrow DA, Antman EM. Evaluation of High-Sensitivity Assays for Cardiac Troponin. *Clin Chem.* 2009;55:5-8.

46. Reichlin T, Hochholzer W, Bassetti S, Steuer S, Stelzig C, Hartwiger S, et al. Early Diagnosis of Myocardial Infarction with Sensitive Cardiac Troponin Assays. *N Engl J Med.* 2009;361:858-67.

47. Januzzi JL Jr, Bamberg F, Lee H, Truong QA, Nichols JH, Karakas M, et al. High-Sensitivity Troponin T Concentrations in Acute Chest Pain Patients Evaluated With Cardiac Computed Tomography. *Circulation.* 2010;121:1227-34.

48. Melanson SEF, Morrow DA, Jarolim P. *Earlier Detection of Myocardial Injury in a Preliminary Evaluation Using a New Troponin I Assay With Improved Sensitivity. Am J Clin Pathol.* 2007;128:282-6.

49. Fesmire FM, Decker WW, Diercks DB, Ghaemmaghami CA, Nazarian D, Brady WJ, et al. Clinical policy: critical issues in the evaluation and management of adult patients with non-ST-segment elevation acute coronary syndromes. *Ann Emerg Med.* 2006;48:270-301.

50. Bassand JP, Hamm CW, Ardissino D, Boersma E, Budaj A, Fernández-Avilés F, et al. Guidelines for the diagnosis and treatment of non-ST-segment elevation acute coronary syndromes. *Eur Heart J.* 2007;28:1598-660.

51. McCord J, Nowak RM, McCullough PA, Foreback C, Borzak S, Tokarski G, et al., Ninety-Minute Exclusion of Acute Myocardial Infarction By Use of Quantitative Point-of-Care Testing of Myoglobin and Troponin I. *Circulation.* 2001;104:1483-8.

52. Jaffe AS, Babuin L, Apple FS. Biomarkers in acute cardiac disease: the present and the future. *J Am Coll Cardiol.* 2006;48:1-11.

53. Christenson RH, Azzazy HME. Biochemical markers of the acute coronary syndromes. *Clin Chem.* 1998;44:1855-64.

54. Herlitz J, Svensson L. The value of biochemical markers for risk stratification prior to hospital admission in acute chest pain. *Acute Card Care.* 2008;10:197-204.

55. Wu AHB, Abbas SA, Green S, Pearsall L, Dhakam S, Azar R, et al. Prognostic value of cardiac troponin T in unstable angina pectoris. *Am J Cardiol.* 1995;76:970-2.

56. Wu AH, Feng YJ, Contois JH, Azar R, Waters D. Prognostic value of cardiac troponin I in patients with chest pain. *Clin Chem.* 1996;42:651-2.

57. Olatidoye AG, Wu AHB, Feng Y-J, Waters D. Prognostic Role of Troponin T Versus Troponin I in Unstable Angina Pectoris for Cardiac Events With Meta-Analysis Comparing Published Studies. *Am J Cardiol.* 1998;81:1405-10.

58. Siriwardena M, Kleffmann T, Ruygrok P, Cameron VA, Yandle TG, Nicholls MG, et al. B-Type Natriuretic Peptide Signal Peptide Circulates in Human Blood: Evaluation as a Potential Biomarker of Cardiac Ischemia. *Circulation.* 2010;122:255-64.

59. de Lemos JA, Peacock WF, McCullough PA. Natriuretic peptides in the prognosis and management of acute coronary syndromes. *Rev Cardiovasc Med.* 2010;11 Suppl 2:S24-34.

60. Sabatine MS, Morrow DA, de Lemos JA, Gibson CM, Murphy SA, Rifai N, et al. Multimarker Approach to Risk Stratification in Non-ST Elevation Acute Coronary Syndromes: Simultaneous Assessment of Troponin I, C-Reactive Protein, and B-Type Natriuretic Peptide. *Circulation.* 2002;105:1760-3.

61. Galvani M, Ottani F, Oltrona L, Ardissino D, Gensini GF, Maggioni AP, et al. N-Terminal Pro-Brain Natriuretic Peptide on Admission Has Prognostic Value Across the Whole Spectrum of Acute Coronary Syndromes. *Circulation.* 2004;110:128-34.

62. Anderson JL, Adams CD, Antman EM, Bridges CR, Califf RM, Casey DE Jr, et al. ACC/ AHA 2007 Guidelines for the Management of Patients With Unstable Angina/Non-ST-Elevation Myocardial Infarction: A Report of the American College of Cardiology/ American Heart Association Task Force on Practice Guidelines (Writing Committee to Revise the 2002 Guidelines for the Management of Patients With Unstable Angina/ Non-ST-Elevation Myocardial Infarction): Developed in Collaboration with the American College of Emergency Physicians, the Society for Cardiovascular Angiography and Interventions, and the Society of Thoracic Surgeons: Endorsed by the American Association of Cardiovascular and Pulmonary Rehabilitation and the Society for Academic Emergency Medicine. *Circulation.* 2007;116:e148-304.

63. Amini B, Patel CB, Lewin MR, Kim T, Fisher RE. Diagnostic nuclear medicine in the ED. *Am J Emerg Med.* 2011;29:91-101.

64. Gibbons RJ, Chatterjee K, Daley J, Douglas JS, Fihn SD, Gardin JM, et al. ACC/AHA/ ACP–ASIM Guidelines for the Management of Patients With Chronic Stable Angina: Executive Summary and Recommendations: A Report of the American College of Cardiology/American Heart Association Task Force on Practice Guidelines (Committee on Management of Patients With Chronic Stable Angina). *Circulation.* 1999;99:2829-48.

65. Ritchie JL, Bateman TM, Bonow RO, Crawford MH, Gibbons RJ, Hall RJ, et al. Guidelines for clinical use of cardiac radionuclide imaging report of the American College of Cardiology/American Heart Association Task Force on Assessment of Diagnostic and Therapeutic Cardiovascular Procedures (Committee on Radionuclide Imaging), developed in collaboration with the American Society of Nuclear Cardiology. *J Am Coll Cardiol.* 1995;25:521-47.

66. Hachamovitch R, Berman DS, Shaw LJ, Kiat H, Cohen I, Cabico JA, et al. Incremental prognostic value of myocardial perfusion single photon emission computed tomography for the prediction of cardiac death: differential stratification for risk of cardiac death and myocardial infarction. *Circulation.* 1998;97:535-43.

67. Ribeiro A, Lindmarker P, Juhlin-Dannfelt A, Johnsson H, Jorfeldt L. Echocardiography Doppler in pulmonary embolism: right ventricular dysfunction as a predictor of mortality rate. *Am Heart J.* 1997;134:479-87.

68. Goldstein JA, Gallagher MJ, O'Neill WW, Ross MA, O'Neil BJ, Raff GL. A randomized controlled trial of multi-slice coronary computed tomography for evaluation of acute chest pain. *J Am Coll Cardiol.* 2007;49:863-71.

69. Hoffmann U, Bamberg F, Chae CU, Nichols JH, Rogers IS, Seneviratne SK, et al. Coronary computed tomography angiography for early triage of patients with acute chest pain: the ROMICAT (Rule Out Myocardial Infarction using Computer Assisted Tomography) trial. *J Am Coll Cardiol.* 2009;53:1642-50.

70. Laudon DA, Behrenbeck TR, Wood CM, Bailey KR, Callahan CM, Breen JF, et al. Computed tomographic coronary artery calcium assessment for evaluating chest pain in the emergency department: long-term outcome of a prospective blind study. *Mayo Clin Proc.* 2010;85:314-22.

71. Fernandez-Friera L, Garcia-Alvarez A, Bagheriannejad-Esfahani F, Malick W, Mirelis JG, Sawit ST, et al. Diagnostic value of coronary artery calcium scoring in low-intermediate risk patients evaluated in the emergency department for acute coronary syndrome. *Am J Cardiol.* 2011;107:17-23.

CHAPTER 4

Laboratory Perspective on Biomarkers for Acute Coronary Syndromes

Alan HB Wu

INTRODUCTION

Clinical laboratory testing plays a critical role in the evaluation of patients who present to the emergency department (ED) with chest pain and symptoms suggestive of acute coronary syndromes (ACS). Clinical laboratory groups, such as the National Academy of Clinical Biochemistry (NACB) and the International Federation of Clinical Chemistry (IFCC), convene regularly to establish national and international laboratory practice guidelines on testing and reporting of cardiac biomarkers[1-4] and quality specifications for the assays themselves.[5,6] Practice guidelines are used by laboratorians for selecting methods and instrumentation and establishing testing goals for their practices. The specifications are used by the *in vitro* diagnostics industry in establishing current and next generation clinical assays of existing markers. In order to best serve the cardiac patient, clinical laboratory leaders must work closely with their clinical colleagues, especially cardiologists and ED physicians, in understanding the changing clinical needs of cardiac patients and industry scientists who create assays.

LABORATORY AND DIAGNOSTIC TEST REGULATIONS

Irrespective of the location of testing, the clinical laboratorian has the overall responsibility of the testing of body fluids for clinical diagnostic purposes. In the United States, clinical testing is mandated under the Clinical Laboratory Improvement Act of 1988 (CLIA 88), and is regulated under the auspices of the Center for Medicare and Medicaid Services (CMS). Similar governmental regulations are being considered and developed in other countries. Under CLIA 88, the laboratory director must be a board-certified pathologist and be responsible for all aspects of testing. All personnel must have minimum qualifications and licensing to conduct the specific tests within their scope. Competency must be assessed on a regular basis. An updated and regularly reviewed standard operating procedure manual must be readily available to technologists at the laboratory bench. There must be a quality control (QC) program where samples of known analyte concentrations in the appropriate matrix are tested each day on each instrument to ensure precision and accuracy relative to previous testing by the laboratory itself. An investigation must be conducted prior to release of test results for QC results that fall outside of the expected range (within pre-established statistical goals). Proficiency testing is also mandated by CLIA 88 to assess accuracy relative to other laboratories using the same commercial instruments or methodology. Samples of unknown analyte concentrations are sent by an agency that has received "deemed status" CMS to be tested and reported by each laboratory. The laboratory is then graded against mean values established by their peers and correctly quantify test results with a score of 80% or better. As an example, table 4-1 illustrates results of the College of American Pathologists Inc. (CAP) cardiac troponin I (cTnI) proficiency testing program. The San Francisco General Hospital (SFGH) laboratory reported a value of 0.70 ng/mL for survey #CR-06 using the Siemens Diagnostics ADVIA Centaur assay. The mean ± standard deviation of the 295 laboratories who reported troponin results on this instrument was 0.69 ± 0.075 ng mL. The SFGH result was within the acceptable reporting range of 0.46–0.92 ng/mL and therefore passed this particular challenge.

Manufacturers of diagnostic tests, instruments and devices in the United States are regulated by the Food and Drug Administration (FDA). New assays and devices are submitted to the FDA for approval under using one of two approval procedures. The "premarket approval" (PMA) is for tests and instruments for which there are not equivalent or predicate devices to compare against. The "510(k)" clearance process is for tests whose analytical and clinical performance is directly compared with a predicate assay. For example, the approval of cardiac troponin was originally based on a comparison with creatine kinase (CK) MB isoenzyme. Once cleared [510(k)] or approved (PMA), the FDA labels all approved tests as being "waived," "moderate complexity," and "high complexity," depending on how the test is performed and how the information from the test is used in clinical practice. Waived tests can be

Table 4-1	Results of the 2010-B CAP Cardiac Marker Proficiency Testing Program			
Instrument	Number of laboratories	Mean (ng/mL)	SD	CV
Abbott Architect®	157	2.006	0.159	7.9
Beckman UniCel Dxl®	133	0.267	0.040	14.9
Siemens ADVIA Centaur®	295	0.694	0.075	10.9
Siemens Dimension HM®	581	0.529	0.068	12.8
Siemens Stratus CS®	116	0.527	0.037	6.9
Vitros ECi®	270	1.049	0.124	11.9
SFGH Result, ADVIA Centaur		0.70		

CAP, College of American Pathologists; SD, standard deviation; CV, coefficient of variance; SFGH, San Francisco General Hospital.
Data used with permission *from* the College of American Pathologists Inc.

performed by general healthcare workers (nurses, respiratory therapists, physician assistants, etc.), whereas moderate and high complex test must be performed by trained clinical laboratory scientists. Most cardiac marker tests are moderately complex, although the Biosite triage assay (Allere Inc., San Diego, CA) for BNP (but not cardiac troponin I) has waived status, and there are two that are listed as high complexity. The FDA maintains a searchable website listing all cleared and approved tests, the manufacturer of the test, the complexity category, and the medical claims made by the manufacturer for use of the test in clinical practice (http://www.accessdata.fda.gov/scripts/cdrh/cfdHYPERLINK "http://www.accessdata.fda.gov/scripts/cdrh/cfdocs/cfCLIA/search.cfm"\t "_parent" ocs/cfCLIA/search.cfm). Recently, the Director of the FDA Division of Chemistry and Toxicology Devices issued a letter to manufacturers indicating the Agency's desire to modernize the performance, labeling, and claims for cardiac troponin assays.[7] This update is particularly relevant to the development and release of next generation or high-sensitivity troponin assays.

LABORATORY OPERATIONS FOR CARDIAC MARKER TESTING

The selection of the scope, instrumentation, location, and test result turnaround time need is especially important and relevant to cardiac biomarkers. The laboratory director or specifically the chemistry division section chief or supervisor must determine how testing is to be conducted within the scope and resources of the division. Particularly important issues for cardiac biomarker testing are turnaround time, analytical sensitivity, and discontinuance of older redundant cardiac biomarker tests.

Turnaround Time

The ED and cardiology departments' turnaround time (TAT) need for cardiac troponin may dictate where testing is to be conducted. The NACB, American College of Cardiology (ACC) and American Heart Association (AHA),[3,8] have opined that results of cardiac marker testing should be made available within 60 minutes from the time of ordering to reporting of results. If an ED has an accelerated acute myocardial infarction (AMI) rule out protocol (i.e., "Chest Pain Center"), a 30-minute turnaround time for test results may be justified. For most clinical laboratories, meeting the 60-minute TAT is possible but requires a streamlined operation for ordering tests, blood collection, transportation to the laboratory, centrifugation, testing, and reporting of results. Table 4-2 enlists variables that can improve or potentially degrade turnaround times by 5–10 minutes for each step. Use of test ordering by the caregivers eliminates the redundancy of reordering the test by the clinical laboratory staff. Samples collected in plasma eliminate the clotting time that

Table 4-2	Variables Affecting TAT for Testing Conducted at the POCT and within a Central Laboratory					
	Ordering	Phlebotomy	Transport	Centrifugation	Testing	Reporting
POCT	ED entry	ED collection	Eliminated	Eliminated	Reduced (~5–15 min)	Direct reporting
Central laboratory						
Favors fast TAT	ED or unit entry	ED or unit collection	Pneumatic tubes	Total automation	Stat mode (~9 min)	Wireless technology
Favors slow TAT	Laboratory entry	Laboratory phlebotomy staff	Manual courier	Manual centrifugation	Routine (~18 min)	Unit printer

TAT, turnaround time; POCT, point-of-care testing.

occurs for serum, enabling samples to be centrifuged immediately. Pneumatic tubes from the ED to the laboratory eliminate human delivery but are expensive to install if they do not preexist within the institution during its initial construction. Reporting of results directly to attending medical staff through wireless communications is becoming an increasingly affordable and attractive option but requires assistance by the information technology staff. These approaches can eliminate or reduce the time needed for some of the steps listed in table 4-2. Significant funding, economic justification, re-engineering, and architectural modifications are needed to facilitate rapid TATs for test results, which are often unavailable. Therefore, if laboratories unable to meet a 60-minute TAT goal, or if important medical or triaging decisions are needed within 30 minutes, then testing should be conducted in a satellite laboratory facility, if available, or through use of point-of-care testing (POCT) devices.

Analytical Sensitivity for Cardiac Troponin

A critical issue for clinical laboratories in the selection of instrumentation and assays is the analytical sensitivity of the commercial troponin test used in the laboratory. Assays with high analytic sensitivity enable an earlier detection of myocardial infarction,[9] and identification of more patients at risk for development of future adverse cardiac events.[10] The clinical value of these next generation assays is discussed in the next chapter. Today, all troponin testing is conducted on automated analyzers using sandwich-type immunoassays (Figure 4-1). There are significant differences in the sensitivity and precision of commercial troponin assays. Instruments that use chemiluminescence signaling technology have higher analytical sensitivity than those based on enzyme or fluorescence-labeled detection. Improved sensitivity can also be achieved by use of more than the traditional two antibodies (to detect troponin whose epitopes may be blocked), and use of longer incubation times and higher sample volumes.

Methodology

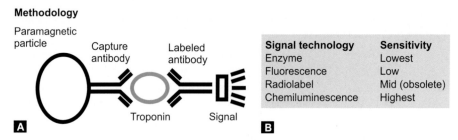

Figure 4-1 **A,** Sandwich-type immunoassays for cardiac troponin. **B,** The sensitivity of various antibody labeling strategies.

Troponin testing is part of the overall menu of immunoassays available on the analyzer. A laboratory director does not select the analyzer based on the performance of any single analyte alone, e.g., troponin. Rather, it is based on an overall contract that a laboratory or hospital has with the vendor for other clinical laboratory testing services. The choice of provider is also based on the reputation of the manufacturer, responsiveness and quality of service, software user-friendliness, any history between the company and the laboratory, and other factors.

The specifications for analytical sensitivity for cardiac troponin were established by NACB, ACC, and AHA guidelines.[3,8] Assays should have analytical sensitivities to reliably detect troponin in a majority of healthy subjects.[11] The cutoff concentration is at the 99th percentile of a healthy population, with assay imprecision of 10% or less.[3,8] Most of the earlier troponin assays do not have the analytical sensitivity to detect troponin in a control population nor do they meet the 10% coefficient of variance (CV) goal.[12] Therefore, use of these older troponin assays may compromise the clinical utility of troponin testing.

Discontinuation of Antiquated Cardiac Markers

Justification for a clinical laboratory to add new cardiac markers to the testing menu can be accomplished in part by the removal of tests that are redundant or antiquated. The development and utilization of next generation troponin assays have obviated the need for testing for myoglobin and CK-MB. The trend for reduced utilization of these tests has been documented in a gradual decline in reporting CAP proficiency survey results for cardiac markers over the past few years.[13] The use of a high sensitive troponin assay and the 99th percentile cuttoff limit enable as early of a detection of AMI as was the case for serum myoglobin.[14] Critics to the removal of CK-MB suggest that this marker is better suited for detection of reinfarction, since troponin remains increased for 7–10 days. While there has not been a clinical trial comparing the utility of CK-MB versus troponin for reinfarction, Apple et al. showed that there is a second release of troponin to detect the presence of new onset myocardial injury.[15] Laboratory directors and administrators must communicate with the medical staff, particularly cardiology and ED medicine to discuss the removal of outdated tests in favor of contemporary troponin assays and the 99th percentile cutoff limit. Such a decision cannot be made by the laboratory alone.

CARDIAC BIOMARKER ASSAY ISSUES

Standardization

A major problem for commercial troponin I assays is the lack of standardization. Results between testing platforms were proportionally biased by as much as 30-fold. As an example, the CAP proficiency survey samples result from table 4-1 shows a 7.5-fold difference between the lowest (Siemens Centaur, Tarrytown, NY) and the highest (Abbott Architect, Abbott Park, IL) results. Therefore, one cannot interpret results of serial testing from the same patient, if different testing platforms are used, without repeating the testing on each platform. The cause for most of this bias is differences in the assignment of the standard used to calibrate the assay. In an attempt to reduced differences between assays, the American Association for Clinical Chemistry established a working committee to create a reference material for use by manufacturers in standardizing their assays.[16] This material is a complex of troponin T, I, and C, and is available through the National Institute of Standards and Technologies (SRM 2921, Gaithersburg, MD). In harmonization studies by this committee, the use of the candidate troponin standard resulted in the reduction of interassay cTnI variability from a median of 88–15.5%.[17] Unfortunately, not all manufacturers have adopted this standard in their assays and biases continue to exist. Even with complete compliance with the NIST standard, variances between assays will continue to exist due to the lack of standardization for the antibodies used in commercial assays. In this regard, the IFCC has established a committee charged to develop a reference assay in hope of establishing a higher degree of assay standardization.

The lack of standardization is not an issue for laboratories who use troponin T as this assay is only available from one manufacturer (Roche Diagnostics), and results and cutoff concentrations are commutable between different Roche testing platforms and between different generations of assays. There is also no universal standardization for assays for myoglobin or CK-MB, although this is becoming less of an issue with these assays being discontinued.

POCT

POCT refers to testing at or near the patient bedside using portable analyzers. This type of testing is widely used for blood glucose testing at home, clinic, or hospital practice. Table 4-3 enlists the advantages and disadvantages of POCT vs central laboratory testing for cardiac markers. POCT eliminates the time and effort needed to transport samples from the patient to the clinical laboratory (Table 4-2). All POCT

Table 4-3	Advantages and Disadvantages of POCT vs the Central Laboratory for Cardiac Marker Testing	
Criteria	Central laboratory	POCT
Instrument cost	Very high ($1000,000)	Very low ($1000–5000)
Reagent costs	Low (< $5.00)	High ($10–$30)
Assay TAT	Long (18 min)	Moderate (5–15 min)
Analytic sensitivity	High (10 ng/mL)	Low (100–500 ng/mL)
Analytic precision	High (5–10%)	Moderate (10–20%)
Centrifugation	Needed (serum or plasma)	Not needed (whole blood)
Testing throughput	High (hundreds per hour)	Low (5–10 per hour)
Assay standardization	None	None

TAT, turnaround time; POCT, point-of-care testing.

devices for cardiac markers test whole blood as the sample thereby eliminating the centrifugation step needed for serum or plasma. Both qualitative and quantitative assays are available for troponin, although qualitative tests were never widely used.

The analytical sensitivity for POCT troponin assays has not kept pace with improvements in central laboratory-based assays. Current POCT devices are 10- to 50-fold less sensitive than central laboratory assays. The consequence of using a less sensitive assay is dependent on the reason for testing. For use in the diagnosis of AMI, the first positive troponin result may occur an hour to so later for POCT assays than for the central laboratory. To rule out of AMI, a longer window of testing may be required (e.g., 0, 3, and 6 hours for the central laboratory vs 0, 4, and 8 hours for POCT). In both situations, the turnaround time advantage for POCT over the central laboratory is somewhat negated. For risk stratification, the use of troponin assays with less analytical sensitivity results in misidentifying patients who have mild myocardial necrosis when assessed against the 99th percentile of a healthy population. A number of studies have shown that patients with minor injury have higher incidence of major adverse cardiac events (cardiac death and AMI) at 30 days.[18] Some laboratories offer both rapid POCT testing by POCT for AMI diagnosis/rule out, and central laboratory testing for risk stratification. In this situation, samples are tested on both platforms, and the reporting is separately listed on the final laboratory report indicating how testing was conducted and the cutoff concentration for the assay used.

Assay Interferences

All clinical assays are subjected to analytical interferences that result in the production of falsely high or low results, with troponin being no exception. Falsely high results can occur with the presence of heterophile antibodies or human antimouse antibodies (HAMA) in the sample. These antibodies can bind both the capture and labeled antibody resulting in an analytical signal in the absence of the analyte. Fibrin strands that remain after incomplete clotting (serum) or incomplete anticoagulation (plasma) can also produce a false-positive result. The laboratory should be contacted if an incorrect result is suspected (e.g., an unexpected rise or fall in troponin results). Repeating the sample on a different troponin testing platform or use of blocking reagents can be useful in determining heterophile antibodies or HAMA. Repeating the sample on the same platform after recentrifugation will often eliminate the fibrin interference.

False-negative results occur in the presence of troponin autoantibodies.[19] These antibodies bind to troponin blocking the epitope from the antibodies used in the troponin assay. The concentration of these antibodies is usually low. Therefore, in cases of acute coronary syndromes, the amount of troponin release overcomes the autoantibody tier resulting in detection of the analyte. For minor myocardial damage, these antibodies may obscure the release of troponin resulting in an inaccurate characterization of future cardiovascular risk. Like HAMA, the degree of the autoantibody effect is variable between different commercial troponin assays.

FUTURE CARDIAC BIOMARKER ASSAYS AND TESTING PLATFORMS

Next Generation Cardiac Troponin Assays

The current "high sensitive troponin assays have a limit of detection (LOD) of about 10 pg/mL and a 99th percentile of about 40 pg/mL. These assays are not able to detect all healthy subjects. A "scorecard" was recently proposed to objectively evaluate troponin assay sensitivity.[11] The next and likely final generation of troponin assays have an LOD of < 1 pg/mL and a 99th percentile of 10 pg/mL.[20] With these assays, it may be possible to detect induced myocardial ischemia, such as with an exercise stress test.[21] These assays require novel analytical detection schemes and have longer assay turnaround times (about 40 minutes). Therefore, they are not currently available on routine automated immunoassay testing platforms.

Novel Biomarkers of Plaque Instability and Myocardial Ischemia

There has been significant research in evaluating other biomarkers of myocardial ischemia, such as free fatty acid, glycogen phosphorylase BB, and ischemia-modified albumin, and the presence of vulnerable plaque within coronary arteries, e.g., high sensitivity C-reactive protein, CD40 ligand, pregnancy associated plasma protein-A, placental growth factor, whole blood choline, myeloperoxidase, among others.[22] The hope was to combine results of these tests with cardiac troponin for early detection of myocardial ischemia and improve risk stratification predictions. Unfortunately, none of these biomarkers have sufficient cardiac specificity to be useful in routine practice and cardiac troponin (T or I) alone remains today as the standard biomarker for AMI diagnosis and risk stratification. Nevertheless, a continued search for novel biomarkers is ongoing.

Multiplex Testing Platforms for the Central Laboratory

While protein-based multiplex biomarker testing is not yet widely used in clinical laboratories, the *in vitro* diagnostics industry and the FDA are anticipating the need for "panel" testing and have begun constructing testing platforms and legislation, respectively. There are two general approaches that have been taken towards multiplex testing for proteins. The Luminex Technology (Austin TX) makes us of multicolored beads and a two-color flow cytometer.[23] Each bead color is a different protein assay and is linked to antibodies directed to a specific analyte. A mixture of beads can be used to simultaneously detect a variety of proteins. The first channel of the flow cytometric analysis identifies the bead color (i.e., which analyte is being measured), and the second channel measures the intensity of the fluorescence label (i.e., the analyte concentration). The luminex detector has been used for multiplex cytokine analysis (for clinical research purposes), and has been incorporated into a clinical multiplex analyzer (Bioplex 2200®, Bio-Rad Laboratories, Hercules, CA) for multiplex autoimmune analysis, infectious disease serology, and cardiac markers (to be released).

The second approach to multiplex analysis is the use of a microchip array. This technology is used for clinical practice for molecular diagnostics testing industry whereby oligonucleotides are linked to silicon-based chips to capture and detect specific DNA sequences. For analysis of proteins, antibodies are used in place of oligonucleotides for capture and detection of proteins. Randox Corporation (Evidence® family of analyzers, Northern Ireland) was among the first to incorporate microchip for multiplex protein analysis including cardiac markers (troponin I, CK-MB, myoglobin, and heart-type fatty acid binding protein).

Next Generation POCT Platforms

Lateral flow is the current testing methodology for most point-of-care immunoassays. A schematic of these assays is shown in figure 4-2A. Samples diffuse via capillary action through filtering layers to separate plasma from red cells and pass through the detection zone where immobilized anti-analyte antibodies capture the target. A second labeled antibody, that is mobile, is also captured by the analyte to complete the sandwich and enable detection. A control zone is used to indicate that sample has pass through the target zone, as it is placed furthest away from the application point. Many lateral flow assays are qualitative, e.g., human chorionic gonadotropin, drugs of abuse, infectious disease serology, etc. For cardiac troponin and B-type natriuretic peptide, the intensity of the signal is measured with a reader to produce a quantitative result. The major disadvantage of the lateral flow technology is lower analytical sensitivity relative to results from an automated immunoassay analyzer. Part of the reason is that high analytical sensitivity is dependent on high analytical precision. In lateral flow, the reproducibility of results between patient samples is due to variation in the plasma viscosity of the samples as well as environmental conditions, such as the temperature, humidity, and atmospheric pressure at the time of testing. Moreover, lateral flow technology is better suited for singleplex analysis, although the Biosite triage device is an exception to this.

A more precise manner to deliver samples to the target zone is the use of microfluidics. As shown in figure 4-2B, microfluidic devices have an onboard pumping mechanism that allows for the precise and positive displacement delivery of samples and reagents to the test zones. This results in higher sample delivery reproducibility, necessary in order to obtain high analytic sensitivity. Microfluidic devices can deliver lower sample volumes and can be adapted for multiplex analysis. Further increases in analytical sensitivity require use of electrochemical signals or novel surface plasmon resonance technology. These detection schemes are more sensitive than the current visual or fluorescence endpoints currently being used. None of these POCT devices are currently FDA cleared, although there are several companies working on these tests for troponin. The costs for these tests may be higher than those for current lateral flow devices.

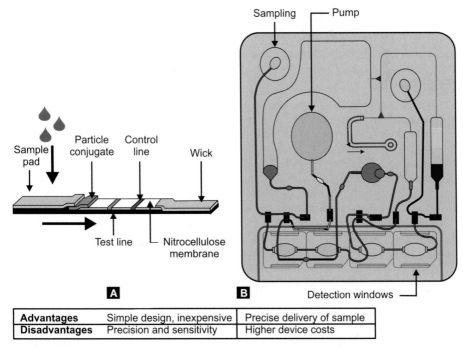

| **Advantages** | Simple design, inexpensive | Precise delivery of sample |
| **Disadvantages** | Precision and sensitivity | Higher device costs |

Figure 4-2 POCT devices with advantages and disadvantages. **A,** Lateral flow. **B,** Microfluidics device and key component parts. Used with permission *from* BioDot Inc., Irvine, CA.

Cardiac Biomarker Discovery Approaches

Because of the high prevalence of cardiac diseases worldwide, there is great interest in discovering new clinical laboratory tests for future clinical practice. There are two approaches towards finding new biomarkers. The "directed" approach involves examining proteins that signify events known to occur in the pathophysiology of acute coronary syndromes. For example, markers of inflammation are consistently positive in evolving cases of AMI. Other important events in ACS include angiogenesis, leukocyte and monocyte infiltration, fibrous cap degradation, platelet activation and thrombogenesis. The "undirected" approach is to compare tissues or blood samples of affected patients with those of healthy subjects or those who have early disease. Proteomic techniques are used to discern differences in the release or absence of proteins in these samples. The identity and function of protein targets can subsequently be conducted. While current cardiac biomarkers are protein-based, genetic expression arrays and metabolomic signatures may also become important. In these situations, a pattern of mRNA expression or metabolites are likely to be more meaningful than individual test results. The interpretation of results will require a higher level of bioinformatics review and interpretation than what is currently being used for cardiac disease. The FDA has indicated that these "*in vitro* diagnostics multivariate indexed assays (IVDMIAs)*"* must themselves be separately validated, reviewed, and approved by the FDA prior to commercialization. It is likely that they will need to go through the PMA route rather than the 510(k). While there are no examples of IVDMIA for cardiac biomarkers, the FDA has approved products for use in breast therapy using indexed assays.

REFERENCES

1. Wu AHB, Apple FS, Gibler WB, et al. National Academy of Clinical Biochemistry Standards of Laboratory Practice: recommendations for use of cardiac markers in coronary artery diseases. *Clin Chem.* 1999;45:1104-21.
2. Morrow DA, Cannon CP, Jesse RL, et al. National Academy of Clinical Biochemistry Laboratory Medicine Practice Guidelines: clinical characteristics and utilization of biochemical markers in acute coronary syndromes. *Circulation.* 2007;115:e356-75.
3. Apple FS, Jesse RL, Newby LK, et al. National Academy of Clinical Biochemistry and IFCC Committee for Standardization of Markers of Cardiac Damage Laboratory Medicine Practice Guidelines: analytical issues for biomarkers of acute coronary syndromes. *Clin Chem.* 2007;53:547-51; *Circulation.* 2007;115:e352-5.
4. Wu AHB, Apple FS, Jaffe AS, et al. National Academy of Clinical Biochemistry Laboratory Medicine Practice Guidelines: use of cardiac troponin and the natriuretic peptides for etiologies other than acute coronary syndromes and heart failure. *Clin Chem.* 2007; 53:2086-96.
5. Panteghini M, Gerhardt W, Apple FS, et al. Quality specifications for cardiac troponin assays. *Clin Chem Lab Med.* 2001;39:174-8.
6. Mair J, Jaffe AS, Ordonez-Llanos J, Christenson RH, et al. Update on quality specifications for cardiac troponin assays: recommendations from the IFCC Committee for Standardization of Markers of Cardiac Damage. *Clin Chem.* 2011;submitted.

7. Letter to Manufacturers of Troponin Assays Listed with the FDA. US Department of Health and Human Services, Food and Drug Administration. http://www.fda.gov/ MedicalDevices/ProductsandMedicalProcedures/InVitroDiagnostics/ucm230118.htm. Accessed January 3, 2011.

8. Anderson JL, Adams CD, Antman EM, et al. ACC/AHA 2007 Guidelines for the management of patients with unstable angina/non–ST-elevation myocardial infarction. *Circulation*. 2007;50:1-157.

9. Melanson SEF, Morrow DA, Jarolim P. Earlier detection of myocardial injury in a preliminary evaluation using a new troponin I assay with improved sensitivity. *Am J Clin Pathol*. 2007;128:282-6.

10. Morrow DA, Cannon CP, Rifai N, et al. Ability of minor elevations of troponins I and T to predict benefit from an early invasive strategy in patients with unstable angina and non-ST elevation myocardial infarction: results from a randomized trial. *JAMA*. 2001;286:2405-12.

11. Apple FS. A new season for cardiac troponin assays: it's time to keep a scorecard. *Clin Chem*. 2009;55:1303-6. Epub 2009 May 28.

12. Panteghini M, Pagani F, Yeo KTJ, et al. Evaluation of the imprecision at low-range concentration of the assays for cardiac troponin determination. *Clin Chem*. 2004;50:327-32.

13. Wu AHB, Lewandrowski KB, Gronowski A, et al. Antiquated tests within the clinical laboratory. *Am J Managed Care*. 2010:16:e220-7.

14. Eggers KM, Oldgren J, Nordenskjold A, et al. Diagnostic value of serial measurement of cardiac markers in patients with chest pain: limited value of adding myoglobin to troponin I for exclusion of myocardial infarction. *Am Heart J*. 2004;148:574-81.

15. Apple FS, Murakami MM. Cardiac troponin and creatine kinase MB monitoring during in-hospital myocardial reinfarction. *Clin Chem*. 2005;51:460-3.

16. Christenson RH, Apple F, Bodor G, et al. Standardization of cardiac troponin I assays, part II: round robin performance of ten candidate reference materials. *Clin Chem*. 2001;47:431-7.

17. Christenson RH, Duh SH, Apple FS, et al. for the American Association for Clinical Chemistry Cardiac Troponin I Standardization Committee. Toward standardization of cardiac troponin I measurements, part II: assessing commutability of candidate reference materials and harmonization of cardiac troponin I assays. *Clin Chem*. 2006;52:1685-92.

18. Wu AHB, Jaffe AS. The clinical need for high sensitivity cardiac troponin assays for ACS and the role for serial testing. *Am Heart J*. 2008;155:208-14.

19. Wu AHB, Fukushima F, Puskas R, et al. Development and preliminary clinical validation of a high sensitivity assay for cardiac troponin using a capillary flow (single molecule) fluorescence detector. *Clin Chem*. 2006;52:2157-9.

20. Pettersson K, Eriksson S, Wittfooth S, et al. Autoantibodies to cardiac troponin associate with higher initial concentrations and longer release of troponin I in acute coronary syndrome patients. *Clin Chem*. 2009;55:938-45.

21. Sabatine MS, Morrow DA, de Lemos JA, et al. Detection of acute changes in circulating troponin in the setting of transient stress test-induced myocardial ischaemia using an ultrasensitive assay: results from TIMI 35. *Eur Heart J*. 2009;30:162-9.

22. Apple FS, Wu AHB, Mair J, et al. Future biomarkers for detection of ischemia and risk stratification in acute coronary syndrome. *Clin Chem*. 2005;51:810-24.

23. Joos TO, Schrenk M, Hopfl P, et al. A microarray enzyme-linked immunosorbent assay for autoimmune diagnostics. *Electrophoresis*. 2000;21:2641-50.

Hypersensitive Troponins

Allan S Jaffe

INTRODUCTION

Increasingly sensitive assays, called here, hypersensitive cardiac troponin (hpscTn) assays, have the potential to markedly improve the diagnosis of cardiac injury and to increase the rapidity with which these diagnoses are appreciated. However, there will be challenges associated with the increase in sensitivity that will need to be addressed. This chapter will review what is known at present concerning the use of these assays. This review builds on present data about how to best use cTn assay values. This in itself is a challenge since there is a relative lack of consistency in the literature about how to use cTn assays. Accordingly, some recapitulation of the basic principles in general may be necessary but will be kept to a minimum. For those who need additional information in this critical area, review articles from several excellent sources are available.[1,2]

DEFINITION OF hpscTn ASSAYS

This is a not an inconsequential issue. Companies who make assays wish to be known as having sensitive assays and some even name their assays to imply high degrees of sensitivity whether they achieve that standard or not. Unfortunately, comparative standards are not universally available. Early studies unmasked a high degree of heterogeneity in regard to both the sensitivity and precision of cTn assays.[3] There may be slightly better harmonization[4] at present but it is far from absolute and true standardization in this area is unlikely in the foreseeable future.

In regard to defining hpscTn assays, the best proposal has been made by Apple[5] (Table 5-1) who suggested hpscTn assays should be defined by the number of normal subjects in whom values are detected. For most assays presently in use, this number is substantially less than 50%. Those presently included as hpscTn assays (Table 5-2) often are said to measure values in over 90% of the patients. The implication is that the detection of more normal subjects means higher sensitivity. This is a reasonable assumption, but it does not necessarily extrapolate to increased clinical sensitivity, which may be unique for a given clinical situation. For example,

Table 5-1	Cardiac Troponin Assay Score-card
Acceptance designation	*Total precision at 99th percentile*
Guideline acceptable	≤10%
Clinically usable	> 10 to ≤ 20%
Not acceptable	> 20%
Assay designation	*Measurable normal values below 99th percentile*
Level 4: third-generation high sensitivity	≥ 95%
Level 3: second-generation high sensitivity	75 to < 95%
Level 2: first-generation high sensitivity	50 to < 75%
Level 1: contemporary	< 50%

Table 5-2	High Sensitivity Assay Score-card			
	99th μg/L	*CV at 99th percentile*		
Beckman Access hs-cTnl	0.0086	10.0	Guideline acceptable	Level 4
Roche Elecsys hs-cTnT	0.013	8.0	Guideline acceptable	Level 4
Nanosphere hs-cTnl	0.0028	9.5	Guideline acceptable	Level 3
Singulex hs-cTnl	0.0101	9.0	Guidelines acceptable	Level 4

one high comparative "high" sensitivity assay, the hscTnT assay was diagnostically equivalent to others in two large recent evaluations of large chest pain cohorts.[6,7] One could argue that cohorts were selective or not ideally characterized and indeed the ROC value in one study[7] for the hscTn assay was superior, but the difference was small and statistically insignificant. Therefore, it may in the long run be necessary to do clinical trials based on clinical accuracy to define the relative sensitivity of these assays.

ANALYTIC AND PREANALYTIC ISSUES

One of the areas, clinicians tend to ignore in the evaluation of blood tests relates to the analytic and preanalytic issues. It used to be as part of clinical training for trainees to understand the biochemical basis for laboratory tests, but it appears that presently, even the basic principles are no longer taught. This is, in the opinion of this author, lamentable, especially for assays that are relied on so frequently. Some understanding of these issues is essential[2] in order to understand potential false-positive and false-negative results. These issues will be even more important with high hpscTn assays.

Several preanalytic and analytic issues have been raised in regard to hpscTn measurements already. The first has to do with hemolysis, which can distort any

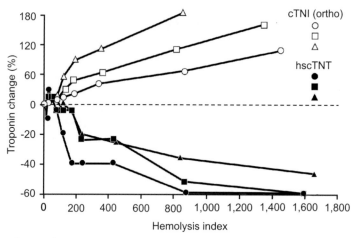

Figure 5-1 Effects of hemolysis on cardiac troponin levels. Note that with the high sensitivity troponin T assay that even modest amounts of hemolysis lowered values. This is in contrast to the response of the ortho assay which is not an hpscTn assay but which shows rises in response to hemolysis. It should be noted that there are some assays that do not respond but many that do. *From* Bais R. The effect of sample hemolysis on cardiac troponin I and T assays. *Clin Chem.* 2010;56:1357-9, with permission.

assay. For cTnI, hemolysis can increase values; with cTnT, values go down.[8] With conventional assays that do not measure near the true normal range, this is probably not a problem. However, with hpscTn assays such issues may be more important since minor increases or decreases could cause one to either exceed or not exceed the 99th percentile URL. Thus, small amounts of hemolysis with hpscTn assays could have marked effects (Figure 5-1).[9] This means that the way in which blood is obtained needs to become more fastidious. Specifically, line draws which are known to markedly accentuate hemolysis and other preanalytic problems[10,11] should be minimized. Laboratories will need to scrutinize samples more carefully to identify those with preanalytic problems.

The most common preanalytic problem is hemolysis, but it is by no means the only one. Another potential issue relates to antibodies directed against the epitopes used for the detection of troponin. This has been best described for cTnI assays.[12] These antibodies usually are to the central portion of the molecule where many of the tag and detection antibodies are targeted because it is a stable region. In general, these antibodies lower values but have not been shown to cause frequent false-negative values.[12] This may be very different with novel hpscTn assays since relatively smaller changes may cause negative results. This issue has been fairly unexplored thus far but is worth consideration. In addition, although we think about this issue as more germane to cTnI assays, recently antibodies to cTnT have also been described presenting healthy blood donors.[13] Their ability to cause problems, however, has not thus far been shown.

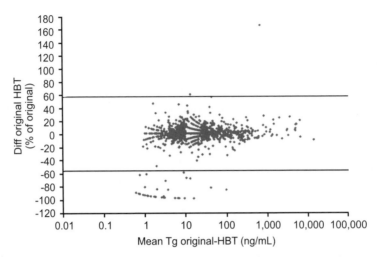

Figure 5-2 The effects of treatment of samples that have heterophilic interference with heterophile blocking antibody tubes. Note the marked reduction in values after treatment.

There are a variety of other analytic confounds that could become problematic as well. For example, all ELISA kits have blocking antibodies to reduce cross-reacting subspecies, be they due to other antibodies or due to existing antibodies against the material that is used to make the detection or tag antibody used in the assay. These are known as heterophilic or cross-reacting antibodies. They are likely ubiquitous but at low levels so they can, although rarely, cause false-positive and/or false-negative results. High levels can occur and cause either elevations or reductions in cTn levels.[12] This is easily unmasked by the laboratory either by adding additional blocking antibodies from so called HBT (heterophile blocking tubes) (Figure 5-2) or with dilution studies.[14] When interferents are present, including antibodies, samples will not dilute until the interferent is totally removed. As assay sensitivity increases, it is likely that ever smaller amounts of antibodies will be able to influence assays and by increasing values push the small distance it may take for a "nonsignificant" value to one that is of concern or to cause false-negative results. Laboratories need to begin to scrutinize samples measuring hpscTn more carefully for such types of problems to detect these potential false-positive and false-negative influences. In addition, there are macrotroponins as well which are recently described.[15] Again, this phenomenon has not heretofore been a problem because of the relative lack of sensitivity of the assays and the fact that whatever changes they induce rarely causes patients to change diagnostic categories. However, with hpscTn assays, where even small amounts could change diagnostic categorization, these confounds may become more important. Only by being prepared and recognizing this as a potential problem and by encouraging clinicians to question results when they do not seem to match the clinical situation will we be able to understand the extent to which these issues are important. The bottom line in this regard is that closer interactions between laboratory personnel and clinicians are going to be essential to develop strategies to deal with these issues in the interest of better patient care.

Finally, as we get more and more hpscTn assays we need to rechallenge the basic assumptions upon which the use of cTn is based. Early studies attempting to detect cTnI and cTnT in skeletal muscle and a variety of other tissues relied on far less sensitivity instruments.[16-18] As our instruments become more sensitive, it is conceivable that this unique specificity of troponins could be challenged.

DIAGNOSIS OF ACUTE MYOCARDIAL INFARCTION

In the long run, it may turn out that a simple change from one hpscTn value to a higher value will be adequate to diagnose an acute myocardial infarction in the appropriate clinical setting even if the values are below the 99th percentile URL. However, in the short-term, the paradigm of insisting on a change and a value above the 99th percentile URL is very likely to persist.[19] However, the optimal way to implement these criteria is unclear. For elevated values, a change of > 20% is considered adequate,[19] however, with lower values, the calculation based on imprecision is more complex and probably best left to the laboratory to report.[2] It may even be that eventually no one will be defined as having unstable coronary artery disease absent an elevated or at least rising pattern of hpscTn values. However, there are real challenges in the implementation of change criteria (see below). The situation is complicated further by the fact that because acute myocardial infarction is such a morbid event with such important prognostic significance, clinicians have a tendency to focus on it differentially. Therefore, when one is unsure, often a diagnosis of MI or possible MI is made. For some clinicians, all elevated cTn values are thought to be indicative of AMI. This further complicates triage because often it is not clear what is causing the cardiac injury and the clinical metrics for defining an "ischemic" presentation vary across age and gender ranges and exceptions are frequent.[20] Thus, clinical studies are necessary to put better metrics around what the clinical presentations should suggest acute ischemic heart disease.[21] Finally, complicating things further, some patients with ischemic heart disease do not present in a time course that allows one to even look for a rising and/or falling pattern. For example, values that are near the peak of the time-concentration curve may not show a rise and fall. Patients who present late can be days after MI and may be on the tail of the time concentration curve and thus also may not manifest a dynamic pattern of values either.

HpscTn assays may provide some assistance with some of the issues that influence this diagnosis. In the past, what constituted differences in values had to be calculated from the precision profiles[19] of the assays because the assessment of conjoint biological and analytical variation requires normal subjects. Now data about biological variation are slowly emerging for these assays. The computation of this change is complex and therefore best done by the laboratories who run the assays. The first study done in this arena was by Wu and colleagues with the hpscTn assay made by Singulex.[22] The so called reference change values (RCVs) of 45% short-term and to 50% longer-term were calculated as values above which a significant change was likely. Similar data are available for the hpscTn Beckman assay.[23] On the other hand, the hpscTnT assay has been studied and is reported to have a RCV of 85%.[24] Thus, in order to know that a value has exceeded the conjoint biologic and analytic variation, one needs to see an 85% change. This is likely because with that assay, low normal values are defined with less precision with the hpscTnT assay than with the Singulex and/or Beckman assays. Studies of normals with higher values achieve lower RCVs.[25] Nonetheless, this metric suggests a much higher value is necessary for the diagnosis of a changing pattern of values. It is conceivable, perhaps even likely, that the key parameter to define in this area is not the mean or even the amount of a rise that exceeds biologic or analytic variation but the minimal value that one needs to see to know that a change is occurring. That number is harder to develop. At present, it is clear that patients who have ST elevation MIs or very overt non-STE AMIs often have big changes in cardiac troponin that are easy to observe.[26] On the other hand, subtle presentations may evoke different levels of change. Indeed, it may be that an absolute change may turn out to be more important than a percentage change because when one gets very high values, one may not be able to have continuing substantial rises of major proportions. Thus, it may turn out that using an absolute change of 6 or 8 or 10 ng/L is a better predictor than a percentage change and this has been suggested for one assay already.[27]

Despite this difficult limitation and the lack of definitive clinical standards, more than a few studies have been done with hpscTn assays. What has been done usually is to utilize contemporary assays, such as the present generation of the cTnT assay[6] or clinically available cTnI assays[28] to make the gold standard diagnosis of AMI. Then investigators evaluate the ability of the newer assays to make the diagnosis in these patients. If these assays are insensitive ones[29] or if the gold standard assays are used at higher than recommended cut off values, it exaggerates the benefit of the novel assays. In general, these assays make the diagnosis earlier[6,28,29] and one can then surmise that all diagnoses can be made that way. However, the novel hpscTn assays will also likely identify additional patients not detected by the contemporary assays.[30] One needs to take these later patients into account to determine the optimal timing to rule in or to exclude AMI rather than the data based on the less than ideal gold standard. A good example of how this might work comes from the work of Wilson and Morrow.[29] They evaluated 50 patients with AMI detected with a relatively insensitive assay with the novel hpscTn nanosphere assay. They showed that there was much more rapid diagnosis with the novel hpscTn assay (Figure 5-3). However, when they evaluated another 50 patients with "unstable angina" based

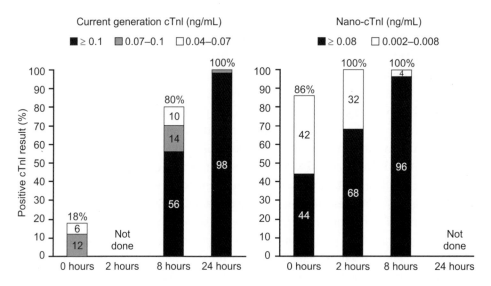

Figure 5-3 Early detection of patients with acute myocardial infarction as documented with a standard generation troponin assay shown on the left. One can appreciate the marked increase in the rapidity of diagnoses utilizing the novel high sensitivity assay whose values are shown in the right panel. *From* Wilson SR, Sabatine MS, Braunwald E, Sloan S, Murphy SA, Morrow DA. Detection of myocardial injury in patients with unstable angina using a novel nanoparticle cardiac troponin I assay: observations from the PROTECT-TIMI 30 Trial. *Am Heart J.* 2009;158:386-91, with permission.

on the less sensitive assay, (Figure 5-4), it became clear that most if not all of these patients had elevations indicative of AMI. Judging from the available literature, it appears that these assays will increase the frequency of AMI by about 15%. We also will need to be prepared to establish different metrics based on gender as with some hpscTn assays, women have lower values[31,32] and with others, they do not.[33] In addition, women have more plaque erosion and endothelial dysfunction and thus may elaborate lesser amounts of hpscTn.[34] These AMIs also can be missed because of the lack of an overt culprit lesions at angiography. However, the diagnosis of MI often can be confirmed with MRI imaging.[35,36]

It is likely the case that most if not all diagnoses of AMI will be achievable within 3 hours.[6,28,29] How long it will take to make sure no one is discharged with an elevated value indicative of AMI may take longer if the ED metric of a 1% or less miss rate is utilized. It is very likely that patients who were present at least 6 hours after the onset of symptoms and those who have very low values with hpscTn asays may be triageable at the time of presentation. This may be as much as 40–50% of the population.[37] If hpscTn assays could be linked to better clinical criteria to define a low-risk subset,[21] one may be able to increase this number substantially. Finally, it is unclear that the incremental value of stress evaluations in those who have had

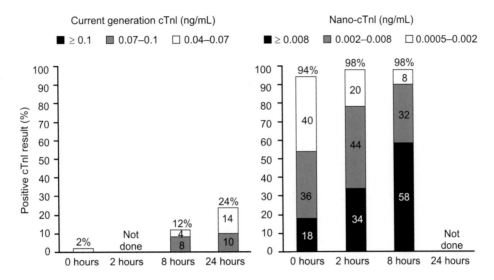

Figure 5-4 Increased detection of elevation troponins in patients previously diagnosed with unstable angina. Note that all of these patients failed to meet criteria for acute myocardial infarction and were designated as having unstable angina. Note that all of them as shown in the right panel had substantial elevations of troponins suggesting that most of these individuals indeed had acute myocardial infarction. *From* Wilson SR, Sabatine MS, Braunwald E, Sloan S, Murphy SA, Morrow DA. Detection of myocardial injury in patients with unstable angina using a novel nanoparticle cardiac troponin I assay: observations from the PROTECT-TIMI 30 Trial. *Am Heart J.* 2009;158:386-91, with permission.

AMI excluded with these hpscTn assays will be achievable. Studies documenting the benefit of this approach used insensitive assays and have not been repeated, but are now a part of the chest pain guidelines.[38] It may be that the incremental value of stress evaluation will not be present with the more sensitive contemporary assays or with hpscTn assays.

The tension that will exist in this area is one that clinicians already are struggling to deal with. The increased sensitivity of the hpscTn assays will inevitably give rise to an increased number of chronic elevations and more acute elevations not due to acute ischemic heart disease as well. Some of those chronic elevations will be in patients with known and putatively stable coronary artery disease. It is already appreciated that many patients with chronic stable angina have elevations in cTn with contemporary assays.[39,40] The subset with such elevations is at an increased risk for subsequent events (Figure 5-5). A recent investigation using an hpscTnI assay was unable to discern diagnostic or prognostic effects in patients undergoing elective angiography for "stable disease,"[41] but it is likely that the number of elevations seen in this group will be better marked with more sensitive assays. This group could be a difficult one since hpscTn values may be elevated but a distinction should be

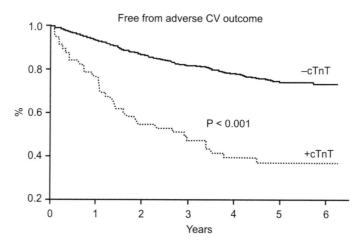

Figure 5-5 Effects of increases in cardiac troponin T using a conventional assay in the heart and sole study. *From* Hsieh BP, Rogers AM, Na B, Wu AH, Schiller NB, Whooley MA. Prevalence and prognostic significance of incidental cardiac troponin T elevation in ambulatory patients with stable coronary artery disease: data from the Heart and Soul study. *Am Heart J.* 2009;158:673-9, with permission.

possible since these values are likely to be stable despite severe disease. However, when these patients have symptoms, it will be difficult not to treat them as having an ACS and recent correlation data in this group point toward the idea that perhaps these patients have troponin values that may rise and fall intermittently.[42] Perhaps then it is correct to consider these patients as having MIs and perhaps this also is the group of putatively stable patients who crossed over in the Courage trial. However, that is a hypothesis at present and not a fact and we are already in an era where the profession is being criticized for too many invasive interventions. This is only one of the multiple challenges in this arena.

In addition, recent data indicate that at least with some assays that have adequate precision at very low values, that what is presently called ischemia during stress testing is associated with tiny increases in hpscTnI values (Figure 5-6) albeit within the normal range.[43] The increases are tiny and thus require high precision to distinguish them from noise which may be why a study using the hpscTnT assay could not recapitulate the findings.[44] If this preliminary experience is confirmed it may be necessary to distinguish such patients from patients who are unstable since it may be that this group requires different therapy from those with ACS. This is an area where additional data are needed. Some would argue that eventually the definition of unstable disease may require rising hpscTn values without an elevation above the 99th percentile URL. However, for now such a value is likely to still be necessary. The other side of this coin is that some patients who have elevations might have significant coronary artery disease but not necessarily unstable disease.

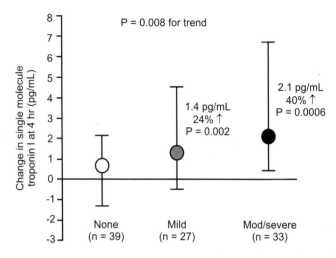

Figure 5-6 Changes in high sensitivity cardiac troponin or hpscTn troponin in patients with positive stress tests. Note the clear rises in patients who had significant stress test abnormalities compared to those who had none. *From* Sabatine MS, Morrow DA, de Lemos JA, Jarolim P, Braunwald E. Detection of acute changes in circulating troponin in the setting of transient stress test-induced myocardial ischaemia using an ultrasensitive assay: results from TIMI 35. *Eur Heart J*. 2009;30:162-9, with permission.

Data to answer these challenges are not totally defined at present and are frequently obfuscated by a literature looking to validate testing of one sort or another and who thus make blanket categorizations of patients that may obfuscate these important issues.[6] It is only with time that data will be developed to answer these critical questions and this is one reason why many of us have advocated the slow approval of these hpscTn assays until we have better information.[45]

In this author's opinion, when we know how to use high sensitivity assays, it is very likely that the diagnosis of MI will be made predicated on a significant change from prior values or a baseline even if they do not exceed the 99th percentile URL. We know even now that values well below that 99th percentile are associated with an increased proclivity to events (Figure 5-7).[46-50] It also it is very likely in this author's opinion that patients will only be considered to be unstable when they have a rising pattern of troponin assuming timing is appropriate. Cut off values will only be necessary for those whose timing is not ideal and must be managed with clinical judgment.

TYPE 1 VERSUS TYPE 2 MI

The most recent guideline defines at least two types of myocardial infarction. The one that receives most of the focus is the one associated with acute plaque rupture. This often is associated with usually ST-T wave changes, substantial elevations in

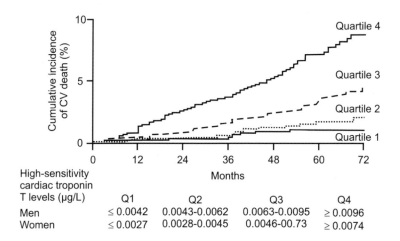

High-sensitivity cardiac troponin T levels (µg/L)	Q1	Q2	Q3	Q4
Men	≤ 0.0042	0.0043-0.0062	0.0063-0.0095	≥ 0.0096
Women	≤ 0.0027	0.0028-0.0045	0.0046-00.73	≥ 0.0074

Figure 5-7 Prognostic effects of values of hpscTn in patients with stable coronary disease are at high risk for coronary disease. Please note that only 11% of these values were above the 99th percentile but note the progressive prognostic effect even for higher values within the normal range. *From* Omland T, de Lemos JA, Sabatine MS, Christophi CA, Rice MM, Jablonski KA, et al. Prevention of events with angiotensin converting enzyme inhibition (PEACE) trial investigators. A sensitive cardiac troponin T assay in stable coronary artery disease. *N Engl J Med.* 2009;361:2538-47, with permission.

troponin, and most studies suggest that those individuals benefit from an invasive strategy, IIB/IIIA glycoprotein antiplatelet agents and an early invasive strategy.[51] However, there are other patients who have a different type of MI, a so called type 2 MI where fixed coronary disease is present or where endothelial dysfunction is present or when microvascular disease is present who may have a rising pattern of troponin elevations.[19] It is thought that the troponin levels in these types of patients may be less markedly elevated.[52] With hpscTn assays, the percentage of these patients in the overall world of patients with AMI may increase substantially but some of these patients may not need acute anticoagulation and early intervention. Those with fixed coronary disease may only require treatment of the underlying exacerbating condition. Those with hypertrophy with subendocardial ischemia or subtle coronary disease that by angiography does not look severe,[53] such as is common particularly in women also may not require aggressive anticoagulant regimens and/or an early invasive strategies. Recent data in those without a significant culprit lesion suggest an excellent prognosis with conservative management since intervention is not possible.[54] This group may become a larger percentage of the patients we diagnose with acute MI as the hpscTn assays come into more use. The consequence of this will be that we will need to develop metrics which are not presently available for distinguishing these different types of events, whether they are by imaging or via clinical presentation. As indicated, it appears that many of these individuals have more subtle elevations of troponin. This group of AMIs is particularly common in the postoperative surgical setting[55] and in patients who are critically ill,[56] where elevations in troponin are commonly seen in association with severe illness.[57-59] These patients need to be distinguished from those with plaque rupture since they probably need different types of therapy. However, this group needs to be distinguished in this author's opinion from patients who have normal coronary anatomy and physiology who may have increased oxygen requirements such as extreme tachycardia in young individuals. These patients may have elevations in troponin due to supply demand imbalance in the absence of coronary heart disease.[60] This author would argue such patients should not be diagnosed with acute MI. Again the criteria to use to make the distinctions necessary to define this group are unclear at present and guidelines need to be developed. This will be a critical issue in regard to hpscTn asays.

NONISCHEMIC ELEVATIONS IN TROPONINS

Just as chronic ischemic heart disease can cause elevations in troponin, it is now clear that a variety of other chronic and acute cardiovascular pathologies can cause elevations as well.[61] This is because in addition to acute ischemia, other stimuli are also capable of causing damage to cardiomyocytes. For example, acute left ventricular stretch is known to proteolyze and cause release of cTnI and it is thought that the cells die due to apoptosis.[62] Similarly, integrin stimulation has been shown to act via similar mechanisms.[63] These other mechanisms are additive to those that are well established with ischemic heart disease. Direct cardiac toxicity due to catecholamines and other drugs can also occur.[64] Since all these mechanisms can cause cTn elevations, clinicians often have difficulties distinguishing these pathophysiologies from those associated with acute ischemic heart disease often leading to unnecessary procedures to clarify the issue. This problem will increase with the hpscTn assays.

Some of these elevations will be acute. For example, it is known that a substantial number of patients with acute illness have cTn elevations and those elevations are prognostic of both short- and long-term outcomes.[57-59] These elevations will become still more common. Whether they will help in defining prognosis still better is unclear. Some of these elevations will be due to supply/demand abnormalities associated with hypotension or hypertension or tachycardia and the like, some will be due to the toxic effect of catecholamines and/or pressor agents or circulating cytokines elaborated during sepsis, reflex changes from the central nervous system, and a variety of other stimuli. Many of these situations will manifest increases that occur acutely. We therefore need to build a better understanding of how to distinguish these sorts of elevations from those associated with plaque rupture and acute myocardial infarction. It may actually be helpful to recognize that many of the elevations even if one thinks they are due to ischemic heart disease can be due to supply/demand imbalance in the absence of an acute coronary event. Thus, fixed coronary artery disease and tachycardia may be responsible in some patients or endothelial dysfunction in others.[53-56] As such, these patients may not necessitate coronary angiography and cardiac intervention. However, the ability to distinguish these two entities will be challenging and it is likely that some patients in each of these groups will have plaque rupture events. There are very few data to clarify these issues but such data will be desperately necessary. Perhaps the renal failure population where elevations in cTnT have been frequent[65] and are thought to be indicative of cardiovascular pathology and have a prognostic significance will be instructive. Recent preliminary data in this subset of patients utilizing the hpscTnT assay suggest that if one follows patients serially then almost every patient on dialysis will have an elevation at some point in time.[66] Whether there are key points in time at which to intervene to reduce morbidity or mortality is unclear but these sorts of findings will obviously further complicate an already complex arena.

One of the areas that may be unmasked in a beneficial way that will help clinicians has to do with cardiovascular drug toxicities. It has already clearly been shown that one can monitor Adriamycin cardiotoxicity with cTn and use it as a way of identifying patients at risk.[64] Once identified it appears that treatment with ACE inhibitors has substantial beneficial effects.[64] A similar ability to monitor toxicity has been shown of late with Herceptin.[67] This is an area that is likely to be facilitated with hpscTn assays. It is conceivable that in the long run finding drugs that are apt to be associated with cardiovascular comorbidities will be something that can be probed utilizing hpscTn assays even during experimental observations when the drugs are being initially developed or during phase 1 or phase 2 trials. This is an area in which the pharmaceutical industry is intensely interested in and which provides a real opportunity for improvement in the detection of drug toxicities.[68]

Finally, there will be more interest and better information about the effects of low levels of cTn that are elaborated during exercise.[69] This is a very controversial area. It appears that such elevations are common and not associated with short-term events.[70] On the other hand, whether there are long-term consequences is something that has not been adequately studied. Recent data suggest that there is, in exercisers, an inducible cardiomyopathy similar to arrhythmogenic right ventricular dysplasia that can occur in well-trained exercise individuals.[71,72] Whether this is the consequence of marked exercise and can be monitored by increases in hpscTn is unclear but it may well turn out that when we have more sensitive assays we will be able to probe this area. It could turn out that some degree of cardiac damage perhaps with a component of repair that we do not appreciate at the present time could occur with all exercise. This is exactly the case with skeletal muscle. If so, it is incumbent on us to figure out when these changes transition from being benign to potentially deleterious. It may also be that we will confirm once we have sufficiently sensitive assays whether or not the speculation the cTn can be released in the absence of overt cardiac injury is correct. This has been hypothesized for some time.[63,73,74] hpscTn assays should allow us to answer that question. It has been thought that the rapid return of values to baseline 24 hours after exercise is indicative of reversible injury since this release comes from a pool that is less tightly structurally bound. It is then argued that since elevations do not persist, they are likely due to this pool and thus reversible injury. hpscTn assays should for the first time allow us to answer this question, albeit indirectly by having very sensitive baseline values and being able to track changes sensitively over longer-term after the exercise episode.

TROPONIN ELEVATIONS IN CHRONIC CARDIOVASCULAR DISEASE

One of the hypotheses that has been expressed over time is that once there are adequately sensitivity of troponin measurements that it was quite likely that one could begin to monitor more chronic disease processes with them. Indeed this researcher has opined frequently that structural comorbidities are often associated with increases in troponin.[75] This has been shown even with conventional assays elevations in cardiac troponin where increase in values are found in association with heart failure, left ventricular hypertrophy, diabetes, and renal dysfunction in a subset of little less than 1% of the population.[76] Recent data looking at larger cohorts suggest hpscTn assays have the ability to detect comorbidities that are subtle and

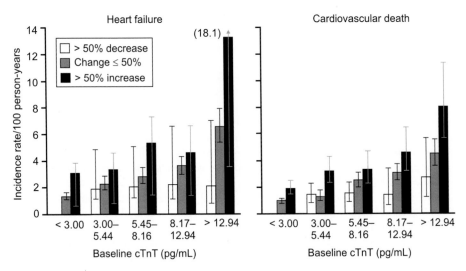

Figure 5-8 Prognostic changes in an older age population in the development of heart failure predicated on the change in cardiac troponin hpscTn over time. *From* deFilippi CR, de Lemos JA, Christenson RH, Gottdiener JS, Kop WJ, Zhan M, et al. Association of serial measures of cardiac troponin T using a sensitive assay with incident heart failure and cardiovascular mortality in older adults. *JAMA*. 2010;304:2494-502, with permission.

unrecognized and that even values are well below the punitive 99th percentile define patients who were at risk for the eventual development of cardiovascular disease.[46-50] For example, in the PEACE trial,[47] patients with higher cardiac troponins even if not formally elevated (below the 99th percentile value) had a markedly increased event rate over time compared to those with lower values. Eleven plus percent of the population had elevations above the 99th percentile and that group had the most adverse prognosis even lower values were associated with long-term adverse findings. These findings and the recent data from de Lemos[48] and Defilippi[49] and from the ARIC trial[50] in patients who initially were deemed to be punitively normal suggest strongly that the paradigm that may exist in the future may be one where one monitors troponins over time and when changes are observed, evaluates patients for progression of cardiovascular comorbidities. This was demonstrated most elegantly by the findings that increases in hpscTn over a four-year period[49] identified a group that was at substantially higher risk than those who simply had elevations at one point in time that remained stable (Figure 5-8).

How far one will be able to take this approach and whether this can be used to all cardiovascular comorbidities, is unclear but it is clearly the next major frontier and the future is now.

REFERENCES

1. Jaffe AS. The 10 commandments of troponin, with special reference to high sensitivity assays. *Heart.* 2011;97:940-6.
2. Thygesen K, Johannes M, Katus H, Plebani M, Venge P, Collinson P, et al. The Study Group on Biomarkers in Cardiology of the ESC Working Group on Acute Cardiac Care Recommendations for the use of cardiac troponin measurement in acute cardiac care. *EHJ.* 2010;31:2197-204.
3. Panteghini M, Pagani F, Yeo KT, Apple FS, Christenson RH, Dati F, et al. Evaluation of imprecision for cardiac troponin assays at low-range concentrations. *Clin Chem.* 2004;50:327-32.
4. Panteghini M, Bunk DM, Christenson RH, Katrukha A, Porter RA, Schimmel H, et al. IFCC Working Group on Standardization of Troponin I. Standardization of troponin I measurements: an update. *Clin Chem Lab Med.* 2008;46:1501-6.
5. Apple FS. A new season for cardiac troponin assays: it's time to keep a scorecard. *Clin Chem.* 2009;55:1303-6.
6. Reichlin T, Hochholzer W, Bassetti S, Steuer S, Stelzig C, Hartwiger S, et al. Early diagnosis of myocardial infarction with sensitive cardiac troponin assays. *N Engl J Med.* 2009;361:858-67.
7. Aldous SJ, Florkowski CM, Crozier IG, Elliott J, Geoarge P, Lainchbury JG, et al. Comparison of high sensitivity and contemporary troponin assays for the early detection of acute myocardial infarction in the emergency department. *Ann Clin Biochem.* 2011; 48:241-8.
8. Snyder A, Rogers MW, King MS, Phillips JC, Chapman JF, Hammett-Stabler CA. The impact of hemolysis on Ortho-Clinical Diagnostic's ECi and Roche's elecsys immunoassay systems. *Clin Chim Acta.* 2008;348:181-7.

9. Bais R. The effect of sample hemolysis on cardiac troponin I and T assays. *Clin Chem.* 2010;56:1357-9.

10. Fernandes CMB, Walker R, Price A, Marsden J, Haley L. Root cause analysis of laboratory delays to an emergency department. *J Emerg Med.* 1997;15:735-9.

11. Ladenson JH. Nonanalytical sources of variation in clinical chemistry results. In: Sonnewirth AC, Jarett L, editors. Gradwohl's Clinical Laboratory Methods and Diagnosis. 8th ed. St. Louis: Mosby Co; 1980. p. 149-92.

12. Eriksson S, Hellman J, Pettersson K. Autoantibodies against cardiac troponins. *N Engl J Med.* 2005;352:98-100.

13. Adamczyk M, Brashear RJ, Mattingly PG. Prevalence of Autoantibodies to Cardiac Troponin T in Healthy Blood Donors. *Clin Chem.* 2009;55:1592-3.

14. Apple FS, Jesse RL, Newby LK, Wu AH, Christenson RH. National Academy of Clinical Biochemistry. IFCC Committee for Standardization of Markers of Cardiac Damage. National Academy of Clinical Biochemistry and IFCC Committee for Standardization of Markers of Cardiac Damage Laboratory Medicine Practice Guidelines: Analytical issues for biochemical markers of acute coronary syndromes. *Circulation.* 2007;115:e352-5.

15. Legendre-Bazydlo LA, Haverstick DM, Kennedy JL, Dent JM, Bruns DE. Persistent increase of cardiac troponin I in plasma without evidence of cardiac injury. *Clin Chem.* 2010;56:702-5.

16. Messner B, Baum H, Fischer P, Quasthoff S, Neumeier D. Expression of Messenger RNA of the Cardiac Isoforms of Troponin T and I in Myopathic Skeletal Muscle. *AJCP.* 2000;114:544-9.

17. Ricchiuti V, Apple FS. RNA Expression of Cardiac Troponin T Isoforms in Diseased Human Skeletal Muscle. *Clin Chem.* 1999;45:2129-35.

18. Haller C, Zehelein J, Remppis A, Muller-Bardorff M, Katus HA. Cardiac troponin T in patients with end-stage renal disease: absence of expression in truncal skeletal muscle. *Clin Chem.* 1998;44:930-8.

19. Thygesen K, Alpert JS, White HD: Joint ESC/ACCF/AHA/WHF Task Force for the Redefinition of Myocardial Infarction. Universal definition of myocardial infarction. *Eur Heart J.* 2007;28:2525-2538; *Circulation.* 2007;116:2634-53; *J Am Coll Cardiol.* 2007;50: 2173-95.

20. Culic V, Eterivuc D, Miric D, Silic N. Symptom presentation of acute myocardial infarction: influence of gender, age and risk factors. *Am Heart J.* 2002;144:1012-7.

21. Hess EP, Perry JJ, Calder LA, Thiruganasambandamoorthy V, Body R, Jaffe AS, et al. Prospective validation of a modified thrombolysis in myocardial infarction risk score in emergency department patients with chest pain and possible acute coronary syndrome. *Acad Emerg Med.* 2010;17:368-75.

22. Wu AH, Lu QA, Todd J, Moecks J, Wians F. Short- and long-term biological variation in cardiac troponin I measured with a high-sensitivity assay: implications for clinical practice. *Clin Chem.* 2009;55:52-8.

23. Vasile VC, Saenger AK, Kroning JM, Klee GG, Jaffe AS. Biologic variation of a novel cardiac troponin I assay. *Clin Chem.* 2011;57:1080-1.

24. Vasile VC, Saenger AK, Kroning JM, Jaffe AS. Biological and Analytical Variability of a Novel High-Sensitivity Cardiac Troponin T Assay. *Clin Chem.* 2010;56:1086-90.

25. Frankenstein L, Wu AHB, Hallermayer K, Wians FH Jr, Giannitsis E, Katus HA. Biological variation and reference change value of high-sensitivity troponin T in healthy individuals during short and intermediate follow-up periods. *Clin Chem.* 2011;57:1068-71.

26. Giannitsis E, Becker M, Kurz K, Hess G, Zdunek D, Katus HA. High-sensitivity cardiac troponin T for early prediction of evolving non-ST-segment elevation myocardial

infarction in patients with suspected acute coronary syndrome and negative troponin results on admission. *Clin Chem.* 2010;56:642-50.

27. Saenger AK, Korpi-Steiner NL, Bryant SC, Karon BS, Jaffe AS. Utilization of a high sensitive troponin T assay optimizes serial sampling in the diagnosis of acute myocardial infarction compared to multiple contemporary troponin assays. *Circulation.* 2010;122:A21588.

28. Keller T, Zeller T, Peetz D, Tzikas S, Roth A, Czyz E, et al. Sensitive troponin I assay in early diagnosis of acute myocardial infarction. *N Engl J Med.* 2009;361:868-77.

29. Wilson SR, Sabatine MS, Braunwald E, Sloan S, Murphy SA, Morrow DA. Detection of myocardial injury in patients with unstable angina using a novel nanoparticle cardiac troponin I assay: observations from the PROTECT-TIMI 30 Trial. *Am Heart J.* 2009;158:386-91.

30. Peter A. Kavsak, Xuesong Wang, Dennis T. Ko, Andrew R. MacRae, and Allan S. Jaffe. Short- and Long-Term Risk Stratification Using a Next-Generation, High-Sensitivity Research Cardiac Troponin I (hs-cTnI) Assay in an Emergency Department Chest Pain Population. *Clin Chem.* 2009;55:1809-15.

31. Apple FS, Simpson PA, Murakami MM. Defining the serum 99th percentile in a normal reference population measured by a high-sensitivity cardiac troponin I assay. *Clin Biochem.* 2010;43:1034-6.

32. Giannitsis E, Kurz K, Hallermayer K, Jarausch J, Jaffe AS, Katus HA. Analytical validation of a high-sensitivity cardiac troponin T assay. *Clin Chem.* 2010;56:254-61.

33. Venge P, Johnston N, Lindahl B, James S. Normal plasma levels of cardiac troponin I measured by the high-sensitivity cardiac troponin I access prototype assay and the impact on the diagnosis of myocardial ischemia. *J Am Coll Cardiol.* 2009;54:1165-72.

34. Wiviott SD, Cannon CP, Morrow DA, Murphy SA, Gibson CM, McCabe CH. Differential expression of cardiac biomarkers by gender in patients with unstable angina/non-ST-elevation myocardial infarction: a TACTICS-TIMI 18 (Treat Angina with Aggrastat and determine Cost of Therapy with an Invasive or Conservative Strategy-Thrombolysis In Myocardial Infarction 18) substudy. *Circulation.* 2004;109:580-6.

35. Martinez MW, Babuin L, Syed IS, Feng DL, Miller WL, Mathew V, et al. Myocardial infarction with normal coronary arteries: a role for MRI? *Clin Chem.* 2007;53:995-6.

36. Assomull RG, Lyne JC, Keenan N, Gulati A, Bunce NH, Davies SW, et al. The role of cardiovascular magnetic resonance in patients presenting with chest pain, raised troponin, and unobstructed coronary arteries. *Eur Heart J.* 2007;28:1242-9.

37. Body R, Carley S, McDowell G, Wibberley C, Nuttall M, France M, et al. Use of low level high sensitivity troponin to rule out acute myocardial infarction in the Emergency Department. JACC in press.

38. Amsterdam EA, Kirk JD, Bluemke DA, Diercks D, Farkouh ME, Garvey JL, et al. American Heart Association Exercise, Cardiac Rehabilitation, and Prevention Committee of the Council on Clinical Cardiology, Council on Cardiovascular Nursing, and Interdisciplinary Council on Quality of Care and Outcomes Research. Testing of low-risk patients presenting to the emergency department with chest pain: a scientific statement from the American Heart Association. [Review][Erratum appears in *Circulation.* 2010;122:e500-1] *Circulation.* 2010;122:1756-76.

39. Hsieh BP, Rogers AM, Na B, Wu AH, Schiller NB, Whooley MA. Prevalence and prognostic significance of incidental cardiac troponin T elevation in ambulatory patients with stable coronary artery disease: data from the Heart and Soul study. *Am Heart J.* 2009;158:673-9.

40. Jeremias A, Kleiman NS, Nassif D, Hsieh WH, Pencina M, Maresh K, et al. Evaluation of Drug Eluting Stents and Ischemic Events (EVENT) Registry Investigators. Prevalence

and prognostic significance of preprocedural cardiac troponin elevation among patients with stable coronary artery disease undergoing percutaneous coronary intervention: results from the evaluation of drug eluting stents and ischemic events registry. *Circulation.* 2008;118:632-8.

41. Schulz O, Reinicke M, Berghoefer GH, Bensch R, Kraemer IS, Jaffe AS. High-sensitive cardiac troponin I (hs-cTnI) values in patients with stable cardiovascular disease: An initial foray. *Clin Chim Acta.* 2010;411:812-7.

42. Korosoglou G, Lehrke S, Mueller D, Hosch W, Kauczor HU, Humpert PM, et al. Determinants of troponin release in patients with stable coronary artery disease: insights from CT angiography characteristics of atherosclerotic plaque. *Heart.* 2011;97:823-31.

43. Sabatine MS, Morrow DA, de Lemos JA, Jarolim P, Braunwald E. Detection of acute changes in circulating troponin in the setting of transient stress test-induced myocardial ischaemia using an ultrasensitive assay: results from TIMI 35. *Eur Heart J.* 2009;30:162-9.

44. Kurz K, Giannitsis E, Zehelein J, Katus HA. Highly sensitive cardiac troponin T values remain constant after brief exercise- or pharmacologic-induced reversible myocardial ischemia. *Clin Chem.* 2008;54:1234-8.

45. Katus HA, Giannitsis E, Jaffe AS, Thygesen K. Higher sensitivity troponin assays: Quo vadis? *Eur Heart J.* 2009;30:127-8.

46. Latini R, Masson S, Anand IS, Missov E, Carlson M, Vago T, et al. Val-HeFT Investigators. Prognostic value of very low plasma concentrations of troponin T in patients with stable chronic heart failure. *Circulation.* 2007;116:1242-9.

47. Omland T, de Lemos JA, Sabatine MS, Christophi CA, Rice MM, Jablonski KA, et al. Prevention of events with angiotensin converting enzyme inhibition (PEACE) trial investigators. A sensitive cardiac troponin T assay in stable coronary artery disease. *N Engl J Med.* 2009;361:2538-47.

48. de Lemos JA, Drazner MH, Omland T, Ayers CR, Khera A, Rohatgi A, et al. Association of troponin T detected with a highly sensitive assay and cardiac structure and mortality risk in the general population. *JAMA.* 2010;304:2503-12.

49. deFilippi CR, de Lemos JA, Christenson RH, Gottdiener JS, Kop WJ, Zhan M, et al. Association of serial measures of cardiac troponin T using a sensitive assay with incident heart failure and cardiovascular mortality in older adults. *JAMA.* 2010;304:2494-502.

50. Saunders JT, Nambi V, de Limos JA, Chambless LE, Virani SS, Boerwinkle E, et al. Cardiac troponin T measured by a highly sensitive assay predicts coronary heart disease, heart failure, and mortality in the atherosclerosis risk in communities study. *Circulation.* 2011;123:1367-76.

51. Anderson JL, Adams CD, Antman EM, Bridges CR, Califf RM, Casey DE Jr, et al. ACC/AHA 2007 guidelines for the management of patients with unstable angina/non ST-elevation myocardial infarction: a report of the American College of Cardiology/American Heart Association Task Force on Practice Guidelines. *Circulation.* 2007;116:e148-304.

52. Wu AH, Jaffe AS. The clinical need for high-sensitivity cardiac troponin assays for acute coronary syndromes and the role for serial testing. *Am Heart J.* 2008;155:208-14.

53. Ong P, Athanasiadis A, Hill S, Vogelsberg H, Voehringer M, Sechtem U. Coronary artery spasm as a frequent cause of acute coronary syndrome: The CASPAR (Coronary Artery Spasm in Patients With Acute Coronary Syndrome) Study. *J Am Coll Cardiol.* 2008;52:523-7.

54. Ong P, Athanasiadis A, Borgulya G, Voehringer M, Sechtem U. 3-year follow-up of patients with coronary artery spasm as cause of acute coronary syndrome: the CASPAR (coronary artery spasm in patients with acute coronary syndrome) study follow-up. *J Am Coll Cardiol.* 2011;57:147-52.

55. Landesberg G, Beattie S, Mosseri M, Jaffe AS, Alpert JS. Perioperative myocardial infarction. *Circulation.* 2009;119:2936-44.

56. Landesberg G, Vesselov Y, Einav S, Goodman S, Sprung CL, Weissman C. Myocardial ischemia, cardiac troponin, and long-term survival of high-cardiac risk critically ill intensive care unit patients. *Crit Care Med.* 2005;33:1281-7.

57. Babuin L, Vasile VC, Rio Perez JA, Alegria JR, Chai HS, Afessa B, et al. Elevated cardiac troponin is an independent risk factor for short- and long-term mortality in medical intensive care unit patients. *Crit Care Med.* 2008;36:759-65.

58. Vasile VC, Babuin L, Rio Perez JA, Alegria JR, Song LM, Chai HS, et al. Long-term prognostic significance of elevated cardiac troponin levels in critically ill patients with acute gastrointestinal bleeding. *Crit Care Med.* 2009;37:140-7.

59. Vasile VC, Chai HS, Khambatta S, Afessa B, Jaffe AS. Significance of elevated cardiac troponin T levels in critically ill patients with acute respiratory disease. *Am J Med.* 2010;123:1049-58.

60. Bukkapatnam RN, Robinson M, Turnipseed S, Tancredi D, Amsterdam E, Srivatsa UN. Relationship of myocardial ischemia and injury to coronary artery disease in patients with supraventricular tachycardia. *Am J Cardiol.* 2010;106:374-7.

61. Jaffe AS, Babuin L, Apple FS. Biomarkers in acute cardiac disease: the present and the future. *J Am Coll Cardiol.* 2006;48:1-11.

62. Feng J, Schaus BJ, Fallavollita JA, Lee TC, Canty JM Jr. Preload induces troponin I degradation independently of myocardial ischemia. *Circulation.* 2001;103:2035-7.

63. Hessel MH, Atsma DE, van der Valk EJ, Bax WH, Schalij MJ, van der Laarse A. Release of cardiac troponin I from viable cardiomyocytes is mediated by integrin stimulation. *Pflugers Arch.* 2008;455:979-86.

64. Cardinale D, Colombo A, Sandri MT, Lamantia G, Colombo N, Civelli M, et al. Prevention of high-dose chemotherapy-induced cardiotoxicity in high-risk patients by angiotensin-converting enzyme inhibition. *Circulation.* 2006;114:2474-81.

65. Apple FS, Murakami MM, Pearce LA, Herzog CA. Predictive value of cardiac troponin I and T for subsequent death in end-stage renal disease. *Circulation.* 2002;106:2941-5.

66. Jacobs LH, van de Kerkhof J, Mingels AM, Kleijnen VW, van der Sande FM, Wodzig WK, et al. Haemodialysis patients longitudinally assessed by highly sensitive cardiac troponin T and commercial cardiac troponin T and cardiac troponin I assays. *Ann Clin Biochem.* 2009;46:283-90.

67. Cardinale D, Colombo A, Torrisi R, Sandri MT, Civelli M, Salvatici M, et al. Trastuzumab-induced cardiotoxicity: clinical and prognostic implications of troponin I evaluation. *J Clin Oncol.* 2010;28:3910-6.

68. Berridge BR, Pettit S, Walker DB, Jaffe AS, Schultze AE, Herman E, et al. A translational approach to detecting drug-induced cardiac injury with cardiac troponins: consensus and recommendations from the cardiac troponins biomarker working group of the health and environmental sciences institute. *Am Heart J.* 2009;158:21-9.

69. Giannitsis E, Roth HJ, Leithauser RM, Scherhag J, Beneke R, Katus HA. New highly sensitive assay used to measure cardiac troponin T concentration changes during a continuous 216-km marathon. *Clin Chem.* 2009;55:590-2.

70. Shave R, Baggish A, George K, Wood M, Scharhag J, Whyte G, et al. Exercise-induced cardiac troponin elevation: evidence, mechanisms, and implications. *J Am Coll Cardiol.* 2010;56:169-76.

71. Heidbüchel H, Hoogsteen J, Fagard R, Vanhees L, Ector H, Willems R, et al. High prevalence of right ventricular involvement in endurance athletes with ventricular

arrhythmias: Role of an electrophysiologic study in risk stratification. *Eur Heart J.* 2003;24:1473-80.

72. Ector J, Ganame J, van der Merwe N, Adriaenssens B, Pison L, Willems R, et al. Reduced right ventricular ejection fraction in endurance athletes presenting with ventricular arrhythmias: a quantitative angiographic assessment. *Eur Heart J.* 2007;28:345-53.

73. Wu AH, Ford L. Release of cardiac troponin in acute coronary syndromes: ischemia or necrosis? *Clin Chim Acta.* 1999;284:161-74.

74. Hickman PE, Potter JM, Aroney C, Koerbin G, Southcott E, Wu AH, et al. Cardiac troponin may be released by ischemia alone, without necrosis. *Clin Chim Acta.* 2010;411:318-23.

75. Jaffe AS. Chasing troponin: how low can you go if you can see the rise? *JACC.* 2006;48: 1763-4.

76. Wallace T, Abdullah S, Drazner M, Das SR, Khera A, McGuire DK, et al. Prevalence and determinants of troponin T elevation in the general population. *Circulation.* 2006;113:1958-65.

6 Evolving Biomarkers for Cardiac Ischemia

Payal Kohli, David A Morrow

INTRODUCTION

Myocardial ischemia is heterogeneous in its clinical presentation and thus is often challenging to recognize. Because of its morbid complications and progressive nature, early diagnosis, risk stratification, and targeted therapy are the focus of contemporary management of ischemic heart disease.[1] These tasks consume a substantial amount of professional and healthcare resources each year. For these reasons, clinicians and researchers remain intensely interested in finding new tools to improve the efficiency, speed, and accuracy of assessing signs and symptoms concerning for myocardial ischemia.

PATHOBIOLOGY OF ISCHEMIA

Myocardial oxygen delivery is closely coupled to coronary blood flow. As such, sudden cessation of perfusion, such as resulting from coronary thrombosis, very quickly leads to anaerobic metabolism, depletion of ATP, and accumulation of catabolites. Following ATP depletion, there is an efflux of potassium into the extracellular space, sarcolemmal damage, and cell swelling. With depletion of ATP, both myocardial relaxation and contraction are impaired as a very early consequence of the ischemic cascade (Figure 6-1). The injury is amplified by entry of leukocytes into the affected area, especially after reperfusion. The onset of irreversible cell damage depends upon the location of the occlusion, the degree of residual flow, and the rate of oxygen consumption, and usually begins within 20 minutes of the occlusion. Occlusion shorter than 20 minutes does not typically cause myocardial necrosis that is detectable via cellular changes visible on electron microscopy but can cause myocardial dysfunction. Evolution of electrocardiographic changes of ischemia is relatively late in onset within this sequence of events.

Over time, the wavefront of infarction travels from the subendocardium to the subepicardium. Within one hour of the occlusion, the subendocardium is irreversibly injured and within four to six hours, a transmural infarction has typically completed.[2] This cascade of events presents multiple opportunities to detect the

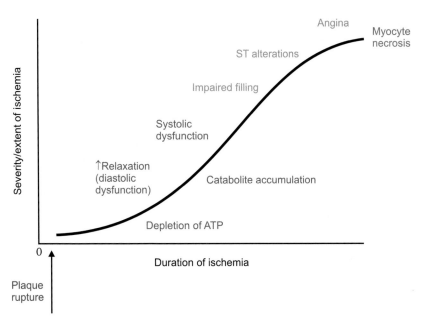

Figure 6-1 Pathobiological and clinical evolution of ischemia. *Adapted from* Cohn PF, Fox KM, Daly C. Silent myocardial ischemia. *Circulation.* 2003;108:1263-77.

onset of ischemia from the point of plaque disruption, early metabolic changes, and hemodynamic stress that precede irreversible cellular injury.

CANDIDATE BIOMARKERS

When used in conjunction with the clinical history, physical examination, ECG, and cardiac imaging, cardiac biomarkers are invaluable tools for diagnostic and prognostic assessment of patients presenting with chest symptoms. The underlying pathobiology of ischemia described in the previous section points towards a varied array of potential candidate biomarkers that may be useful for this assessment. In particular, this list includes several candidate markers which may permit the detection of ischemia before the onset of irreversible injury is occurred. These biomarkers can be broadly categorized into markers of inflammation/plaque rupture, markers of metabolic stress, markers of hemodynamic perturbation, or markers of tissue injury or necrosis (Table 6-1). Only some of these biomarkers are specific to ischemia *per se*, but they nevertheless may permit detection of processes contributing to ischemia.

The challenges for developing a new biomarker to the point of routine use in clinical practice are stiff (Table 6-2). The majority of candidate markers that are investigated will never enter clinical practice. In this chapter, we will focus on selected biomarkers that have attracted interest, because of their potential

Table 6-1	Candidate Biomarkers	
	Description	*Additional details*
	Markers of plaque vulnerability or rupture	
High-sensitivity CRP (hs-CRP)	Acute phase protein produced by hepatocytes	Binds LDL, allowing it to be taken up by macrophages Induces cytokine/chemokine release, adhesion molecule expression
Myeloperoxidase (MPO)	Released by activated neutrophils and macrophages; concentrated in culprit lesions	Oxidizes lipids Depletes NO, leading to dysregulation of coronary blood flow
Pregnancy-associated plasma protein A (PAPP-A)	Present in human fibroblasts and released during atherosclerotic plaque rupture	IGF-like IGF-binding protein-4 metalloproteinase
Matrix metalloproteinase-9 (MMP-9)	Found in most tissues but localized in shoulder of a plaque, leads to thin fibrous cap	Regulates ECM and participates in vascular remodeling Leads to plaque instability Involved in ventricular remodeling
Soluble CD40 ligand (sCD40L)	Released from activated platelets and interacts with inflammatory cells to destabilize plaques	Stimulates release of chemokines and cytokines Induces release of metalloproteinases from inflammatory cells
Placental growth factor (PIGF)	Platelet-derived protein involved in initiation of inflammatory process and atheroma formation	Chemoattractant for monocytes, up-regulated chemokines Regulation of vascular endothelial growth and stimulation of smooth muscle
Growth differentiation factor 15 (GDF-15)	Transforming growth factor-β family member; secreted by cardiomyocytes in setting of ischemia and reperfusion	Regulation of inflammatory and apoptotic pathways for tissue repair
Choline	Released from membrane phospholipids after activation of cell receptors following plaque destabilization and ischemia	Released into plasma with secondary uptake into blood cells
SCUBE1	Protein associated with platelet-endothelial interactions; may be indicative of platelet activation during acute ischemia	Detectable as early as 6 hours after symptom onset Can remain elevated for up to 84 hours

Continued

Continued

Markers of hemodynamic stress		
Natriuretic peptides (BNP, NT-proBNP, ANP, proANP)	Released from myocardium in response to stretch; ANP released from atrium	Results in balanced vasodilation, natriuresis and inhibition of sympathetic and renin-angiotensin responses
Copeptin	C-terminal fragment of vasopressin precursor molecule; mirrors vasopressin production	Longer half-life than vasopressin
Unbound free fatty acids (FFA$_u$)	Catecholamines lead to increase in adipose lipolysis	Rises early after cardiac ischemia
Mid-regional proadrenomedullin (MR proADM)	Precursor to adrenomedullin, a vasodilator important for endothelial function; 52 amino acid peptide that is highly expressed in endothelial cells and is homologous to calcitonin gene-related peptide	Leads to an increase in cyclic AMP and results in vasodilation and hypotension, increased cardiac output and natriuresis and diuresis. More stable in blood than its precursor, adrenomedullin. Increased in heart failure and inversely related to ejection fraction
Markers of tissue ischemia/necrosis		
Creatine kinase-MB	Creatine kinase is an enzyme found in cardiac and skeletal; the MB fraction has a higher concentration in cardiac muscle	Detectable 4–6 h after symptom onset. Peaks at 24 h. Returns to baseline after 48–72 h
Troponin I or T	Regulatory proteins found in cardiac muscle, distinct from skeletal muscle troponin	Elevated within three hours of symptom onset. Remains elevated in blood for 7–10 days (Troponin I) or up to 14 days (Troponin T)
Myoglobin	Protein found in cardiac and skeletal muscle; involved in oxygen binding	Detectable in 2–4 h. Peaks at 6–12 h. Returns to normal at 24–36 h
Heart-type fatty acid binding protein (H-FABP)	Involved in intracellular uptake and buffering of free fatty acids in the myocardium	Rapidly released from the cytosol into circulation after myocardial ischemia and necrosis
Glycogen phosphorylase isoenzyme BB (GPBB)	Glycolytic enzyme that is converted to a soluble form following tissue hypoxia and glycogenolysis; diffuses out of cell	Released 2–4 h after the onset of ischemia in parallel with myoglobin

Continued

Continued

Markers of catabolism/oxidation		
Ischemia-modified albumin (IMA)	Oxidative modification of albumin in setting of ischemia alters binding of cobalt	Used with caution when albumin concentrations are < 20 g/L or > 55 g/L

hs-CRP, high-sensitivity C-reactive protein; LDL, low density lipoprotein; MPO, myeloperoxidase; NO, nitric oxide; PAPP-A, pregnancy-associated plasma protein A; IGF, insulin-like growth factor; MMP-9, matrix metalloproteinase-9; ECM, extracelluar matrix; sCD40L, soluble CD40 ligand; PIGF, placental insulin-like growth factor; GDF-15, growth differentiation factor 15; BNP, NT-proBNP, ANP, proANP, natriuretic peptides; FFA$_u$, unbound free fatty acids; MR proADM, mid-regional proadrenomedullin; H-FABP, heart-type fatty acid binding protein; GPBB, glycogen phosphorylase isoenzyme BB; IMA, ischemia-modified albumin.

Table 6-2   Challenges with Adapting a New Marker into Routine Clinical Use

Sample collection

Assays are not always commercially available and non-standardized

Collection method, type of sample (blood, serum, or plasma), and time of collection can affect marker levels and results

Storage

Stability and storage options for many markers are unknown

Interpretation

Cutoff values used for interpretation are different between studies

Reference ranges are presented differently (i.e., threshold versus quartiles)

Comparison is made to older troponin assays, which are now clinically obsolete

Publishing bias favors positive over negative results, leading to an imbalanced collection of studies

Clinical validation

Clinical validation requires more than one suitably sized clinical study with well-characterized patients and adjudicated outcomes

Clinical integration is dependent on large trials demonstrating that the biomarker actually enhances clinical decision-making

---

to improve diagnosis and/or risk stratification in patients with suspected acute coronary syndromes (ACS), and that are able to serve as examples of other evolving biomarkers of ischemia. In addition, we will conclude briefly with the potential use of biomarkers during stress testing. Several biomarkers of significant interest are discussed in other chapters (sensitive assays for troponin, ST2, midregion-proadrenomedullin) and will not be presented here.

CLINICAL APPLICATIONS OF CARDIAC BIOMARKERS

Evaluation of the Patient with Suspected ACS

Cardiac troponin is the cornerstone for diagnosis and risk assessment, because of its high sensitivity and myocardial tissue specificity.[1-5] Because of a large molecular size and location within the contractile apparatus of the cardiac myocyte, there are inherent limits to the rapidity of release of troponin release, potentially diminishing its sensitivity in patients presenting early after the onset of symptoms.[6] However, the advent of more sensitive assays (see chapter 5) has enabled progressively earlier detection, and raised the possibility of identifying ischemic injury when it is reversible.[6,7] Nevertheless, the search for very early biomarkers of necrosis and ischemia has remained of high interest.

BIOMARKERS OF ISCHEMIC INJURY

Heart-type Fatty Acid Binding Protein (H-FABP)

Alongside increasing the sensitivity of assays for cardiac troponin, an alternative approach to earlier detection is to seek cellular components released earlier than troponin based on a smaller molecular size. H-FABP is a small molecule (14 kDa, compared with 21–27 kDa for troponin) involved in fatty acid transport, and contained in the cytoplasm of the cardiac myocyte.[6] H-FABP is approximately ten times more abundant in the cardiac myocyte than skeletal muscle and is released into the blood as early as 30 minutes after injury, detectable in the circulation as early as 1–3 hours, returning to baseline within 12–24 hours.[8,9] H-FABP has also been found in urine as early as 1–2 hours following an ischemic insult.[8]

Diagnosis

Several studies have suggested that H-FABP is a useful aid for diagnosis of MI and performs better than myoglobin, CK-MB, or older less sensitive troponin assays.[10-13] In a study of 264 patients with chest pain presenting for emergency evaluation, H-FABP was found to have a sensitivity of 92.9%, compared with 88.6% for myoglobin and 18.6% for CK-MB; the specificity of H-FABP was 67.3% compared with 57.1% and 98.0% for myoglobin and CK-MB, respectively.[12] The overall diagnostic accuracy of H-FABP quantified by the area under the receiver operating characteristic curve (AUC) was superior (0.921) to that for myoglobin (0.843) and CK-MB (0.654). When stratified according to time after symptom onset, H-FABP has shown an advantage over older assays for troponin for diagnosis < 4 hours after symptom-onset. When combined with troponin, H-FABP increases the positive predictive value of biomarker testing (Figure 6-2). One study suggested better accuracy of H-FABP when compared with a prior generation assay for troponin T.[13] Together, these studies have supported a potential clinical role for H-FABP, particularly for the diagnosis of patients presenting early after onset of symptoms. However, evaluation of H-FABP in conjunction with newer, sensitive troponin assays is still ongoing.

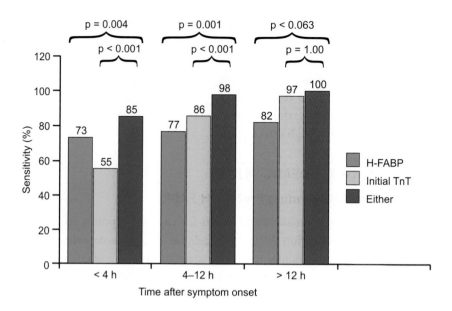

Figure 6-2 Sensitivity for the diagnosis of acute myocardial infarction of H-FABP, cardiac troponin T or elevation of either, stratified by time after symptom onset. *Adapted from* McCann CJ, Glover BM, Menown IB, Moore MJ, McEneny J, Owens CG, et al. Novel biomarkers in early diagnosis of acute myocardial infarction compared with cardiac troponin T. *Eur Heart J.* 2008;29:2843-50.

Prognosis

Similar to troponin, the concentration of H-FABP in patients with ACS is associated with the risk for major adverse cardiovascular events, including death, congestive heart failure, and recurrent myocardial infarction.[14] Moreover, in a study of 1,448 patients with ACS, H-FABP was an independent marker of risk when evaluated along with troponin and B-type natriuretic peptide (BNP). Although the troponin assay in that study was poorly sensitive, a subsequent study using a contemporary assay confirmed the independent relationship of H-FABP with mortality, including in the setting of normal troponin values.[15]

Summary

- Commercially available for clinical use in some countries in Europe and Asia
- Can be measured in whole blood, serum, citrate-plasma, EDTA-plasma, or heparin-plasma
- May be useful for diagnosis of MI very early after presentation in combination with troponin
- Appears to complement troponin for risk stratification in suspected ACS.

BIOMARKERS OF INFLAMMATION AND PLAQUE RUPTURE

Biomarkers reflecting myocardial necrosis are useful for diagnosis when myocyte destruction has already occurred. Markers that reflect the increased inflammatory state that contributes to acute plaque rupture or its vulnerability to do so have been avidly sought as potential early indicators of atherothrombosis. Of this group of markers, high sensitivity C-reactive protein (hs-CRP) is the best studied and will serve to illustrate the strengths and limitations of this group of biomarkers. In particular, although sometimes cited as biomarkers of ischemia, this group is not tied directly to ischemia but rather to causes of vascular inflammation and thus may be elevated in a variety of nonischemic settings. We will also discuss myeloperoxidase (MPO) as the first inflammatory biomarker to be specifically approved by the Food and Drug Administration (FDA) for identifying patients presenting with chest pain, who are at high risk for major adverse cardiac events. In addition, pregnancy-associated protein A (PAPP-A) will be reviewed as an example of an evolving biomarker that is a potential direct participant in the pathogenesis of ACS.

hs C-reactive Protein (hs-CRP)

The role of inflammation in atherosclerosis and plaque rupture has been well established.[16] Produced by hepatocytes in response to IL-6 and tumor necrosis factor-α, CRP is an inflammatory molecule and a nonspecific acute phase reactant. It is enriched in atherosclerotic plaques and binds to LDL, allowing LDL to be taken up into macrophages without modification.[17] Infusion in animal models leads to increases in atherosclerotic plaque area, adhesion molecule expression, coagulation, decreased nitric oxide activity and recruitment of monocytes and lymphocytes.[18,19]

Diagnosis

Although hs-CRP is associated with underlying CAD, its specificity for ACS is poor. Compared to controls, hs-CRP is elevated in patients with documented CAD and previous MI,[20] with even higher concentrations in patients with non-ST-elevation ACS.[21] However, as a nonspecific acute phase reactant, hs-CRP can be elevated in any state of inflammatory hyperresponsiveness.[22] In addition, inflammatory markers can have diurnal variation and vary with age, race, gender, and ethnicity. As an example, on the basis observed associations in a published study,[23] if one were to take a 100 hypothetical patients presenting with non-traumatic chest pain, only 9 patients with ACS would have elevated CRP, compared with 18 patients without ACS. Therefore, twice the number of patients with a positive result would have something other than ACS as the final diagnosis (positive predictive value only 33%). For this reason, hs-CRP is not recommended for use as a diagnostic marker; moreover, its performance forecasts the limitations of other inflammatory markers without any base for vascular specificity.

Prognosis

In contrast, the prognostic capacity of hs-CRP is extremely well validated. The blood concentration of hs-CRP is associated with outcomes across the entire spectrum of patients at risk for and with established ischemic heart disease.[24-36] In particular, in patients with ACS, hs-CRP identifies those at higher mortality risk independently of cardiac troponin.[31-33,36] Despite this clear association with outcomes, the incremental value of hs-CRP for clinically meaningful reclassification of risk and for directing therapy is debated. In the acute setting, there are no clear therapeutic implications and thus while use of hs-CRP is reasonable when the clinician desires additional risk information,[37,38] routine clinical application is very infrequent. Testing of hs-CRP in patients who have been stabilized post-ACS, however, may be useful for directing the intensity of statin therapy as suggested in the PROVE-IT TIMI 22 trials, where an achieved concentration of hs-CRP < 1 mg/L in ACS patients were randomized to intensive statin therapy was associated with lowest risk of recurrent events, regardless of lipid levels.[39] Although other therapies, such as aspirin, abciximab, thiazolidinediones, and beta blockers can reduce levels of CRP, it is not known whether that modification is useful for directing treatment.[40-45]

Summary

- High throughput, commercial assays are widely available
- hs-CRP is a nonspecific acute phase reactant that can be elevated in other inflammatory states and thus is not useful for diagnosis of ACS
- hs-CRP is strongly associated with short and long-term mortality after ACS that is complementary to other biomarkers
- In patients stabilized after ACS, achieved hs-CRP concentration on statin therapy is correlated with outcomes and may be useful to guide the use of intensive statin therapy.

MPO

A hallmark of atherosclerosis is the infiltration of inflammatory cells leading to a necrotic core and vulnerability of the plaque to rupture.[16] MPO is released by activated neutrophils, monocytes, and tissue macrophages and is found to be up-regulated in culprit plaques in ACS.[46-49] It is a member of the heme peroxidase superfamily and is involved in lipid peroxidation, post-translational modification of multiple target proteins and depletion of endothelium-derived nitric oxide.[48,50,51] Individuals who are completely or partially deficient in this enzyme are less likely to develop cardiovascular disease.[52-55] Conversely, those that have CAD[56] or chronic heart failure[57] are more likely to have higher levels of MPO. Furthermore, increased concentrations of this enzyme are associated with an increased risk of CAD in healthy individuals.[58]

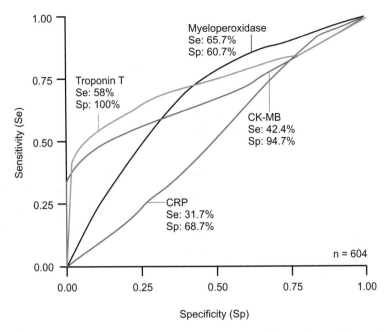

Figure 6-3 Receiver-operating-characteristic (ROC) curve analysis of biomarker performance for the diagnosis of acute coronary syndromes. Using a cutoff point for myeloperoxidase (≥ 198 pM) that was derived from the ROC curve for the entire cohort and established cutoff points for the other biologic markers, sensitivity and specificity for each marker was calculated. *Adapted from* Brennan ML, Penn MS, van Lente F, Nambi V, Shishehbor MH, Aviles RJ, et al. Prognostic value of myeloperoxidase in patients with chest pain. *N Engl J Med.* 2003;349:1595-604.

Diagnosis

It has been suggested that MPO is released prior to the sentinel event and may identify patients at increased cardiovascular risk, before vascular occlusion has occurred.[59] MPO has a superior performance to hs-CRP for diagnosis of ACS (Figure 6-3). However, when compared to established biomarkers of necrosis, such as troponin and CK-MB, MPO exhibits a trade-off between higher sensitivity and lower specificity. Using a cut-point (≥ 198 pM) for MPO derived from ROC analysis, Brennan and colleagues calculated the following values for the sensitivity, specificity, positive predictive values, and negative predictive values, respectively: MPO (65.7%, 60.7%, 53.3%, and 72.2%) versus troponin T (58.0%, 100%, 100%, and 77.7%), and CRP (31.7%, 68.7%, 40.6%, and 60.0%).[60]

Prognosis

In a study of all-comers with chest pain presenting to the emergency room, MPO concentration at presentation was associated with the risk of major adverse cardiac

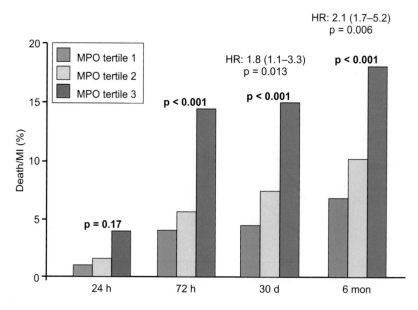

Figure 6-4 Risk of death or MI at 24 hours, 72 hours, 30 days, and 6 months, stratified by tertiles of (MPO). *p*-values shown are for differences in event rates across MPO tertiles. Multivariate cox proportional hazard-adjusted ratios for dichotomized MPO value, 95% CIs and *p*-values are also listed at 30 days and 6 months. *Data from* Baldus S, Heeschen C, Meinertz T, Zeiher AM, Eiserich JP, Munzel T, et al. Myeloperoxidase serum levels predict risk in patients with acute coronary syndromes. *Circulation.* 2003;108:1440-5.

events (MI, need for revascularization, or death) within 30 days and at 6 months, including in the subset of patients with negative troponin T results (using a high cut-point).[60] Similarly, in a cohort of 1,090 patients presenting with ACS, serum MPO levels were predictive of risk for death and MI at 6 months (Figure 6-4), including in the subgroup of patients that had troponin T levels below 0.01 µg/L.[59] On the basis of these data, MPO was approved by the FDA for risk stratification in conjunction with clinical history, ECG findings and troponin in patients presenting with chest pain.[59-62] However, clinical use has been somewhat limited[63-65] and, as for hsCRP, subsequent studies have not established a clearly meaningful reclassification of risk over troponin and a natriuretic peptide, or clear therapeutic implications.[66] Lastly, the influence of heparin on the serum concentration of MPO remains of uncertain clinical consequence, and the marker can be nonspecifically elevated in noncardiac diseases.

Summary

- High throughput commercial assays are available in the US with a clinical indication for risk stratification in patients with chest pain

- Heparin anticoagulation may increase the concentration of MPO
- Insufficient specificity as a diagnostic marker for ACS
- Independent predictor of the risk of major cardiovascular events in suspected ACS.

Pregnancy-associated Plasma Protein (PAPP-A)

PAPP-A is a promising investigational marker of risk in patients with suspected ACS. A group of metalloproteinases have been strongly implicated in disruption of vulnerable plaques via disruption of the protective fibrous cap.[67-71] PAPP-A, a zinc-binding matrix metalloproteinase, exists in high concentration during pregnancy and is diagnostic of fetal Down syndrome when elevated in maternal blood. It is also found in healthy men and women.[72-76] It is an activator of insulin-like growth factor 1 (IGF-1) and degrades insulin-like growth factor binding proteins. Secreted by fibroblasts and osteoblasts, PAPP-A is enriched in plaque cells and the extracellular matrix of ruptured and eroded unstable plaques.[75]

PAPP-A is found circulating predominantly in an inactive complexed form of two PAPP-A subunits plus two eosinophilic major basic proteins (proMBP).[77-79] Commercial assays exist for PAPP-A that can detect both the complexed PAPP-A/proMBP and the free PAPP-A fractions.[80] In ACS, the "cardiac PAPP-A" appears to exist as a homodimer and is not complexed to proMBP.

Diagnosis

PAPP-A concentration is increased in patients with unstable angina or acute MI, compared to controls and those with stable angina.[39] Evaluated as a diagnostic marker for ACS at a threshold level of 10 mIU per liter, PAPP-A was found to have a sensitivity of 89.2% and a specificity of 81.3%.[39] However, in a subsequent study in patients with ACS symptoms presenting to the emergency room, the test had a poor sensitivity of 66.7% and specificity of 51.1% at a cutoff value of 0.22 mIU per liter.[81] As would be expected, PAPP-A correlated with markers of inflammation, such as CRP, but did not have an association with markers of myocardial injury (troponin I, CK-MB and CK). Similar to MPO, heparin may influence PAPP-A concentration by increasing release of the enzyme.[82,84] Finally the effect of renal dysfunction and/or dialysis on levels of PAPP-A needs to be explored further.[84]

Prognosis

As a prognostic marker, PAPP-A was studied in 200 ACS patients, of which 136 remained troponin-negative patients in the first 24 hours of admission. In this troponin-negative cohort, PAPP-A levels above 2.9 mIU per liter during early admission were predictive of 4.6-fold higher risk of cardiovascular death, myocardial infarction, or revascularization and levels above 4.5 mIU per liter conferred a 6.9-fold risk.[85]

Summary

- Among available commercial assays, most measure PAPP-A/pro-MBP hetero-dimers (found in pregnancy) in addition to PAPP-A homodimers. Assays for "cardiac PAPP-A" are for investigational use only as of early 2011
- Only serum should be used; heparin and EDTA can affect concentrations of PAPP-A
- An interesting investigational marker with good diagnostic performance in two studies and preliminary evidence suggest an association with risk of recurrent cardiovascular events
- Preanalytical influences remain to be completely defined.

BIOMARKERS OF HEMODYNAMIC STRESS

Once plaque rupture has occurred and ATP is depleted, cardiomyocyte dysfunction rapidly leads to an increase in intracardiac pressures and increased wall stress simultaneous with the onset of clinical symptoms (Figure 6-1). Potential biomarkers of this process are listed in table 6-1. The natriuretic peptides, which are the most advanced in clinical practice, are discussed here along with copeptin, which has been approved in some countries in Europe to aid in the rapid exclusion of acute myocardial infarction in patients presenting with chest pain.[86] Adrenomedulin and ST-2 are discussed elsewhere in this text.

Natriuretic Peptides (BNP, NT-proBNP)

BNP is secreted as a prohormone following myocardial stretch and cleaved by peptidases into the active C-terminal hormone.[87] Both the N-terminal fragments as well as the bioactive C-terminal hormones have been studied extensively. BNP induces vasodilatation, natriuresis, inhibition of the sympathetic and renin-angiotensin systems.[88] Plasma levels are elevated in patients with congestive heart failure and correlate with the degree of left ventricular dysfunction.[89,90] Evidence suggests that transient ischemia, which increases wall stress, can result in BNP synthesis or release; BNP also correlates with left ventricular end diastolic volume and therefore, pulmonary capillary wedge pressure.[88]

Diagnosis

Because of the onset of hemodynamic stress during ischemia, the natriuretic peptides have been considered as potential diagnostic markers. Indeed, after onset of ACS, BNP concentration rises and peaks within 14–40 hours.[91-93] As ventricular remodeling occurs, particularly in large infarcts, a second peak is seen in some patients with a subsequent decline in levels over the next several weeks.[91] In a cohort of patients with stable angina, unstable angina and non-ST-elevation ACS, BNP levels were directly correlated with disease burden. Patients with multivessel disease had significantly higher levels than patients with one or two vessel disease.[94] Natriuretic peptides are released during ischemia even in the absence of cardiac necrosis and levels correlate with size or severity of the ischemic insult.[88] Nevertheless, because natriuretic peptides are increased in a variety of non-ischemic conditions associated with an increase in wall stress, their specificity as diagnostic biomarkers of ischemia does not appear adequate. However, these biomarkers are widely used for the evaluation of chest symptoms potentially because of their relationship with ischemia or heart failure.

Prognosis

Early observations that BNP measured 1–7 days post-MI is predictive of LV dysfunction, heart failure and death has prompted researchers to assess BNP across the spectrum of ACS.[95,96] In 755 patients presenting with chest pain, NT-proBNP was independently associated with prognosis.[97] A larger pooled analysis of six studies, with > 12,000 non-ST-elevation MI patients showed that NT-proBNP was strongly predictive of death and future risk of CHF,[98] independent of left ventricular function (Figure 6-5a).[95,96,99] This association has been confirmed in multiple studies and shown to be independent of elevated troponin I, ECG changes, and the presenting syndrome (MI versus unstable angina).[97,100,101] Moreover, in stable patients four months after ACS, BNP was predictive of death or new CHF (Figure 6-5b).[102] In an unselected patient population, NT-proBNP levels drawn three days after ACS correlated with outcomes over an average follow-up period of more than four years.[103] Together, these data have shown natriuretic peptides to be among the strongest predictors of death or heart failure after ACS and been recommended as reasonable to measure along with troponin when the clinician desires addition information for risk assessment.[37,38] BNP is well validated at a cut-point of 80 or 100 pg/mL. Studies of NTproBNP have not used a single cut-point consistently but have suggested ≥ 400 pg/mL to be a reasonable threshold for risk stratification in patients with ischemic heart disease.[66,104-106]

BNP has also been suggested to identify high-risk patients who may benefit most from specific therapies. In the FRISC II trial of early invasive versus conservative therapy for patients with non-ST-elevation ACS, NT-proBNP (third tertile, > 906 pg/mL) identified a subset of patients who had particular benefit from the early invasive strategy.[107] In addition, in the MERLIN-TIMI 36 trial of 4,543 patients with non-ST-elevation ACS randomized to the anti-ischemic agent ranolazine, those with elevated BNP had more extensive CAD and higher risk of recurrent ischemia and appeared to benefit from treatment with ranolazine, whereas those with low levels of BNP did not.[108] Similarly, in the PROVE IT-TIMI 22 trial, patients with the highest concentrations of BNP following ACS benefitted the most from intensive statin therapy.[109]

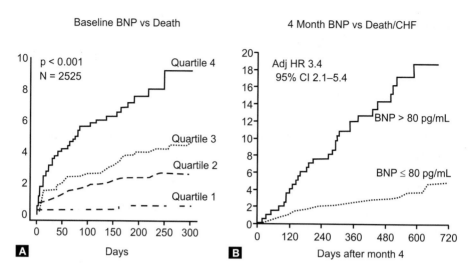

Figure 6-5 BNP and outcomes in ACS. **A,** Kaplan-Meier analysis of incidence of death according to baseline level of BNP at presentation with unstable angina, or myocardial infarction. *Adapted from* de Lemos JA, Morrow DA, Bentley JH, Omland T, Sabatine MS, McCabe CH, et al. The prognostic value of B-type natriuretic peptide in patients with acute coronary syndromes. *N Engl J Med.* 2001;345:1014-21. **B,** Kaplan-Meier analysis of incidence of death or congestive heart failure according to BNP result when clinically stable 4 months after non-ST-elevation acute coronary syndrome. *Adapted from* Morrow DA, de Lemos JA, Blazing MA, Sabatine MS, Murphy SA, Jarolim P, et al. Prognostic value of serial B-type natriuretic peptide testing during follow-up of patients with unstable coronary artery disease. *JAMA.* 2005;294:2866-71.

Summary

- High throughput, commercial assays widely available, with clinical indications for risk stratification in ACS for some assays
- BNP should be measured in plastic tubes using plasma. NTproBNP may be measured in serum or plasma and is less sensitive to the timing of measurement relative to sample collection
- The natriuretic peptides appear useful for the detection of underlying structural heart disease and increased wall stress but are not specific for myocardial ischemia
- Natriuretic peptides are among the strongest predictors of death or heart failure after ACS both in the short- and long-term
- Elevated BNP may identify high-risk ACS subsets that benefit from specific medical therapies, in particular, early invasive evaluation.

Copeptin

Copeptin is an emerging biomarker of cardiac stress that is now available in Europe as an aid, together with troponin and other clinical findings, to rule out acute myocardial infarction. This marker is discussed in detail in Chapter 15 but warrants brief discussion here because of its place as the newest clinically available (Europe) biomarker of ischemia. This glycosylated C-terminal fragment of the vasopressin precursor hormone (preprovasopressin) is secreted in an equimolar ratio with its sister compound, vasopressin.[110] Vasopressin is a stress hormone, regulated by hyperosmolality, hypotension, low blood volume, temperature, cytokines, and hypoxemia.[110,111] Vasopressin has an important role in the pathogenesis of congestive heart failure and remodeling following acute myocardial infarction.[112-114] Routine measurement of vasopressin, however, is not possible in clinical practice because of its short half-life of 5-15 minutes, its platelet binding effects and variations in assays.[110,115] In contrast, copeptin has a longer half-life in the circulation, which makes it easier to measure using a commercial assay.[116,117]

Diagnosis

The diagnostic utility of copeptin has been recently demonstrated. As an example, in a cohort of 487 patients presenting with chest pain to the emergency room, copeptin was found to be higher in those patients who had an acute MI compared to those having other diagnoses.[118] Although the marker alone was diagnostic of ACS, the combination of a non-necrotic marker (copeptin) with a necrotic marker (troponin T) significantly improved the area under the ROC curve and increased the negative predictive value to > 99% for those patients presenting with a negative troponin test and a copeptin level < 14 pmol/L. This increase in sensitivity came at the cost of decreased specificity from 93 to 77% and a fall in positive predictive value from 72 to 46%.[118] The use of copeptin in emergency rooms to rapidly rule out myocardial infarction may lower the cost of treatment by 30%[119] (see chapter 15 for discussion of additional studies). Because copeptin is plausibly elevated in the setting of other changes in volume or stress, the specificity for diagnostic use in broader populations and the clinical implications of testing remains to be fully defined.

Prognosis

The prognostic utility of copeptin has also been demonstrated. For example, in a post-MI patient population of 980 patients in a prospective single-center study, patients who had elevated levels of copeptin at presentation (> 7 pmol/L) carried a significantly higher risk of death or heart failure at 60 days.[120] Combining this marker with NT-proBNP further increased its positive predictive value.[120] In a head-to-head comparison of copeptin and BNP or NT-proBNP in patients with heart failure after an MI, copeptin was a stronger predictor of mortality (AUC 0.81 vs 0.66 or 0.0063, respectively).[121] It remains to be determined whether copeptin is simply a marker of a heightened stress response or whether it plays a pathological role in the acute changes that follow an MI including alterations in coronary blood flow that lead to adverse cardiovascular outcomes.[122]

Summary

- Commercially available in Europe
- May be measured in serum or plasma (EDTA and heparin)
- Appears to be most valuable for its negative predictive value or to supplement the sensitivity of troponin when measured very early after symptom onset.

STRESS TESTING

Stress testing with exercise electrocardiography has been the mainstay for noninvasive diagnosis and risk stratification for CAD. Nevertheless, exercise-induced ECG changes and chest symptoms have only moderate sensitivity and specificity for flow-limiting CAD. Perfusion imaging improves diagnostic accuracy but is expensive. Recently, researchers have assessed incorporating biochemical data to improve the diagnostic yield of stress testing.

As an example, our group studied the effects of transient myocardial ischemia-induced stress testing on levels of circulating natriuretic peptides and found that baseline concentration was correlated to the subsequent severity of inducible ischemia, both for BNP as well as the N-terminal of the BNP prohormone (NT-proBNP).[123] Following exercise, there was an immediate increase in these peptides and the degree of increase was proportional to the degree of ischemia for BNP and, to a lesser extent, NT-proBNP (Figure 6-6). When added to traditional markers of cardiac ischemia, a BNP level ≥ 80 pg/mL was a strong and independent predictor of inducible myocardial ischemia. Similar to our findings, the Heart and Soul Study investigators also found that resting pro-NT-proBNP levels are independently associated with inducible ischemia in a cross-sectional study of 901 patients with stable CAD after exercise stress testing.[124] The overall utility of BNP and other biomarkers with respect to increasing the yield of the diagnostic utility of stress testing is still under investigation.

SUMMARY

Although there are a burgeoning number of biomarkers studied as tools for diagnosis of cardiac ischemia, few have become available for clinical application,[125] and none have yet become fully integrated into routine clinical testing along with cardiac troponin. It remains highly appealing to detect myocardial ischemia in the absence of myocardial necrosis. However, most biomarkers studied for this purpose have failed to deliver the specificity desired in order to provide a high positive predictive value in community-based emergency populations where ACS comprises < 20% of the cases presenting with nontraumatic chest pain. Several biomarkers,

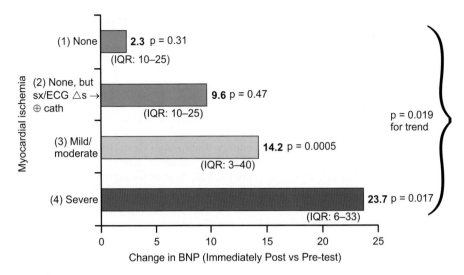

Figure 6-6 Median changes in BNP levels in response to exercise stress testing in patients with (1) no ischemia, (2) no ischemia on perfusion imaging but shown to have critical coronary disease during cardiac catheterization, (3) mild-to-moderate ischemia, and (4) severe ischemia. The p-value at the far right is for the trend across ischemic categories. Cath, cardiac catheterization; ECG, electrocardiography; IQR, interquartile range; sx, symptoms. *Data from* Sabatine MS, Morrow DA, de Lemos JA, Omland T, Desai MY, Tanasijevic M, et al. Acute changes in circulating natriuretic peptide levels in relation to myocardial ischemia. *J Am Coll Cardiol.* 2004;44:1988-95.

such as H-FABP and copeptin, may offer clinical value because of their very high negative predictive value in the emergency setting. Others, such as the inflammatory biomarkers, appear to offer prognostic but not useful diagnostic value and are likely to require specific links to therapy to justify routine clinical use. To date, the natriuretic peptides have the best support for clinical use as a prognostic marker that assists with diagnosis when heart failure is being considered and can point to an increased absolute benefit from early revascularization in patients with unstable ischemic heart disease.

Acknowledgments and Disclosures

Payal Kohli has no disclosures other than research grant support to the TIMI Study Group.

David A Morrow has received consulting fees from Beckman-Coulter, Boehringher Ingelheim, Cardiokinetix, Gilead, Instrumentation Laboratory, Ikaria, Menarini, Merck, OrthoClinical Diagnostics, Roche Diagnostics, and Siemens and remuneration from AstraZeneca for adjudication as a member of a Clinical Events Committee.

The TIMI Study Group has received significant research grant support from Accumetrics, Amgen, AstraZeneca, Beckman Coulter, BRAHMS (ThermoFisher), Bristol-Myers Squibb, Buhlmann, CV Therapeutics, Daiichi Sankyo Co Ltd, Eli Lilly and Co, GlaxoSmithKline, Integrated Therapeutics, Merck and Co, Nanosphere, Novartis Pharmaceuticals, Nuvelo,

OrthoClinical Diagnostics, Pfizer, Randox, Roche Diagnostics, Sanofi-Aventis, Sanofi-Synthelabo, Siemens Medical Solutions, and Singulex.

REFERENCES

1. Morrow DA, Cannon CP, Jesse RL, Newby LK, Ravkilde J, Storrow AB, et al. National Academy of Clinical Biochemistry Laboratory Medicine practice guidelines: clinical characteristics and utilization of biochemical markers in acute coronary syndromes. *Circulation.* 2007;115:e356-75.

2. Libby P, Bonow R, Mann D, Zipes D, editors. Braunwald's Heart Disease: A Textbook of Cardiovascular Medicine. 8th ed. Philadelphia: Saunders; 2008.

3. Keller T, Zeller T, Peetz D, Tzikas S, Roth A, Czyz E, et al. Sensitive troponin I assay in early diagnosis of acute myocardial infarction. *N Engl J Med.* 2009;361:868-77.

4. Reichlin T, Hochholzer W, Bassetti S, Steuer S, Stelzig C, Hartwiger S, et al. Early diagnosis of myocardial infarction with sensitive cardiac troponin assays. *N Engl J Med.* 2009;361:858-67.

5. Kavsak PA, Wang X, Ko DT, MacRae AR, Jaffe AS. Short- and long-term risk stratification using a next-generation, high-sensitivity research cardiac troponin I (hs-cTnI) assay in an emergency department chest pain population. *Clin Chem.* 2009;55:1809-15.

6. de Lemos JA, O'Donoghue M. The skinny on fatty acid-binding protein. *J Am Coll Cardiol.* 2007;50:2068-70.

7. Omland T, de Lemos JA, Sabatine MS, Christophi CA, Rice MM, Jablonski KA, et al. A sensitive cardiac troponin T assay in stable coronary artery disease. *N Engl J Med.* 2009;361:2538-47.

8. Tanaka T, Hirota Y, Sohmiya K, Nishimura S, Kawamura K. Serum and urinary human heart fatty acid-binding protein in acute myocardial infarction. *Clin Biochem.* 1991;24:195-201.

9. Kleine AH, Glatz JF, van Nieuwenhoven FA, van der Vusse GJ. Release of heart fatty acid-binding protein into plasma after acute myocardial infarction in man. *Mol Cell Biochem.* 1992;116:155-62.

10. Glatz JF, van der Vusse GJ, Simoons ML, Kragten JA, van Dieijen-Visser MP, Hermens WT. Fatty acid-binding protein and the early detection of acute myocardial infarction. *Clin Chim Acta.* 1998;272:87-92.

11. Seino Y, Ogata K, Takano T, Ishii J, Hishida H, Morita H, et al. Use of a whole blood rapid panel test for heart-type fatty acid-binding protein in patients with acute chest pain: comparison with rapid troponin T and myoglobin tests. *Am J Med.* 2003;115:185-90.

12. Okamoto F, Sohmiya K, Ohkaru Y, Kawamura K, Asayama K, Kimura H, et al. Human heart-type cytoplasmic fatty acid-binding protein (H-FABP) for the diagnosis of acute myocardial infarction. Clinical evaluation of H-FABP in comparison with myoglobin and creatine kinase isoenzyme MB. *Clin Chem Lab Med.* 2000;38:231-8.

13. Ishii J, Ozaki Y, Lu J, Kitagawa F, Kuno T, Nakano T, et al. Prognostic value of serum concentration of heart-type fatty acid-binding protein relative to cardiac troponin T on admission in the early hours of acute coronary syndrome. *Clin Chem.* 2005;51:1397-404.

14. O'Donoghue M, de Lemos JA, Morrow DA, Murphy SA, Buros JL, Cannon CP, et al. Prognostic utility of heart-type fatty acid binding protein in patients with acute coronary syndromes. *Circulation.* 2006;114:550-7.

15. Kilcullen N, Viswanathan K, Das R, Morrell C, Farrin A, Barth JH, et al. Heart-type fatty acid-binding protein predicts long-term mortality after acute coronary syndrome and identifies high-risk patients across the range of troponin values. *J Am Coll Cardiol.* 2007;50:2061-7.

16. Libby P. Inflammation in atherosclerosis. *Nature.* 2002;420:868-74.
17. Zwaka TP, Hombach V, Torzewski J. C-reactive protein-mediated low density lipoprotein uptake by macrophages: implications for atherosclerosis. *Circulation.* 2001;103:1194-7.
18. Bisoendial RJ, Kastelein JJ, Levels JH, Zwaginga JJ, van den Bogaard B, Reitsma PH, et al. Activation of inflammation and coagulation after infusion of C-reactive protein in humans. *Circ Res.* 2005;96:714-6.
19. Schwedler SB, Amann K, Wernicke K, Krebs A, Nauck M, Wanner C, et al. Native C-reactive protein increases whereas modified C-reactive protein reduces atherosclerosis in apolipoprotein E-knockout mice. *Circulation.* 2005;112:1016-23.
20. Anderson JL, Carlquist JF, Muhlestein JB, Horne BD, Elmer SP. Evaluation of C-reactive protein, an inflammatory marker, and infectious serology as risk factors for coronary artery disease and myocardial infarction. *J Am Coll Cardiol.* 1998;32:35-41.
21. Arroyo-Espliguero R, Avanzas P, Cosin-Sales J, Aldama G, Pizzi C, Kaski JC. C-reactive protein elevation and disease activity in patients with coronary artery disease. *Eur Heart J.* 2004;25:401-8.
22. Liuzzo G, Buffon A, Biasucci LM, Gallimore JR, Caligiuri G, Vitelli A, et al. Enhanced inflammatory response to coronary angioplasty in patients with severe unstable angina. *Circulation.* 1998;98:2370-6.
23. Berk BC, Weintraub WS, Alexander RW. Elevation of C-reactive protein in "active" coronary artery disease. *Am J Cardiol.* 1990;65:168-72.
24. Tomoda H, Aoki N. Prognostic value of C-reactive protein levels within six hours after the onset of acute myocardial infarction. *Am Heart J.* 2000;140:324-8.
25. Chew DP, Bhatt DL, Robbins MA, Penn MS, Schneider JP, Lauer MS, et al. Incremental prognostic value of elevated baseline C-reactive protein among established markers of risk in percutaneous coronary intervention. *Circulation.* 2001;104:992-7.
26. Mueller C, Buettner HJ, Hodgson JM, Marsch S, Perruchoud AP, Roskamm H, et al. Inflammation and long-term mortality after non-ST elevation acute coronary syndrome treated with a very early invasive strategy in 1,042 consecutive patients. *Circulation.* 2002;105:1412-5.
27. Walter DH, Fichtlscherer S, Sellwig M, Auch-Schwelk W, Schachinger V, Zeiher AM. Preprocedural C-reactive protein levels and cardiovascular events after coronary stent implantation. *J Am Coll Cardiol.* 2001;37:839-46.
28. Zairis MN, Ambrose JA, Manousakis SJ, Stefanidis AS, Papadaki OA, Bilianou HI, et al. The impact of plasma levels of C-reactive protein, lipoprotein (a) and homocysteine on the long-term prognosis after successful coronary stenting: The Global Evaluation of New Events and Restenosis after Stent Implantation Study. *J Am Coll Cardiol.* 2002; 40:1375-82.
29. de Winter RJ, Koch KT, van Straalen JP, Heyde G, Bax M, Schotborgh CE, et al. C-reactive protein and coronary events following percutaneous coronary angioplasty. *Am J Med.* 2003;115:85-90.
30. Liuzzo G, Biasucci LM, Gallimore JR, Grillo RL, Rebuzzi AG, Pepys MB, et al. The prognostic value of C-reactive protein and serum amyloid a protein in severe unstable angina. *N Engl J Med.* 1994;331:417-24.
31. Morrow DA, Rifai N, Antman EM, Weiner DL, McCabe CH, Cannon CP, et al. C-reactive protein is a potent predictor of mortality independently of and in combination with troponin T in acute coronary syndromes: a TIMI 11A substudy. Thrombolysis in Myocardial Infarction. *J Am Coll Cardiol.* 1998;31:1460-5.
32. Toss H, Lindahl B, Siegbahn A, Wallentin L. Prognostic influence of increased fibrinogen and C-reactive protein levels in unstable coronary artery disease. FRISC Study Group. Fragmin during Instability in Coronary Artery Disease. *Circulation.* 1997;96:4204-10.

33. Lindahl B, Toss H, Siegbahn A, Venge P, Wallentin L. Markers of myocardial damage and inflammation in relation to long-term mortality in unstable coronary artery disease. FRISC Study Group. Fragmin during Instability in Coronary Artery Disease. *N Engl J Med.* 2000;343:1139-47.

34. Heeschen C, Hamm CW, Bruemmer J, Simoons ML. Predictive value of C-reactive protein and troponin T in patients with unstable angina: a comparative analysis. CAPTURE investigators. Chimeric c7E3 antiplatelet therapy in unstable angina refractory to standard treatment trial. *J Am Coll Cardiol.* 2000;35:1535-42.

35. Biasucci LM, Liuzzo G, Grillo RL, Caligiuri G, Rebuzzi AG, Buffon A, et al. Elevated levels of C-reactive protein at discharge in patients with unstable angina predict recurrent instability. *Circulation.* 1999;99:855-60.

36. James SK, Armstrong P, Barnathan E, Califf R, Lindahl B, Siegbahn A, et al. Troponin and C-reactive protein have different relations to subsequent mortality and myocardial infarction after acute coronary syndrome: a GUSTO-IV substudy. *J Am Coll Cardiol.* 2003;41:916-24.

37. Tang WH, Francis GS, Morrow DA, Newby LK, Cannon CP, Jesse RL, et al. National Academy of Clinical Biochemistry Laboratory Medicine Practice Guidelines: clinical utilization of cardiac biomarker testing in heart failure. *Clin Biochem.* 2008;41:210-21.

38. Wu AH, Jaffe AS, Apple FS, Jesse RL, Francis GL, Morrow DA, et al. National Academy of Clinical Biochemistry laboratory medicine practice guidelines: use of cardiac troponin and B-type natriuretic peptide or N-terminal proB-type natriuretic peptide for etiologies other than acute coronary syndromes and heart failure. *Clin Chem.* 2007;53:2086-96.

39. Bayes-Genis A, Conover CA, Overgaard MT, Bailey KR, Christiansen M, Holmes DR Jr, et al. Pregnancy-associated plasma protein A as a marker of acute coronary syndromes. *N Engl J Med.* 2001;345:1022-9.

40. Lincoff AM, Kereiakes DJ, Mascelli MA, Deckelbaum LI, Barnathan ES, Patel KK, et al. Abciximab suppresses the rise in levels of circulating inflammatory markers after percutaneous coronary revascularization. *Circulation.* 2001;104:163-7.

41. Haffner SM, Greenberg AS, Weston WM, Chen H, Williams K, Freed MI. Effect of rosiglitazone treatment on nontraditional markers of cardiovascular disease in patients with type 2 diabetes mellitus. *Circulation.* 2002;106:679-84.

42. Pfutzner A, Marx N, Lubben G, Langenfeld M, Walcher D, Konrad T, et al. Improvement of cardiovascular risk markers by pioglitazone is independent from glycemic control: results from the pioneer study. *J Am Coll Cardiol.* 2005;45:1925-31.

43. Hanefeld M, Marx N, Pfutzner A, Baurecht W, Lubben G, Karagiannis E, et al. Anti-inflammatory effects of pioglitazone and/or simvastatin in high cardiovascular risk patients with elevated high sensitivity C-reactive protein: the PIOSTAT study. *J Am Coll Cardiol.* 2007;49:290-7.

44. Jenkins NP, Keevil BG, Hutchinson IV, Brooks NH. Beta-blockers are associated with lower C-reactive protein concentrations in patients with coronary artery disease. *Am J Med.* 2002;112:269-74.

45. Ikonomidis I, Andreotti F, Economou E, Stefanadis C, Toutouzas P, Nihoyannopoulos P. Increased proinflammatory cytokines in patients with chronic stable angina and their reduction by aspirin. *Circulation.* 1999;100:793-8.

46. Schultz J, Kaminker K. Myeloperoxidase of the leucocyte of normal human blood. I. Content and localization. *Arch Biochem Biophys.* 1962;96:465-7.

47. Bos A, Wever R, Roos D. Characterization and quantification of the peroxidase in human monocytes. *Biochim Biophys Acta.* 1978;525:37-44.

48. Daugherty A, Dunn JL, Rateri DL, Heinecke JW. Myeloperoxidase, a catalyst for lipo-protein oxidation, is expressed in human atherosclerotic lesions. *J Clin Invest.* 1994; 94:437-44.

49. Naruko T, Ueda M, Haze K, van der Wal AC, van der Loos CM, Itoh A, et al. Neutrophil infiltration of culprit lesions in acute coronary syndromes. *Circulation.* 2002;106:2894-900.

50. Nicholls SJ, Hazen SL. Myeloperoxidase and cardiovascular disease. *Arterioscler Thromb Vasc Biol.* 2005;25:1102-11.

51. Podrez EA, Abu-Soud HM, Hazen SL. Myeloperoxidase-generated oxidants and atherosclerosis. *Free Radic Biol Med.* 2000;28:1717-25.

52. Asselbergs FW, Reynolds WF, Cohen-Tervaert JW, Jessurun GA, Tio RA. Myeloperoxidase polymorphism related to cardiovascular events in coronary artery disease. *Am J Med.* 2004;116:429-30.

53. Asselbergs FW, Tervaert JW, Tio RA. Prognostic value of myeloperoxidase in patients with chest pain. *N Engl J Med.* 2004;350:516-8; author reply 516-8.

54. Kutter D, Devaquet P, Vanderstocken G, Paulus JM, Marchal V, Gothot A. Consequences of total and subtotal myeloperoxidase deficiency: risk or benefit? *Acta Haematol.* 2000; 104:10-5.

55. Nikpoor B, Turecki G, Fournier C, Theroux P, Rouleau GA. A functional myeloperoxidase polymorphic variant is associated with coronary artery disease in French-Canadians. *Am Heart J.* 2001;142:336-9.

56. Zhang R, Brennan ML, Fu X, Aviles RJ, Pearce GL, Penn MS, et al. Association between myeloperoxidase levels and risk of coronary artery disease. *JAMA.* 2001; 286:2136-42.

57. Tang WH, Brennan ML, Philip K, Tong W, Mann S, Van Lente F, et al. Plasma myeloper-oxidase levels in patients with chronic heart failure. *Am J Cardiol.* 2006;98:796-9.

58. Meuwese MC, Stroes ES, Hazen SL, van Miert JN, Kuivenhoven JA, Schaub RG, et al. Serum myeloperoxidase levels are associated with the future risk of coronary artery disease in apparently healthy individuals: the EPIC-Norfolk prospective population study. *J Am Coll Cardiol.* 2007;50:159-65.

59. Baldus S, Heeschen C, Meinertz T, Zeiher AM, Eiserich JP, Munzel T, et al. Myeloper-oxidase serum levels predict risk in patients with acute coronary syndromes. *Circulation.* 2003;108:1440-5.

60. Brennan ML, Penn MS, van Lente F, Nambi V, Shishehbor MH, Aviles RJ, et al. Prognostic value of myeloperoxidase in patients with chest pain. *N Engl J Med.* 2003; 349:1595-604.

61. Cavusoglu E, Ruwende C, Eng C, Chopra V, Yanamadala S, Clark LT, et al. Usefulness of baseline plasma myeloperoxidase levels as an independent predictor of myocardial infarction at two years in patients presenting with acute coronary syndrome. *Am J Cardiol.* 2007;99:1364-8.

62. FDA Approvals: PLAC, CardioMPO, HemosIL2005: Available from: http://www.medscape.com/viewarticle/507691.

63. de Azevedo Lucio E, Goncalves SC, Ribeiro JP, Nunes GL, de Oliveira JR, Araujo GN, et al. Lack of association between plasma myeloperoxidase levels and angiographic severity of coronary artery disease in patients with acute coronary syndrome. *Inflamm Res.* 2011;60:137-42.

64. Borges FK, Stella SF, Souza JF, Wendland AE, Werres Junior LC, Ribeiro JP, et al. Serial analyses of C-reactive protein and myeloperoxidase in acute coronary syndrome. *Clin Cardiol.* 2009;32:E58-62.

65. Roman RM, Wendland AE, Polanczyk CA. Myeloperoxidase and coronary arterial disease: from research to clinical practice. *Arq Bras Cardiol.* 2008;91:e11-9.

66. Scirica BM, Sabatine MS, Jarolim P, Murphy SA, de Lemos JL, Braunwald E, et al. Assessment of multiple cardiac biomarkers in non-ST-segment elevation acute coronary syndromes: observations from the MERLIN-TIMI 36 Trial. *Eur Heart J.* 2011;32:697-705.

67. Inokubo Y, Hanada H, Ishizaka H, Fukushi T, Kamada T, Okumura K. Plasma levels of matrix metalloproteinase-9 and tissue inhibitor of metalloproteinase-1 are increased in the coronary circulation in patients with acute coronary syndrome. *Am Heart J.* 2001; 141:211-7.

68. Lee RT, Schoen FJ, Loree HM, Lark MW, Libby P. Circumferential stress and matrix metalloproteinase 1 in human coronary atherosclerosis. Implications for plaque rupture. *Arterioscler Thromb Vasc Biol.* 1996;16:1070-3.

69. Shah PK, Galis ZS. Matrix metalloproteinase hypothesis of plaque rupture: players keep piling up but questions remain. *Circulation.* 2001;104:1878-80.

70. Okamoto Y, Satomura K, Ohsuzu F, Nakamura H, Takeuchi K, Yoshioka M. Expression of matrix metalloproteinase 3 in experimental atherosclerotic plaques. *J Atheroscler Thromb.* 2001;8:50-4.

71. Uzui H, Harpf A, Liu M, Doherty TM, Shukla A, Chai NN, et al. Increased expression of membrane type 3-matrix metalloproteinase in human atherosclerotic plaque: role of activated macrophages and inflammatory cytokines. *Circulation.* 2002;106:3024-30.

72. Laursen LS, Overgaard MT, Nielsen CG, Boldt HB, Hopmann KH, Conover CA, et al. Substrate specificity of the metalloproteinase pregnancy-associated plasma protein-A (PAPP-A) assessed by mutagenesis and analysis of synthetic peptides: substrate residues distant from the scissile bond are critical for proteolysis. *Biochem J.* 2002;367:31-40.

73. Bayes-Genis A, Schwartz RS, Lewis DA, Overgaard MT, Christiansen M, Oxvig C, et al. Insulin-like growth factor binding protein-4 protease produced by smooth muscle cells increases in the coronary artery after angioplasty. *Arterioscler Thromb Vasc Biol.* 2001; 21:335-41.

74. Gerard N, Delpuech T, Oxvig C, Overgaard MT, Monget P. Proteolytic degradation of IGF-binding protein (IGFBP)-2 in equine ovarian follicles: involvement of pregnancy-associated plasma protein-A (PAPP-A) and association with dominant but not subordi-nated follicles. *J Endocrinol.* 2004;182:457-66.

75. Lawrence JB, Oxvig C, Overgaard MT, Sottrup-Jensen L, Gleich GJ, Hays LG, et al. The insulin-like growth factor (IGF)-dependent IGF binding protein-4 protease secreted by human fibroblasts is pregnancy-associated plasma protein-A. *Proc Natl Acad Sci U S A.* 1999;96:3149-53.

76. Laursen LS, Overgaard MT, Soe R, Boldt HB, Sottrup-Jensen L, Giudice LC, et al. Pregnancy-associated plasma protein-A (PAPP-A) cleaves insulin-like growth factor binding protein (IGFBP)-5 independent of IGF: implications for the mechanism of IGFBP-4 proteolysis by PAPP-A. *FEBS Lett.* 2001;504:36-40.

77. Wittfooth S, Qin QP, Lund J, Tierala I, Pulkki K, Takalo H, et al. Immunofluorometric point-of-care assays for the detection of acute coronary syndrome-related noncomplexed pregnancy-associated plasma protein A. *Clin Chem.* 2006;52:1794-801.

78. Oxvig C, Sand O, Kristensen T, Gleich GJ, Sottrup-Jensen L. Circulating human pregnancy-associated plasma protein-A is disulfide-bridged to the proform of eosinophil major basic protein. *J Biol Chem.* 1993;268:12243-6.

79. Overgaard MT, Haaning J, Boldt HB, Olsen IM, Laursen LS, Christiansen M, et al. Expression of recombinant human pregnancy-associated plasma protein-A and identi-fication of the proform of eosinophil major basic protein as its physiological inhibitor. *J Biol Chem.* 2000;275:31128-33.

80. Lund J, Wittfooth S, Qin QP, Ilva T, Porela P, Pulkki K, et al. Free vs total pregnancy-associated plasma protein A (PAPP-A) as a predictor of 1-year outcome in patients

presenting with non-ST-elevation acute coronary syndrome. *Clin Chem.* 2010;56: 1158-65.

81. Laterza OF, Cameron SJ, Chappell D, Sokoll LJ, Green GB. Evaluation of pregnancy-associated plasma protein A as a prognostic indicator in acute coronary syndrome patients. *Clin Chim Acta.* 2004;348:163-9.

82. Terkelsen CJ, Oxvig C, Norgaard BL, Glerup S, Poulsen TS, Lassen JF, et al. Temporal course of pregnancy-associated plasma protein-A in angioplasty-treated ST-elevation myocardial infarction patients and potential significance of concomitant heparin administration. *Am J Cardiol.* 2009;103:29-35.

83. Tertti R, Wittfooth S, Porela P, Airaksinen KE, Metsarinne K, Pettersson K. Intravenous administration of low molecular weight and unfractionated heparin elicits a rapid increase in serum pregnancy-associated plasma protein A. *Clin Chem.* 2009;55:1214-7.

84. Fialova L, Kalousova M, Soukupova J, Sulkova S, Merta M, Jelinkova E, et al. Relationship of pregnancy-associated plasma protein-a to renal function and dialysis modalities. *Kidney Blood Press Res.* 2004;27:88-95.

85. Lund J, Qin QP, Ilva T, Pettersson K, Voipio-Pulkki LM, Porela P, et al. Circulating pregnancy-associated plasma protein a predicts outcome in patients with acute coronary syndrome but no troponin I elevation. *Circulation.* 2003;108:1924-6.

86. BRAHMS copeptin assay to aid the rapid exclusion of acute myocardial infarction in patients with acute chest pain2011: Available from: http://www.nice.org.uk/nicemedia/ live/13257/53391/53391.pdf.

87. Levin ER, Gardner DG, Samson WK. Natriuretic peptides. *N Engl J Med.* 1998;339:321-8.

88. de Lemos JA, Morrow DA. Brain natriuretic peptide measurement in acute coronary syndromes: ready for clinical application? *Circulation.* 2002;106:2868-70.

89. Yasue H, Yoshimura M, Sumida H, Kikuta K, Kugiyama K, Jougasaki M, et al. Localization and mechanism of secretion of B-type natriuretic peptide in comparison with those of A-type natriuretic peptide in normal subjects and patients with heart failure. *Circulation.* 1994;90:195-203.

90. Omland T, Aakvaag A, Vik-Mo H. Plasma cardiac natriuretic peptide determination as a screening test for the detection of patients with mild left ventricular impairment. *Heart.* 1996;76:232-7.

91. Morita E, Yasue H, Yoshimura M, Ogawa H, Jougasaki M, Matsumura T, et al. Increased plasma levels of brain natriuretic peptide in patients with acute myocardial infarction. *Circulation.* 1993;88:82-91.

92. Talwar S, Squire IB, Downie PF, Davies JE, Ng LL. Plasma N terminal pro-brain natriuretic peptide and cardiotrophin 1 are raised in unstable angina. *Heart.* 2000;84:421-4.

93. Wiese S, Breyer T, Dragu A, Wakili R, Burkard T, Schmidt-Schweda S, et al. Gene expression of brain natriuretic peptide in isolated atrial and ventricular human myocardium: influence of angiotensin II and diastolic fiber length. *Circulation.* 2000;102:3074-9.

94. Palazzuoli A, Maisel A, Caputo M, Fineschi M, Quatrini I, Calabro A, et al. B-type natriuretic peptide levels predict extent and severity of coronary disease in non-ST elevation coronary syndromes and normal left ventricular systolic function. *Regul Pept.* 2011;167:129-33.

95. Omland T, Aakvaag A, Bonarjee VV, Caidahl K, Lie RT, Nilsen DW, et al. Plasma brain natriuretic peptide as an indicator of left ventricular systolic function and long-term survival after acute myocardial infarction. Comparison with plasma atrial natriuretic peptide and N-terminal proatrial natriuretic peptide. *Circulation.* 1996;93:1963-9.

96. Richards AM, Nicholls MG, Yandle TG, Frampton C, Espiner EA, Turner JG, et al. Plasma N-terminal pro-brain natriuretic peptide and adrenomedullin: new neurohormonal

predictors of left ventricular function and prognosis after myocardial infarction. *Circulation.* 1998;97:1921-9.

97. Jernberg T, Stridsberg M, Venge P, Lindahl B. N-terminal pro brain natriuretic peptide on admission for early risk stratification of patients with chest pain and no ST-segment elevation. *J Am Coll Cardiol.* 2002;40:437-45.

98. Jernberg T, James S, Lindahl B, Stridsberg M, Venge P, Wallentin L. NT-ProBNP in non-ST-elevation acute coronary syndrome. *J Card Fail.* 2005;11:S54-8.

99. Arakawa N, Nakamura M, Aoki H, Hiramori K. Plasma brain natriuretic peptide concentrations predict survival after acute myocardial infarction. *J Am Coll Cardiol.* 1996; 27:1656-61.

100. de Lemos JA, Morrow DA, Bentley JH, Omland T, Sabatine MS, McCabe CH, et al. The prognostic value of B-type natriuretic peptide in patients with acute coronary syndromes. *N Engl J Med.* 2001;345:1014-21.

101. Morrow DA, de Lemos JA, Sabatine MS, Murphy SA, Demopoulos LA, DiBattiste PM, et al. Evaluation of B-type natriuretic peptide for risk assessment in unstable angina/non-ST-elevation myocardial infarction: B-type natriuretic peptide and prognosis in TACTICS-TIMI 18. *J Am Coll Cardiol.* 2003;41:1264-72.

102. Morrow DA, de Lemos JA, Blazing MA, Sabatine MS, Murphy SA, Jarolim P, et al. Prognostic value of serial B-type natriuretic peptide testing during follow-up of patients with unstable coronary artery disease. *JAMA.* 2005;294:2866-71.

103. Omland T, de Lemos JA, Morrow DA, Antman EM, Cannon CP, Hall C, et al. Prognostic value of N-terminal pro-atrial and pro-brain natriuretic peptide in patients with acute coronary syndromes. *Am J Cardiol.* 2002;89:463-5.

104. Sabatine MS, Morrow DA, Higgins LJ, MacGillivray C, Guo W, Bode C, et al. Complementary roles for biomarkers of biomechanical strain ST2 and N-terminal prohormone B-type natriuretic peptide in patients with ST-elevation myocardial infarction. *Circulation.* 2008;117:1936-44.

105. James SK, Lindahl B, Siegbahn A, Stridsberg M, Venge P, Armstrong P, et al. N-terminal pro-brain natriuretic peptide and other risk markers for the separate prediction of mortality and subsequent myocardial infarction in patients with unstable coronary artery disease: a Global Utilization of Strategies To Open occluded arteries (GUSTO)-IV substudy. *Circulation.* 2003;108:275-81.

106. Heeschen C, Hamm CW, Mitrovic V, Lantelme NH, White HD. N-terminal pro-B-type natriuretic peptide levels for dynamic risk stratification of patients with acute coronary syndromes. *Circulation.* 2004;110:3206-12.

107. Jernberg T, Lindahl B, Siegbahn A, Andren B, Frostfeldt G, Lagerqvist B, et al. N-terminal pro-brain natriuretic peptide in relation to inflammation, myocardial necrosis, and the effect of an invasive strategy in unstable coronary artery disease. *J Am Coll Cardiol.* 2003;42:1909-16.

108. Morrow DA, Scirica BM, Sabatine MS, de Lemos JA, Murphy SA, Jarolim P, et al. B-type natriuretic peptide and the effect of ranolazine in patients with non-ST-segment elevation acute coronary syndromes: observations from the MERLIN-TIMI 36 (Metabolic Efficiency With Ranolazine for Less Ischemia in Non-ST Elevation Acute Coronary-Thrombolysis in Myocardial Infarction 36) trial. *J Am Coll Cardiol.* 2010;55:1189-96.

109. Scirica BM, Morrow DA, Cannon CP, Ray KK, Sabatine MS, Jarolim P, et al. Intensive statin therapy and the risk of hospitalization for heart failure after an acute coronary syndrome in the PROVE IT-TIMI 22 study. *J Am Coll Cardiol.* 2006;47:2326-31.

110. Keller T, Tzikas S, Zeller T, Czyz E, Lillpopp L, Ojeda FM, et al. Copeptin improves early diagnosis of acute myocardial infarction. *J Am Coll Cardiol.* 2010;55:2096-106.

111. Hochholzer W, Morrow DA, Giugliano RP. Novel biomarkers in cardiovascular disease: update 2010. *Am Heart J.* 2010;160:583-94.

112. Kelly D, Squire IB, Khan SQ, Quinn P, Struck J, Morgenthaler NG, et al. C-terminal provasopressin (copeptin) is associated with left ventricular dysfunction, remodeling, and clinical heart failure in survivors of myocardial infarction. *J Card Fail.* 2008;14: 739-45.

113. Francis GS, Benedict C, Johnstone DE, Kirlin PC, Nicklas J, Liang CS, et al. Comparison of neuroendocrine activation in patients with left ventricular dysfunction with and without congestive heart failure. A substudy of the Studies of Left Ventricular Dysfunction (SOLVD). *Circulation.* 1990;82:1724-9.

114. Goldsmith SR, Francis GS, Cowley A Jr, Levine TB, Cohn JN. Increased plasma arginine vasopressin levels in patients with congestive heart failure. *J Am Coll Cardiol.* 1983;1:1385-90.

115. Kluge M, Riedl S, Erhart-Hofmann B, Hartmann J, Waldhauser F. Improved extraction procedure and RIA for determination of arginine 8-vasopressin in plasma: role of premeasurement sample treatment and reference values in children. *Clin Chem.* 1999; 45:98-103.

116. Morgenthaler NG, Struck J, Alonso C, Bergmann A. Assay for the measurement of copeptin, a stable peptide derived from the precursor of vasopressin. *Clin Chem.* 2006; 52:112-9.

117. Struck J, Morgenthaler NG, Bergmann A. Copeptin, a stable peptide derived from the vasopressin precursor, is elevated in serum of sepsis patients. *Peptides.* 2005;26:2500-4.

118. Reichlin T, Hochholzer W, Stelzig C, Laule K, Freidank H, Morgenthaler NG, et al. Incremental value of copeptin for rapid rule out of acute myocardial infarction. *J Am Coll Cardiol.* 2009;54:60-8.

119. Twerenbold R, Reichlin T, Reiter M, Meissner J, Heinisch C, Socrates T, et al., editors. Economic Benefit of Copeptin for Rapid Rule Out of Acute Myocardial Infarction. Congress of the European Society of Cardiology: Stockholm, Sweden. 2010.

120. Khan SQ, Dhillon OS, O'Brien RJ, Struck J, Quinn PA, Morgenthaler NG, et al. C-terminal provasopressin (copeptin) as a novel and prognostic marker in acute myocardial infarction: Leicester Acute Myocardial Infarction Peptide (LAMP) study. *Circulation.* 2007;115:2103-10.

121. Voors AA, von Haehling S, Anker SD, Hillege HL, Struck J, Hartmann O, et al. C-terminal provasopressin (copeptin) is a strong prognostic marker in patients with heart failure after an acute myocardial infarction: results from the OPTIMAAL study. *Eur Heart J.* 2009;30:1187-94.

122. Holmes CL, Landry DW, Granton JT. Science review: vasopressin and the cardiovascular system part 2 - clinical physiology. *Crit Care.* 2004;8:15-23.

123. Sabatine MS, Morrow DA, de Lemos JA, Omland T, Desai MY, Tanasijevic M, et al. Acute changes in circulating natriuretic peptide levels in relation to myocardial ischemia. *J Am Coll Cardiol.* 2004;44:1988-95.

124. Singh HS, Bibbins-Domingo K, Ali S, Wu AH, Schiller NB, Whooley MA. N-terminal pro-B-type natriuretic peptide and inducible ischemia in the Heart and Soul Study. *Clin Cardiol.* 2009;32:447-53.

125. Apple FS, Wu AH, Mair J, Ravkilde J, Panteghini M, Tate J, et al. Future biomarkers for detection of ischemia and risk stratification in acute coronary syndrome. *Clin Chem.* 2005;51:810-24.

CHAPTER 7

Natriuretic Peptides in Patients with Acute Shortness of Breath

Yang Xue, Navaid Iqbal,
Arrash Fard, Alan S Maisel

INTRODUCTION

Heart failure is a serious healthcare challenge with 5.8 million heart failure patients in the United States alone.[1] Heart failure is the leading diagnosis among hospitalized patients in the United States and the number is increasing.[2] Clinically, heart failure is a complex disease process that results from a variety of conditions that prevent the left ventricle from properly filling and ejecting blood. Exacerbations of chronic heart failure are associated with high morbidity and mortality. In spite of major advances in the medical management of heart failure, challenges still remain in the timely diagnosis of acute heart failure. The use of biomarkers in acute heart failure stemmed from the need for a fast, objective and reliable test with high specificity and sensitivity to aide the diagnostic work-up of patients with acute dyspnea. Differentiating between pulmonary and cardiac causes of acute dyspnea has traditionally been a challenge as the history, physical examination, laboratory and radiographic findings of the two conditions have significant overlap. Delayed or erroneous diagnosis for acute heart failure not only increases morbidity and cost but also leads to increased mortality, making the accurate diagnosis imperative. Biomarkers with their objectivity, reproducibility and widespread availability have an indispensible role in assisting heart failure diagnosis and management.

Among the biomarkers available today, natriuretic peptides are probably the most validated and accepted in the diagnostic evaluation for acute heart failure. The relevant biomarkers in this peptide family are B-type natriuretic peptide (BNP), N-terminal pro-B-type natriuretic peptide (NT-proBNP), atrial natriuretic peptide (ANP), and mid-region proatrial natriuretic peptide (MR-proANP). BNP was first isolated from the porcine brain, leading to its original name "brain natriuretic peptide". BNP is a 32 amino acid peptide hormone with an *in vivo* half-life of 20 minutes. It is a cleavage product of NT-proBNP, which is a 76 amino acid peptide with an *in vivo* half-life of 120 minutes. NT-proBNP is a cleavage product of 134 amino acid pro-B-type natriuretic peptide. ANP is a 28 amino acid peptide hormone first isolated from the atrial tissue of rats. ANP is a cleavage product of the 126 amino acid precursor prohormone ANP (proANP).[3] MR-proANP is a cleavage fragment of proANP. ANP is made in the atria as well as the ventricles in humans, while BNP is made predominantly in the ventricles.[4] Among the four, BNP and NT-proBNP are more validated by clinical trials and more widely used in today's clinical practice. Physiologically, natriuretic peptides are protective hormones that counteract the physiologic abnormalities of heart failure. Their functions include increasing glomerular filtration rate, sodium and water excretion, vasodilation by relaxing arterioles and venules, diastolic relaxation, decreasing myocardial fibrosis, inhibiting cardiac hypertrophy, and inhibiting renin and aldosterone secretion. Natriuretic pepides are removed from circulation by receptor mediated degradation, proteolytic degradation by neutral endopeptidases and excretion by the kidneys. In general, BNP has much slower clearance than ANP. The circulating half-life of ANP is 3–5 minutes while the circulating half-life of BNP is about 20–30 minutes. NT-proBNP has a circulating half-life of 60–90 minutes. Comparing to ANP, MR-proANP is much more resistant to cleavage and has a considerably longer half-life.

Natriuretic peptides are released by the cardiac myocytes in response to increased wall stress caused by the volume expansion and pressure overload that accompanies heart failure. There were extensive studies correlating elevations of natriuretic peptide concentrations with increased central venous pressure, elevated pulmonary capillary wedge pressure (PCWP), and increased left ventricular wall stress.[5-8] For example, in a study by Ikeda et al., which examined patients undergoing aortic valve replacement for aortic stenosis, BNP concentrations correlated very well with left ventricular wall stress in both pre- and postoperative patients, demonstrating that BNP was a good biomarker for left ventricular wall stress. In a separate study by Yoshimura et al., significantly elevated natriuretic peptide levels were seen in patients with dilated cardiomyopathy. Furthermore, BNP levels correlated very well with PCWP, which was a direct measurement of left ventricular preload. Elevated PCWP has been associated with increased mortality in patients with dilated cardiomyopathy.[9] The reason BNP levels correlate so well with increased left ventricular wall stress and preload lies in its origin. BNP is produced mostly by the ventricles, with the left ventricle being the predominant source. Increased ventricular wall stress leads to upregulation of BNP and increased BNP production by ventricular myocytes. This upregulation can be seen histologically in patients with hypertrophic cardiomyopathy. Furthermore, the correlation between BNP and PCWP has been demonstrated clinically in patients treated for acute heart failure[10] (Figure 7-1). The strong correlation between elevated natriuretic peptides and PCWP provides the physiological basis for using natriuretic peptides in the diagnostic evaluation of patients with acute heart failure.

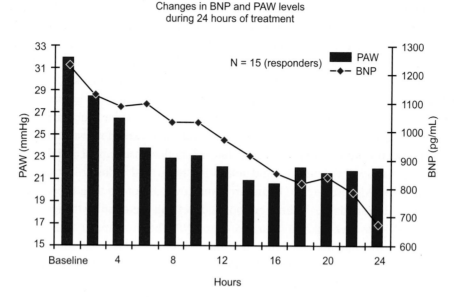

Figure 7-1 Correlation between BNP and pulmonary artery wedge pressure. BNP, B-type nitriuretic peptides; PAW, pulmonary artery wedge. *Adapted from* Kazanegra R, Cheng V, Garcia A, Krishnaswamy P, Gardetto N, Clopton P, et al. A rapid test for B-type natriuretic peptide correlates with falling wedge pressures in patients treated for decompensated heart failure: a pilot study. *J Card Fail.* 2001;7:21-9.

B-TYPE NATRIURETIC PEPTIDE

Although BNP was first isolated by Sudoh et al. in 1988, its role as a biomarker in acute heart failure was not established until 2002. The multicentre Breathing Not Properly trial by Maisel et al. was the first study to validate the effectiveness of BNP in the diagnostic work-up of patients presenting to the emergency department with acute dyspnea.[11] In this study, 1,586 patients with acute dyspnea as their chief complaint were enrolled from 7 international sites. Patients with cardiac temponade, myocardial infarction and renal failure were excluded. Blood samples were obtained during the time of initial presentation for BNP measurement. Patient clinical data including history, physical examination, laboratory data, chest roentgenogram, echocardiogram and other imaging studies were also collected at the time of enrollment. Initial diagnosis was made by emergency room physicians who were blinded to BNP measurements. Each case was reviewed by two cardiologists who were blinded to BNP measurements and the diagnosis by emergency department physicians. The cardiology reviewers determined if the dyspnea was due to acute heart failure or other causes based on the clinical information collected. There were 883 male and 773 female patients in this study. Acute heart failure was diagnosed in 744 patients.

In patients with acute heart failure, BNP levels were 675 ± 450 pg/mL while patients without heart failure had BNP levels of 110 ± 225 pg/mL. In this cohort, BNP was the single most accurate predictor of acute heart failure with an area under the receiver-operating characteristic curve (AUC) of 0.91 (95% confidence interval (CI): 0.90–0.93, $p < 0.001$). A BNP cutoff of 100 pg/mL had a sensitivity of 90%, specificity of 75%, and diagnostic accuracy of 83%. For the diagnosis of acute heart failure, BNP cutoff of 100 pg/mL was more accurate than MHANES criteria and Framingham criteria (67% and 73% respectively). BNP levels less than 50 pg/mL were associated with a negative predictive value of 96%. In multiple logistic-regression analysis, BNP with a cutoff of 100 pg/mL was the strongest independent predictor of acute heart failure with an odds ratio of 29.6. In this model, BNP also added significant additional prognostic information when it was entered after other clinical predictors of acute heart failure ($p < 0.001$) (Figure 7-2).

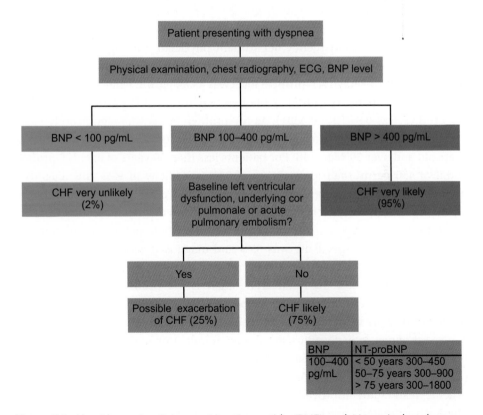

Figure 7-2 Algorithm using B-type natriuretic peptide (BNP) and N-terminal prohormone B-type natriuretic peptide (NT-proBNP) levels to rule in and rule out congestive heart failure (CHF). *Adapted from* Maisel A, et al. B-Type natriuretic peptide measurements in diagnosing congestive heart failure in the dyspneic emergency department patient. *Rev Cardiovasc Med.* 2002;3:S10-7.

N-TERMINAL PRO-B-TYPE NATRIURETIC PEPTIDE

Besides BNP, NT-proBNP was also studied extensively for the diagnostic evaluation of patients with acute dyspnea. In the PRIDE study by Januzzi et al., NT-proBNP was shown to be an effective biomarker for the diagnosis of acute heart failure.[12] This study included 599 patients presenting to a single medical center with the chief complaint of acute dyspnea. The study design was very similar to the Breathing Not Properly trial. Patients with severe renal insufficiency, dyspnea due to severe coronary ischemia, more than 2 hour delay after administration of urgent intravenous loop diuretics, and unblended natriuretic peptide measurements were excluded. Patient clinical information was recorded at the time of the initial evaluation. Blood samples were also collected from the initial visit for NT-proBNP measurement. The initial clinical assessment for the likelihood of acute heart failure was made by the emergency department physician, who was blinded to NT-proBNP measurements. The diagnosis of acute heart failure was confirmed by two cardiology reviewers who were blinded to NT-proBNP measurements and the diagnosis of the emergency department physician. Among the 599 patients enrolled, 209 had a final diagnosis of acute heart failure. Among patients with acute heart failure, the average NT-proBNP level was 4,054 pg/mL while the average NT-proBNP level in patients without acute heart failure was 131 pg/mL. The AUC for NT-proBNP was 0.94 (p < 0.0001). As NT-proBNP levels vary significantly based on age, optimal cutpoints for NT-proBNP were selected for patients less than 50 years old and over 50 years old. For patients less than 50 years of age, NT-proBNP cutoff of 450 pg/mL had a sensitivity of 93%, specificity of 95% and diagnostic accuracy of 95%. For patients over 50 years of age, a NT-proBNP cutoff of 900 pg/mL had a sensitivity of 91%, specificity of 80% and diagnostic accuracy of 85%. When the cutoff of 900 pg/mL was applied to the whole patient population, the sensitivity was 90%, specificity was 85% and diagnostic accuracy was 87%. NT-proBNP concentration less than 300 pg/mL had a sensitivity of 99% and negative predictive value of 99%. By multivariate analysis, NT-proBNP was the strongest predictor of acute HF with an odds ratio of 44.0 (p < 0.0001). Other independent predictors of acute heart failure in this cohort included pulmonary edema on chest X-ray, orthopnea, loop diuretic use, rales on examination and age. NT-proBNP was better than clinician estimated likelihood for the diagnosis of acute heart failure (AUC = 0.94 vs AUC = 0.90). Adding NT-proBNP to clinician estimated likelihood of acute heart failure improved the AUC from 0.90 to 0.96. Among patients with the physician estimated acute heart failure likelihood between 0% and 25%, NT-proBNP by optimal cutpoint had a sensitivity of 96% and specificity of 88% for acute heart failure. Among patients with physician estimated acute heart failure likelihood of 25–75%, NT-proBNP had a sensitivity of 93% and specificity of 85% for acute heart failure. In patients with physician estimated acute heart failure likelihood range of

> 75%, the sensitivity of NT-proBNP was 93% and specificity was 84% for acute heart failure.

ATRIAL NATRIURETIC PEPTIDE AND MID-REGION PROATRIAL NATRIURETIC PEPTIDE

Although both elevations of BNP and ANP have been associated with acute heart failure, ANP was inferior to BNP in head to head studies. For example, in one study by Cowie et al. in 1997, ANP was compared to BNP in 122 patients with new diagnosis of heart failure. The diagnosis of heart failure was made by cardiologists who took a standardized medical history and clinically examined each patient. The cardiologist also had access to electrocardiography, chest radiography, and transthoracic echocardiography. Blood samples were collected at the initial visit for standardized measurements of biomarkers. Out of the 122 patients there were 35 cases of acute heart failure. The AUC acute heart failure was 0.96 for BNP and 0.93 for ANP. The sensitivity for ANP was 97%, specificity 72%, and positive predictive value 55%. In comparison, the sensitivity of BNP was 97%, specificity 84%, and positive predictive value 70%.[13] The suboptimal result for ANP was due in part to its rapid clearance, which made reliable measurements difficult in typical clinical settings, thus limiting ANP's clinical application.

Recently, biochemical assays targeting a stable mid-region fragment of proANP, MR-proANP became available. MR-proANP is a much more stable and degradation resistant molecule than the active ANP with substantially longer serum half-life. The diagnostic utility of MR-proANP in acute heart failure was demonstrated in a large scale multinational study, Biomarker in Acute Heart Failure (BACH) trial, by Maisel et al. in 2008. The BACH trial was designed as a noninferiority study comparing MR-proANP to BNP for the diagnosis of acute heart failure.[14] One thousand six hundred and forty-one patients from 15 multinational centers in the United States, Europe and New Zealand with the chief complaint of acute dyspnea were enrolled in the study. Patients with myocardial infarction, renal failure and hemodialysis were excluded. The initial diagnosis was made prospectively by the emergency department physician who assessed the likelihood of acute heart failure on a visual analog scale. The gold standard diagnosis of acute heart failure was made retrospectively by two cardiologists who had full access to emergency department report forms, laboratory, imaging studies and diagnostic procedure reports. All blood samples for study biomarkers were collected at the time of initial enrollment and measured at a central laboratory. Among the 1,641 patients enrolled in the study, 568 had a final diagnosis of acute heart failure. The correlation between MR-proANP and both BNP and NT-proBNP was 0.92. The study was designed to show that MR-proANP at a predefined cutpoint of 120 pmol/L was noninferior to BNP at a predefined cutpoint of 100 pg/mL for the diagnosis of acute heart failure. BNP at

Table 7-1	MR-proANP vs BNP for Diagnosis of Acute Heart Failure in the Biomarkers in Acute Heart Failure (BACH) Trial		
Measure	*Sensitivity*	*Specificity*	*Accuracy*
MR-proANP 120 pmol/L	95.56	59.85	72.64
BNP 100 pg/mL	96.98	61.90	73.50
Difference	1.42	2.05	0.86
Upper 95% limit	2.82	3.84	2.10
Noninferiority p	<0.0001	<0.0001	<0.0001

Adapted from Maisel A, Mueller C, Nowak R, et al. Mid-region prohormone markers for diagnosis and prognosis in acute dyspnea: results from the BACH (Biomarkers in Acute Heart Failure) trial. *J Am Coll Cardiol.* 2010;55:2062-76.

the 100 pg/mL cutpoint had a sensitivity of 95.6%, specificity of 61.9%, diagnostic accuracy of 73.6%, positive predictive value of 57%, and a negative predictive value of 96.4%. In comparison, MR-proANP with a cutpoint of 120 pmol/L had a sensitivity of 97%, specificity of 59.9%, diagnostic accuracy of 72.7%, positive predictive value of 56%, and a negative predictive value of 97.4. MR-proANP was determined to be noninferior to BNP by preset criteria of 10% (Table 7-1). Furthermore, elevated MR-proANP added significantly to elevated BNP, increasing the C-statistic from 0.787 to 0.816 (p < 0.001). Requiring both MR-proANP and BNP to be elevated increased the overall diagnostic accuracy from 73.6% for BNP alone to 76.6% for the combined diagnosis. In patients with intermediate BNP levels and obesity, MR-proANP added incremental predictive value to a logistic regression model with BNP for the prediction of acute heart failure. In patients with intermediate NT-proBNP levels, renal insufficiency (creatinine > 1.6 mg/dL), obesity, age > 70 years and edema, MR-proANP added incremental predictive value to a logistic regression model with NT-proBNP for the prediction of acute heart failure. In the subgroup of patients where the emergency department physicians were uncertain of the diagnosis, defined as 20–80% probability of acute heart failure on the visual analog scale, the addition of MR-proANP reduced indecision by 29%. In summary, in this large scale study, MR-proANP was noninferior to BNP for the diagnosis of acute HF and added to the diagnostic utility of BNP and NT-proBNP in patients with intermediate BNP or NT-proBNP levels, renal insufficiency, obesity, age > 70 and edema.

CONCLUSION

Natriuretic peptides with their low cost, objectivity, reproducibility and accessibility are excellent adjuncts to physical examination, standard laboratory and imaging studies in diagnosing acute heart failure. By providing us with insight into one of the most important pathophysiologic processes in acute heart failure, natriuretic peptides have revolutionized the evaluation of the patients with acute dyspnea, improving diagnostic accuracy and efficiency of acute heart failure in a variety of clinical settings. With more experience in their clinical application, natriuretic peptides will undoubtedly continue to play a significant role in the evaluation and management of heart failure patients in the future.

REFERENCES

1. American Heart Association, Heart Disease and Stroke Statistics: 2010 Update, American Heart Association, Dallas, TX; 2010.
2. Haldeman GA, Croft JB, Giles WH, et al. Hospitalization of patients with heart failure: National Hospital Discharge Survey, 1985 to 1995. *Am Heart J.* 1999;137:352-60.
3. Xu-Cai YO, Wu Q. Molecular forms of natriuretic peptides in heart failure and their implications. *Heart.* 2010;96:419-24.
4. Yasue H, Yoshimura M, Sumida H, et al. Localization and mechanism of secretion of B-type natriuretic peptide in comparison with those of A-type natriuretic peptide in normal subjects and patients with heart failure. *Circulation.* 1994;90:195-203.
5. Ikeda T, Matsuda K, Itoh H, et al. Plasma levels of brain and atrial natriuretic peptides elevate in proportion to left ventricular end-systolic wall stress in patients with aortic stenosis. *Am Heart J.* 1997;133:307-14.
6. Yoshimura M, Yasue H, Okumura K, et al. Different secretion patterns of atrial natriuretic peptide and brain natriuretic peptide in patients with congestive heart failure. *Circulation.* 1993;87:464-9.
7. Lang CC, Choy AM, Turner K, et al. The effect of intravenous saline loading on plasma levels of brain natriuretic peptide in man. *J Hypertens.* 1993;11:737-41.
8. Haug C, Metzele A, Kochs M, et al. Plasma brain natriuretic peptide concentrations correlate with left ventricular end-diastolic pressure. *Clin Cardiol.* 1993;16:553-7.
9. Massie B, Ports T, Chatterjee K, et al. Long-term vasodilator therapy for heart failure: clinical response and its relationship to hemodynamic measurements. *Circulation.* 1981;63:269-78.
10. Kazanegra R, Cheng V, Garcia A, Krishnaswamy P, Gardetto N, Clopton P, et al. A rapid test for B-type natriuretic peptide correlates with falling wedge pressures in patients treated for decompensated heart failure: a pilot study. *J Card Fail.* 2001;7:21-9.
11. Maisel AS, Krishnaswamy P, Nowak RM, et al. Rapid measurement of B-type natriuretic peptide in the emergency diagnosis of heart failure. *N Engl J Med.* 2002;347:161-7.
12. Januzzi JL Jr, Camargo CA, Anwaruddin S, et al. The N-terminal Pro-BNP investigation of dyspnea in the emergency department (PRIDE) study. *Am J Cardiol.* 2005;95:948-54.
13. Cowie MR, Struthers AD, Wood DA, et al. Value of natriuretic peptides in assessment of patients with possible new heart failure in primary care. *Lancet.* 1997;350:1349-53.
14. Maisel A, Mueller C, Nowak R, et al. Mid-region pro-hormone markers for diagnosis and prognosis in acute dyspnea: results from the BACH (Biomarkers in Acute Heart Failure) trial. *J Am Coll Cardiol.* 2010;55:2062-76.

CHAPTER 8

Natriuretic Peptides in the Hospital: Risk Stratification and Treatment Titration

Arrash Fard, Pam R Taub,
Navaid Iqbal, Alan S Maisel

INTRODUCTION

Heart failure (HF) continues to place a tremendous burden on healthcare system. It is the leading cause of hospital admission in the US and the combined direct and indirect cost of heart failure to the US healthcare system was estimated to be \$34.8 billion in 2008.[1] Over the past few decades there have been major developments in the diagnosis, risk stratification and management of patients with heart failure. However, despite these efforts, the overall prognosis of these patients remains poor. This reflects the difficulties that arise when attempting to manage a condition with such a complex pathophysiology, variety of etiologies, and exacerbating factors.

Natriuretic peptides (NP), such as B-type natriuretic peptide (BNP) and N-terminal proBNP (NT-proBNP) have been at the forefront of the recent advances in HF management. These biomarkers have provided a diagnostic tool to reliably identify patients with acute dyspnea due to HF exacerbations and differentiate these patients from those with similar presenting complaints, such as chronic obstructive pulmonary disease (COPD). Since their adoption into the clinical practice of diagnosing HF, the roles of these two peptides have evolved into broader areas, such as prognosis and NP-guided treatment strategies.

The rationale in using NP levels to determine disease severity, guide treatment decisions, and assess treatment success lies in their physiology. NPs are released by the ventricular myocytes in response to wall stress caused by volume expansion or pressure overload that accompanies a variety of pathological processes. This knowledge is based on several studies that have correlated a rise in NP levels with elevated pulmonary capillary wedge pressure (PCWP), increased central venous pressure and increased left ventricular wall stress.[2-6] These peptides work to counteract the physiological abnormalities of HF and thus serve a protective purpose. Their functions include increasing glomerular filtration rate, increasing sodium and water excretion, increasing vasodilation by relaxing arterioles and venules, inhibiting cardiac hypertrophy, and inhibiting renin and aldosterone secretion.[7,8] In patients with heart failure, elevated PCWP is an important objective marker of fluid overload, especially of left ventricular preload. In fact, elevated PCWP is associated with increased mortality in this cohort.[9] The strong correlation between elevations of BNP and left ventricular wall stress and preload highlights the role of BNP as a surrogate marker for these processes, which are crucial pathophysiologic components of congestive heart failure.[10] From these relationships one can infer that because these biomarkers reflect the state and severity of disease, they can be used beyond diagnosis and into areas, such as prognosis and treatment.

This chapter will focus on the versatile role of natriuretic peptides in the inpatient setting. We will examine their ability to help distinguish those with more severe disease from milder cases at both admission and discharge. We will also consider ways in which NPs are incorporated into treatment titration. The evidence presented here will demonstrate the expanding uses of these peptides beyond diagnosis and highlight future applications.

NATRIURETIC PEPTIDES IN HOSPITAL: RISK STRATIFICATION AT PRESENTATION AND ADMISSION

The nature of chronic diseases, such as HF make it difficult to manage patients as outpatients for extended periods of time; due to periodic deterioration or exacerbation which results in readmission.[11] Therefore, there is an urgent need for simple measurements that allow for better risk stratification of those at risk for HF exacerbations. The NPs have proven useful as an adjunct tool to clinical judgment in the risk stratification of these HF patients. The ability to risk stratify patients early in their hospital stay can allow the clinician to construct a unique treatment plan tailored to fit each patient's disease process. These individualized treatments could not only decrease morbidity and mortality to the overall patient population but also alleviate superfluous costs to the overall health system. In practice, lower risk patients would need less intensive therapies and monitoring; thus they could remain in a standard ward or telemetry unit while those with a higher risk may be placed immediately in an intensive care unit bed with more aggressive therapies. Both BNP and NT-proBNP have shown the ability to enable such risk stratification strategies.

BNP

Numerous studies have been conducted recently to assess the ability of NPs to risk stratify patients at presentation and admission. A systematic review performed by Doust et al. demonstrated that BNP levels are better suited to predict mortality than other more traditional factors, such as age, left ventricular ejection fraction, New York Heart Association (NYHA) classification, and serum creatinine levels.[12] In fact, in 9 of the 35 multivariable models they analyzed, NPs were the only predictors that reached significance. In these studies, other prognostic markers provided no information beyond that given by NPs.[12] This paper also noted that even low concentrations of NPs (BNP > 20 pg/mL) in asymptomatic patients were associated with a twofold increase in relative risk of death during a four- to five-year follow-up period.[12] This implies that even subclinical NP elevation signifies some degree of hemodynamic stress leading to worse clinical outcomes. Therefore, even mild elevations of NPs at admission should get clinicians thinking of the diverse etiologies that can cause hemodynamic stress in patients with a variety of presenting complaints. This differential diagnosis should be formulated in the context of the multiple caveats in interpreting NP levels, such as obesity, poor renal function, and advancing age.

The Acute Decompensated Heart Failure National Registry (ADHERE) database of 65,275 ADHF patients showed that initial emergency department (ED) NP values can identify the risk of death or readmission within 30 days and that inpatient mortality can be related to admission BNP in a linear fashion.[13] The same registry showed that patients with a BNP at presentation > 1730 pg/mL had an inhospital mortality rate over three times greater than those with a BNP < 430 pg/mL (Figure 8-1). Interestingly, the ADHERE database analysis also showed the additive value of other markers, such as cardiac troponins. When combined with a positive troponin

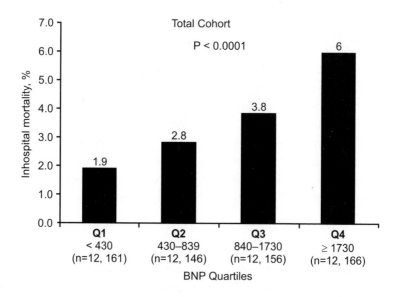

Figure 8-1 Inhospital mortality risk by initial BNP levels in the ADHERE registry database. 48,629 (63%) out of 77,467 patient episodes had BNP assessment at initial evalution. *From* Fonarow GC, Peacock WF, Phillips CO, Givertz MM, Lopatin M. Admission B-type natriuretic peptide levels and in-hospital mortality in acute decompensated heart failure. *J Am Coll Cardiol.* 2007;49:1943-50, with permission.

test, a BNP value > 840 pg/mL showed a 10.2% mortality rate while a negative troponin and BNP value < 840 pg/mL displayed a 2.2% mortality rate (or 5.10, p < 0.0001).[14] Findings, such as this help support not only the prognostic power of natriuretic peptides but also the evolving role of a multimarker approach for the management of HF.

NT-proBNP

NT-proBNP has also shown similar predictive abilities at patient presentation. Januzzi et al. demonstrated that an ED level of NT-proBNP > 986 pg/mL is indicative of severe heart failure and an adverse prognosis.[15] The IMPROVE-CHF study showed that knowing a patient's NT-proBNP level had benefits, including decreasing duration of the ED visit by 21% and rehospitalizations over 60 days by 35%, in addition to reducing overall medical costs.[16] Again we see that by making an accurate diagnosis and subsequently administering appropriate therapies, patient outcomes are improved.

These studies are just a few that show how powerful even a single measurement of NPs can be to correctly risk stratify patients presenting with decompensated HF. Therefore, in practice, a clinician should be aware that patient presenting with an elevated NP level is more likely have a worse outcome than one with a lower value with similar treatment. The use of NPs to identify high-risk patients will lead to better triaging and allocation of resources. This NP-guided approach provides a cost-effective and individually tailored approach to the HF patient.[17]

NATRIURETIC PEPTIDES IN HOSPITAL: TREATMENT TITRATION AND POST-DISCHARGE PROGNOSIS

In addition to helping risk stratify HF patients, NPs are important in determining optimal inpatient treatment strategies and therefore guide a patient's overall hospital course. Indeed, there is a growing pool of evidence to suggest that NPs should be used to direct treatment in acute HF and that NP values at discharge can predict the prognosis in this cohort of patients. If integrated into standard clinical practice, use of NPs could emerge as powerful tool to reduce hospital readmissions and overall mortality.

Study designs and results have varied as to what NP values to aim for while titrating therapy: some have focused on cut points that maximize their predictive properties while others have examined certain percentages of change from admission or baseline NP values. Despite the different focuses, many have found the predischarge NP level to be the best indicator of subsequent cardiac events, including readmission and mortality.[7] Both BNP and NT-proBNP have had favorable results in these studies, just as they did in admission risk stratification.

BNP

Strong evidence for the use of BNP-guided therapy came from a retrospective study of 186 patients by Valle et al. This study involved NYHA class III and IV HF patients admitted with acute exacerbations and included patients of both systolic and diastolic dysfunctions. After treatment utilizing standard guidelines, those deemed clinically stable and with BNP values < 250 pg/mL were discharged within 24 hours of that measurement. Those with clinical stability but with BNP values > 250 pg/mL were given more intensive therapy with prolonged intravenous diuretics, maximum ACE inhibitor doses and vasodilators (unless they showed signs of dehydration or kidney injury).[18] These patients were then discharged when deemed clinically stable despite what their new BNP values were at that time and followed up for six months for cardiac events. They found that BNP levels on admission and discharge were both significantly lower in those patients who did not have cardiac events. In fact, those with predischarge BNP values of < 250 pg/mL showed a much lower event rate (16%) than those with BNP values higher than that amount (57%, p = 0.0001). Overall, the BNP value on discharge had a receiver operating characteristics curve-area under curve (ROC-AUC) of 0.79 to discriminate between patients with events and those who were event-free in the six month window.[18]

Cheng et al. also used BNP and found that in patients admitted with decompensated HF, changes in BNP levels during treatment were strong predictors for mortality and early readmission. This study suggested that BNP levels might be utilized to effectively guide treatment of inpatients being that those who left with BNP < 430 pg/mL had a negative predictive value of 0.96 for readmission in 30 days. They also found that predischarge BNP concentrations predicted 30-day readmissions with a ROC-AUC of 0.73.[19]

Cournot and colleagues were one of the groups to analyze change in BNP in their study of 61 consecutive patients aged 70 and over presenting with acute decompensated heart failure. In a group with median BNP level of 1136 pg/mL at admission, they found their average change to be −32% during the course of hospitalization. The change in BNP values after in-hospital treatment was the strongest predictor of cardiac death or readmission. In fact, those patients who did not reach a decrease of at least −40% change from admission BNP had the worst prognosis (HR 4.03, 95% CI: 1.5–10.84 in multivariate analysis).[20] Overall, studies using BNP to guide treatment during hospitalization and risk stratify patients at discharge had favorable results whether they used cutoff values or percent change in NP concentration with treatment.

In another study, predischarge BNP levels in decompensated HF patients have been shown to be useful in predicting post-discharge outcomes. An elevated predischarge BNP level (> 700 pg/mL), an indication of subclinical pulmonary

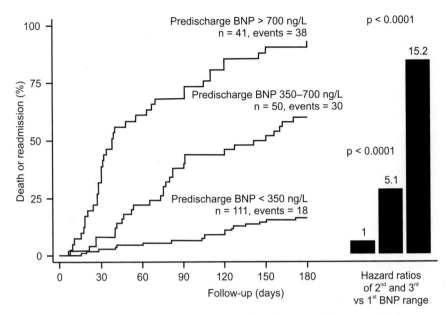

Figure 8-2 Cumulative incidence of death or readmission according to predischarge BNP. *From* Logeart D, Thabut G, Jourdain P, Chavelas C, Beyne P, Beauvais F, et al. Predischarge B-type natriuretic peptide assay for identifying patients at high risk of re-admission after decompensated heart failure. *J Am Coll Cardiol*. 2004;43:635-41, with permission.

congestion was an independent predictor of readmission and death. Patients with lower discharge BNP levels (< 350 pg/mL) were found to have a lower incidence of death and readmission (Figure 8-2).[21] Logeart et al. found predischarge BNP to have an AUC of 0.80 to reach this endpoint while remaining the only significant variable in multivariate analysis with a hazard ratio of 1.14 (95% CI: 1.02–1.28, p = 0.027). Furthermore, the adjusted hazard ratios for those with predischarge BNP values between 350 and 700 ng/mL and above 700 ng/mL were 5.1 (95% CI: 2.8–9.1) and 15.2 (95% CI: 8.5–27), respectively.[21] This study found very strong evidence of predischarge BNP's value as a prognostic and risk stratifying marker even more so than clinical or echocardiographic criteria.

NT-proBNP

Similar promising results have been found in studies centered around NT-proBNP as well. Bettencourt et al. demonstrated that admission and discharge NT-proBNP had the ability to predict subsequent hazard, including readmission for AHF or death. The strongest indicator was a post-treatment NT-proBNP value of 4137 ng/L; the data suggested an 8% increase in the likelihood of hazard over six months per every 1000 ng/L over this critical number.[22] In a later analysis, Bettencourt and Januzzi suggest that whenever possible to aim for a reduction in NT-proBNP of

≥ 30% from the admission level after treatment of AHF as these patients fared the best.[23] They found that those with a < 30% decrease in NT-proBNP had intermediate outcomes, while those with increased in their NP concentrations had very poor prognoses.[23]

Another study, this time by Bayes-Genis et al. also looked at NT-proBNP and focused on the degree of NP change from admission to discharge to predict outcomes. Their work indicated that those patients with larger changes in their NT-proBNP values during hospitalization (e.g., ≥ 50%) had fewer complications than those with smaller degrees of change (e.g., ≤ 15%). The AUC for the change in NT-proBNP in this study was a strong 0.78 (p = 0.002).[24]

THE CONCEPT OF "DRY" VERSUS "WET" NP IN HF

Patients with decompensated HF have a NP level that can be interpreted as having a baseline and a volume overloaded component: a "dry" and "wet" component, respectively.[25] The "dry" NP value represents the total baseline cardiac pathologies that a HF patient lives with day-to-day while "wet" value is the "dry" value plus the additional strain put on the myocardium during the decompensation episode[23] (Table 8-1). Having a "dry" NP level for a patient when their heart failure is stable can be extremely helpful in diagnosing decompensation episodes, assessing a patient's morbidity and mortality risks and providing treatment titration goals. In comparing decompensated ("wet") NP values to their stable baseline values, a clinician can determine how severe the current deterioration is and adjust the aggressiveness of therapy accordingly. NP levels that fail to decrease with appropriate therapy at discharge have been linked with a poor prognosis and these patients need to be treated as higher risk and be closely monitored going forward.[23]

NP LEVELS IN HOSPITAL: TRANSLATING LITERATURE INTO PRACTICE

The current general consensus in NP-guided treatment of heart failure in the hospital is to obtain a NP value with admission and again prior to discharge when

Table 8-1 "Wet" versus "Optivolemic" NP Levels	
Wet NP level	*Optivolemic NP level*
Any NP level 25–50% over what the patients optivolemic BNP level is	NP level once optimum fluid status is reached
If patient comes to ER, often > 600 pg/mL for BNP and > 900 pg/mL for NT-proBNP	Correlated with functional class and prognosis
Falls rapidly with treatment	May be 20–2,000 pg/mL-depending on severity of disease
	Falls slowly with treatment

the patient is deemed to be clinically optivolemic. Repeat NP levels are suggested if there is clinical deterioration in the patient or to perhaps evaluate the effectiveness of the current regimen.[23] Natriuretic peptides, while important in initiating and titrating therapy, seem to have their greatest powers of prediction and subsequent risk stratification in predischarge values.

While some trials have shown that the lower the discharge "dry" NP level, the lower the risk of readmission and death,[18] and the body of literature has been inconsistent. Still, an as low as possible NP level is a reasonable goal for a clinician to aim for, as this usually indicates a stable and compensated case of heart failure, because of the pathophysiologic properties mentioned above. Overall, the evidence indicates that a BNP level < 350–400 pg/mL or NT-proBNP level < 4000 pg/mL at discharge is generally linked to a stable post-hospital course. This is especially true if the patient is clinically optivolemic.[7] It is important to emphasize that NP levels should only be an adjunct to clinical acumen when treating heart failure and the physician's clinical skills are still as important as ever in managing these difficult patients. While these peptides can serve to aid clinicians in treating their patients, they are of course not meant to replace them. That being said, there are important caveats and special cases that will be discussed below.

Caveats and Nonresponders

In order to optimally use NPs in practice, the clinician must be aware of important properties that may alter their interpretation or limit their use. More specifically, the differential diagnosis of NP elevation (Table 8-2) and caveats of NP use (Table 8-3) should always be considered.

- *Obesity:* NP levels are lower in obese patients both with and without HF. The reason for this is that it may have to do with increased NP receptor-C clearance receptors on adipocytes. This is supported by the fact that obese patients have been shown to still have elevated levels of BNP and NT-proBNP's precursor proBNP despite having low levels of the active NPs. NP levels in obese patients should be doubled or even tripled to account for this discrepancy.[7]

- *Gray zone:* Often times moderate increases in NPs fall into the "gray zone" where the evidence is not as strong in supporting an acute HF diagnosis. In these cases, clinical acumen is especially important, and other causes of myocardial stress need to be considered, such as pulmonary hypertension, pulmonary embolism, arrhythmias, acute coronary syndrome, pneumonia, or COPD with cor pulmonale. In cases such as this, knowing a patient's optivolemic NP levels can greatly aid a clinician in determining the occurrence and severity of an acute exacerbation.

- *Renal disease:* Renal disease can influence NP values through several mechanisms, including decreased clearance from low GFR or even counter-regulatory

Table 8-2	Differential Diagnosis of Elevated NP Levels
Acute and chronic heart failure	Pulomonary heart disease/right heart dysfunction
Acute coronary syndrome	Pulmonary embolism

Valvular diseases
  Aortic stenosis
  Mitral stenosis
	Pulmonary hypertension
	Obstructive sleep apnea

Atrial fibrillation	Primary pulmonary diseases COPD

Myocardial diseases
  Hypertrophic cardiomyopathy
  Infiltrative cardiomyopathy
  Apical ballooning syndrome
  Inflammatory disease, including
    myocarditis and chemotherapy
	Asthma
	ARDS
	
	Congenital heart disease
	Stroke

High-output
  Sepsis
  Burns
  Hyperthyroidism
  Cirrhosis	

Table 8-3	Caveats in Using NP Levels	
Low NP levels	*Normal NP levels*	*Factors increasing baseline NP levels*
Anemia	Flash pulmonary edema	Advancing age
Obesity	Acute mitral valve rupture	Female gender
	Constrictive pericarditis	Chronic kidney disease
	Cardiac tamponade	

responses from the cardiorenal syndrome. It has been suggested that NP cutoffs for patients with a GFR < 60 mL/min may need to be raised. Detailed knowledge of a patient's renal function is important with any NP assessment.

The possibility remains that even with recommended inhospital treatment; a patient's NP value could remain elevated. There could be multiple reasons for this situation. First, the high NP value could reflect the patient's optivolemic or "dry" NP level caused by chronic HF and therefore constantly increased ventricular wall stress. Second, excessive treatment with diuretics may have caused the patient to enter a prerenal state leading to acute kidney injury and a decreased glomerular filtration rate (GFR). Because NPs are partly cleared by the kidney, the decreased GFR can lead to increased serum concentrations of the peptides. Another possibility could involve the patient with concurrent right heart failure leading to significant edema and even ascites. This third space fluid accretion would allow the clinician to diurese large amounts of fluid before intravascular pressure would be reduced and thus ventricular wall stress would remain elevated for a longer duration of therapy. Finally, there is of course the possibility that the treatment does not work properly and cardiovascular pressures are not adequately reduced.[7]

CONCLUSION

Utilization of NP levels in the inpatient setting is a valuable tool to risk stratify HF patients and determine whether inpatients' hospital stay should be lengthened or if more aggressive treatment is warranted.

Currently, the mainstay of treatment for HF revolves around lifestyle modifications (e.g., decreased salt intake), pharmacological and device therapies. The pharmacological treatment for heart failure involves combinations of medications with proven mortality benefit, such as angiotensin-converting enzyme inhibitors, angiotensin II receptor blockers (ARBs), beta blockers, and aldosterone antagonists; as well as those with symptomatic benefits, e.g., diuretics and vasodilators [SOURCE POSS GUIDELINES]. The manner in which these drugs are used and titrated is a matter of the clinician's personal preference because much of the patient assessment is done in a subjective manner. Therefore, this assessment and its subsequent therapies can vary from clinician to clinician. With the use of biomarkers to guide therapies, these patient evaluations can take a more objective route. This could lead to more effective therapies by helping standardized patient analysis yet still offer personalized medical care based on the degree of biomarker elevations added to clinical decompensation assessments.

With a complex condition, such as heart failure, inherent difficulties will arise in risk stratification and therapy titration. The medical community worldwide truly needs assistance in tackling these challenges due to both the increased mortality and financial burden attributed to the disease. Ideally, a cost-effective and standardized biomarker could help provide added clinical assessment as well as directing treatments that are as unique as each patient dealing with the condition. While still more research needs to be performed, there is a strong indication that we may already have powerful tools with the NPs to help solve this dilemma. Indeed, the natriuretic peptides have shown an early ability to be exactly the biomarkers that we require.

REFERENCES

1. American Heart Association. *Heart Disease and Stroke Statistics- 2008 Update.* Dallas, Texas: American Heart Association; 2008.
2. Ikeda T, Matsuda K, Itoh H, Shirakami G, Miyamoto Y, Yoshimasa T, et al. Plasma levels of brain and atrial natriuretic peptides elevate in proportion to left ventricular endsystolic wall stress in patients with aortic stenosis. *Am Heart J.* 1997;133:307-14.
3. Yoshimura M, Yasue H, Okumura K, Ogawa H, Jougasaki M, Mukoyama M, et al. Different secretion patterns of atrial natriuretic peptide and brain natriuretic peptide in patients with congestive heart failure. *Circulation.* 1993;87:464-9.

4. Yasue H, Yoshimura M, Sumida H, Kikuta K, Kugiyama K, Jougasaki M, et al. Localization and mechanism of secretion of B-type natriuretic peptide in comparison with those of A-type natriuretic peptide in normal subjects and patients with heart failure. *Circulation.* 1994;90:195-203.

5. Lang CC, Choy AM, Turner K, Tobin R, Coutie W, Struthers AD. The effect of intravenous saline loading on plasma levels of brain natriuretic peptide in man. *J Hypertens.* 1993; 11:737-41.

6. Haug C, Metzele A, Kochs M, Hombach V, Grünert A. Plasma brain natriuretic peptide concentrations correlate with left ventricular end-diastolic pressure. *Clin Cardiol.* 1993; 16:553-7.

7. Maisel A, Mueller C, Adams K Jr, Anker SD, Aspromonte N, Cleland JG, et al. State of the art: using natriuretic peptide levels in clinical practice. *Eur J Heart Fail.* 2008;10:824-39. Epub 2008 Aug 29. Review.

8. Xue Y, Chan J, Sakariya S, Maisel A. Biomarker-guided treatment of congestive heart failure. *Congest Heart Fail.* 2010;16:S62-7.

9. Massie B, Ports T, Chatterjee K, Parmley W, Ostland J, O'Young J, et al. Longterm vasodilator therapy for heart failure: clinical response and its relationship to hemo-dynamic measurements. *Circulation.* 1981;63:269-78.

10. Yamamoto K, Burnet JC Jr, Jougasaki M, Nishimura RA, Bailey KR, Saito Y, et al. Superiority of brain natriuretic peptide as a hormonal marker of ventricular systolic and diastolic dysfunction and ventricular hypertrophy. *Hypertension.* 1996;28:988-94.

11. Westert GP, Lagoe RJ, Keskimäki I, Leyland A, Murphy M. An international study of hospital readmissions and related utilization in Europe and the USA. *Health Policy.* 2002;61:269-78.

12. Doust JA, Pietrzak E, Dobson A, Glasziou P. How well does B-type natriuretic peptide predict death and cardiac events in patients with heart failure: a systematic review. *BMJ.* 2005;330:625-34.

13. Fonarow GC, Peacock WF, Phillips CO, Givertz MM, Lopatin M. Admission B-type natriuretic peptide levels and in-hospital mortality in acute decompensated heart failure. *J Am Coll Cardiol.* 2007;49:1943-50.

14. Fonarow GC, Peacock WF, Horwich TB, Phillips CO, Givertz MM, Lopatin M, et al. Usefulness of B-type natriuretic peptide and cardiac troponin levels to predict in-hospital mortality from ADHERE. *Am J Cardiol.* 2008;101:231-7.

15. Januzzi JL Jr, Sakhuja R, O'donoghue M, Baggish AL, Anwaruddin S, Chae CU, et al. Utility of amino-terminal pro-brain natriuretic peptide testing for prediction of 1-year mortality in patients with dyspnea treated in the emergency department. *Arch Intern Med.* 2006;166:315-20.

16. Moe GW, Howlett J, Januzzi JL, Zowall H. N-terminal pro-B-type natriuretic peptide testing improves the management of patients with suspected acute heart failure: primary results of the Canadian prospective randomized multicenter IMPROVE-CHF study. *Circulation.* 2007;115:3103-10.

17. Mueller C, Laule-Kilian K, Schindler C, Klima T, Frana B, Rodriguez D, et al. Cost-effectiveness of B-type natriuretic peptide testing in patients with acute dyspnea. *Arch Intern Med.* 2006;166:1081-7.

18. Valle R, Aspromonte N, Giovinazzo P, Carbonieri E, Chiatto M, di Tano G, et al. B-type natriuretic Peptide-guided treatment for predicting outcome in patients hospitalized in sub-intensive care unit with acute heart failure. *J Card Fail.* 2008;14:219-24.

19. Cheng V, Kazanagra R, Garcia A, Lenert L, Krishnaswamy P, Gardetto N, et al. A rapid bedside test for B-type peptide predicts treatment outcomes in patients admitted for decompensated heart failure: a pilot study. *J Am Coll Cardiol.* 2001;37:386-91.

20. Cournot M, Leprince P, Destrac S, Ferrières J. Usefulness of in-hospital change in B-type natriuretic peptide levels in predicting long-term outcome in elderly patients admitted for decompensated heart failure. *Am J Geriatr Cardiol.* 2007;16:8-14.

21. Logeart D, Thabut G, Jourdain P, Chavelas C, Beyne P, Beauvais F, et al. Predischarge B-type natriuretic peptide assay for identifying patients at high risk of re-admission after decompensated heart failure. *J Am Coll Cardiol.* 2004;43:635-41.

22. Bettencourt P, Azevedo A, Pimenta J, Frioes F, Ferreira S, Ferreira A. N-terminal-pro-brain natriuretic peptide predicts outcome after hospital discharge in heart failure patients. *Circulation.* 2004;110:2168-74.

23. Bettencourt P, Januzzi JL Jr. Amino-terminal pro-B-type natriuretic peptide testing for inpatient monitoring and treatment guidance of acute destabilized heart failure. *Am J Cardiol.* 2008;101:67-71.

24. Bayes-Genis A, Santalo-Bel M, Zapico-Muniz E, Lopez L, Cotes C, Bellido J, et al. N-terminal probrain natriuretic peptide (NT-proBNP) in the emergency diagnosis and inhospital monitoring of patients with dyspnoea and ventricular dysfunction. *Eur J Heart Fail.* 2004;6:301-8.

25. Maisel AS. Use of BNP Levels in monitoring hospitalized heart failure patients with heart failure. *Heart Fail Rev.* 2003;8:339-44.

Natriuretic Peptides in the Outpatient Setting

Anna McDivit, Leo Slavin,
Mark Richards, Alan S Maisel

INTRODUCTION

Despite many advances, heart failure (HF) remains a leading cause of death, hospitalization, and rehospitalization. The use of natriuretic peptides (NP) has gained widespread acceptance for diagnosis and prognosis in the emergency department and hospital setting.[1-4] Whether clinicians need a biomarker to guide outpatient heart failure therapy continues to be an issue of considerable debate.

RATIONALE FOR USE OF BIOMARKERS TO GUIDE HF THERAPY

On an individual level, both B-type natriuretic peptide (BNP) and N-terminal-pro-BNP (NT-proBNP) are reasonable correlates of wedge pressure and NYHA class association, and are superior to ejection fraction for risk stratification.[3,5,6] In the Val-HeFT (Valsartan Heart Failure Trial) neurohormonal substudy,[7,8] comparison of BNP and NT-proBNP demonstrated that both were powerfully and similarly related to mortality and risk of admission with acute decompensated HF. Change in BNP or NT-proBNP over time was more predictive of outcomes than single values of NPs. Heart failure therapies proven to have beneficial long-term effects on mortality, such as ACE inhibitors (ACE-I), angiotensin receptor blockers (ARB), beta blockers, aldosterone antagonists, and cardiac resynchronization therapy generally decrease natriuretic peptide levels over time.[9-12] As patients with falling NP levels have a better outcome than those whose levels do not fall over time, it is intuitive to titrate HF therapy guided by NP levels.

NP-GUIDED THERAPY TRIALS

The efficacy of measuring serial NPs to guide the titration of standard HF therapy has been the subject of several randomized control trials. The first studies using BNP and NT-proBNP to tailor HF treatment came out in the late 1990s.[9,13] Since then, there have been several other studies with variable study designs, patient populations, and end-points (Table 9-1). Many of these studies were relatively small and some had

Table 9-1 Summary of NP-guided Therapy Trials

	Troughton[13]	STARS-BNP[14]	STAR-BRITE[15]	TIME-CHF[16]	BATTLE-SCARRED[17]	PRIMA[18]	Berger[19]	PROTECT[20]	NORTH-STAR[22]
N	69	220	137	499	364	345	278	151	407
NP	NT-proBNP*	BNP	BNP	NT-proBNP	NT-proBNP	NT-proBNP	BNP	NT-proBNP	NT-proBNP
Strategy for NP-group	Target NT-proBNP < 1,692 pg/mL	Target BNP < 100 pg/mL	Target BNP value chosen at hospital discharge	Target NT-proBNP < 400 pg/mL for age < 75; < 800 pg/mL for age ≥ 75	Target NT-proBNP < 1,270 pg/mL	NT-proBNP at discharge from hospital	HF specialist target BNP < 2,200 pg/mL before nurse-supervised therapy	Target NT-proBNP ≤ 1000 pg/mL	Stable outpatients with NT-proBNP ≥ 1,000 pg/mL, if > 30%, titration protocol
Control	Heart failure score	Usual care, BNP measurement not allowed	Congestion score	Target symptoms NYHA class II	Usual care or intensive clinical care base on heart failure score	Usual care	Usual care	Usual care	Usual care, half with routine NT-proBNP, half without
Follow-up	9.6 mon	15 mon	3 mon	18 mon	≥ 12 mon	≥ 12 mon	12 mon	10 mon	2.5 yr
Primary endpoint	Death + cardiovascular hospitalization + outpatient HF event	HF death + HF hospitalization	Total days alive and out of hospital	Death + all cause mortality	All-cause mortality	Days alive and out of hospital	Death + HF readmission	Cardiovascular events	All-cause mortality + cardiovascular hospitalization

Continued

Continued

	Troughton[13]	STARS-BNP[14]	STAR-BRITE[15]	TIME-CHF[16]	BATTLE-SCARRED[17]	PRIMA[18]	Berger[19]	PROTECT[20]	NORTH-STAR[22]
Age (mean, yr)	70	66	61	77	76	72	71	63	68
LVEF	27%	31%	20%	30%	37%	33%	Majority < 35%	28%	32%
Result	Statistically significant difference in primary endpoint in favor of NP-guided therapy	Statistically significant difference in primary endpoint in favor of NP-guided therapy	No significant difference in primary endpoint	No significant difference in primary endpoint; mortality benefit < 75 years in NP-guided group	Statistically significant difference in primary endpoint in favor of NP-guided therapy in ≤ 75-year olds at 3 years	No significant difference in primary endpoint	Statistically significant difference in primary endpoint in favor of NP-guided therapy	Statistically significant difference in primary endpoint in favor of NP-guided therapy	No significant difference in primary endpoint

*BNP, 100 pg/mL ~ 22 pmol/L; NT-proBNP, 300 pg/mL ~ 35 pmol/L.

nonsignificant results, but in aggregate, as seen in two recent meta-analyses, they show a trend towards mortality benefit and reduction in HF hospitalization with use of NP-guided outpatient therapy. This trend was seen particularly in patients who are < 75 years old and have depressed left ventricular function.

The first study to examine NP-guided therapy in HF patients was performed by Troughton et al.[13] in Christchurch, New Zealand. They recruited 69 patients with a left ventricular ejection fraction (LVEF) < 40% and a hospital admission for acute decompensated HF. Patients were randomized to NP-guided therapy or to a clinical-guided group. The NP-guided group used NT-proBNP < 1691 pg/mL as a cut-point for therapy titration, while the clinical-guided group used an objective HF score to guide treatment. Drug treatment was intensified according to an algorithm, which did not include beta blockers, as they were not standard of care at that time. The primary end-point was total cardiovascular events (cardiovascular death plus hospital admission for any cardiovascular event), which occurred less in the NP-guided group (19 vs 54 events, p = 0.02). Follow-up was an average of 9.6 months. The mean age was 70 years and the mean LVEF was 27%. After multivariate regression analysis, biomarker-guided therapy demonstrated a beneficial effect on the primary end-point (p < 0.001). Although the event rate of this study was low, the findings prompted several further interventional trials.

STARS-BNP[14] was a study conducted at 17 centers and included 220 patients with NYHA class II-III HF with an LVEF of < 45%. Patients were randomized to NP-guided versus clinical-guided therapy. The goal in patients randomized to the NP-guided arm was to intensify medical therapy until the BNP was < 100 pg/mL. Patients in the clinical-guided group had therapy titrated based on standardized clinical examinations. Patients were seen every month for the first three months, and then every four months afterward. They were followed for a total of 15 months. The mean age was 65 years. The primary composite endpoint of HF hospitalization or HF death was observed in 25 of 110 (24%) in the NP-guided group versus 57 of 110 (52%) in the clinical-guided group (p < 0.001). Furthermore, BNP guidance resulted in more frequent changes (134 vs 66) and intensification of neurohormal therapy. This study suggested that NP-guided therapy may result in improved utilization of evidence-based therapy, in turn associated with better outcomes.

The STARBRITE (Strategies for Tailoring Advanced Heart Failure Regimens in the Outpatient Setting: Brain Natriuretic Peptide versus the Clinical Congestion Score) trial[15] examined the effect of titrating therapy to individualized serial BNPs with point-of-care testing. In this study of 137 patients, a target BNP value was chosen for each patient at hospital discharge and standard HF therapy was up-titrated to achieve a reduction in BNP. The NP-guided arm was compared to a clinical-guided arm that used a congestion score to guide up-titration of therapy. The mean age was 61 years. At 3 months, there was no significant difference in the primary endpoint, which was number of days alive and outside of the hospital (NP-guided group 85 ± 12 days versus clinical-guided group 80 ± 21 days; HR 0.72, 95% CI: 0.47–1.27, p = 0.25), however, there was a favorable trend. Importantly, the NP-guided arm achieved higher doses of ACE inhibitors (p = 0.03) and beta-blockers (p = 0.08), as target doses reported in clinical trials are routinely not achieved in real practice. The low event rate and short follow-up period may have prevented a detectable difference in the primary endpoint between the two groups.

TIME-CHF (Trial of Intensified versus Standard Medical Therapy in Elderly Patients with Congestive Heart Failure)[16] was a European trial of 499 patients, including those with preserved and reduced LVEF. The patients were > 60 years old with a mean age of 76 years, and reflective of a typical HF population with a high prevalence of ischemic heart disease, hypertension, and diabetes. Patients were stratified by age and randomized to HF therapy guided by NT-proBNP < 400 pg/mL, if they were < 75 years, and < 800 pg/mL, if ≥ 75 years, or to symptom-guided therapy. Patients were followed for 18 months. So far, only data from the subset of patients with reduced systolic function have been published. The primary endpoints were all-cause hospital admissions, and quality of life. There was no significant difference between groups in either of the primary endpoints, however, the secondary endpoint, survival free from hospitalization, was higher in the NP-guided group (HR 0.68; 95% CI: 0.50–0.92, p = 0.01). Of note, NP-guided therapy improved survival free from hospitalization in patients 60–75 years but not those ≥ 75 years (p = 0.02 for interaction).

BATTLESCARRED (NT-proBNP-Assisted Treatment to Lessen Serial Cardiac Readmissions and Death)[17] was a trial of 364 outpatients with HF randomized to one of three treatment strategies: usual care, or intensified care either with or without NP. The goal was to drive NT-proBNP below 1,270 pg/mL. The mean age of patients in this study was 76 years, and patients with both preserved and reduced systolic ejection fraction were included. Patients were followed for three years. The 1-year mortality was less in both the NP-guided (9.1%) and clinical-guided groups (9.1%) versus the usual care group (18.9%, p = 0.03). The 3-year mortality was reduced only in patients ≤ 75 years in the NP-guided group (15.5%) compared to the clinically-guided group (30.9%, p = 0.048) or usual care (31.3%, p = 0.021). BATTLESCARRED did not show any difference in ACE inhibitor or beta blocker doses achieved, but frequency of drug dose changes was significantly greater in the NP-guided group. Similar to the observation in TIME-CHF, younger patients (60–75 years) had a mortality benefit with NP-guided therapy compared to those > 75 years old.

PRIMA (Can Pro-brain-natriuretic Peptide Guided Therapy of Chronic Heart Failure Improve Heart Failure Morbidity and Mortality?)[18] was a study with a unique trial design from the Netherlands, of 345 patients recruited after admission to the hospital for acute decompensated HF and elevated NT-proBNP (> 1700 pg/mL) with a fall of at least 10% and 850 pg/mL during hospitalization. Patients were randomized to clinical-guided therapy or an individually set BNP level identified as the lowest level obtained between discharge and the following two weeks. The median target BNP was 2,491 pg/mL. The median follow-up was 702 days. There was a trend towards a significant reduction in the primary endpoint, which was days alive and out of the hospital: 685 in the NP-guided group versus 664 in the clinical-guided group (p = 0.49). There was also a trend towards reduced mortality with NP-guided therapy [46 (26%) vs 57 (33%), p = 0.206]. The trend towards fever deaths in the NP-guided group was seen particularly in a subgroup of patients who were < 75 years and with LVEF < 45%. More patients in the NP-guided group had higher doses ACE inhibitors and beta blockers.

Berger et al.[19] recently published a study of 278 patients who were randomized in eight Viennese hospitals to one of three groups: usual care, nurse-supervised management, or specialist-supervised management with frequent initial visits for titration of treatment. In the latter group, the goal was for the specialist's intensive titration of therapy to achieve a BNP < 2,200 pg/mL before the transfer to nurse-guided care. After 12 months, the NP-guided group had less days of HF hospitalization (488 days) compared with nurse-guided care (1,254 days) and usual care (1,588 days) groups (p < 0.0001). The combined endpoint of death or HF readmission was also lower in the NP-guided (37%) than in the nurse-guided group (50%; p < 0.05) and in the nurse-guided than in the usual care group (65%; p < 0.04). Death rates were similar between NP-guided (22%) and nurse-guided (22%) groups and both were lower than in usual care (39%; p < 0.02 compared with both other groups). The NP-guided group had the highest proportion of individuals receiving triple-therapy with ACEI or ARB, beta blocker and aldosterone antagonists.

PROTECT (Pro-B Type Natriuretic Peptide Outpatient Tailored Chronic Heart Failure Therapy)[20,21] was a single center, open-label trial including 151 patients with LVEF ≤ 40%. Patients were randomized to standard guideline-driven HF therapy or NP-guided therapy with a target NT-proBNP of ≤ 1,000 pg/mL. Patients were followed for ten months. The primary composite endpoint of total cardiovascular events was seen less in the NP-guided group compared to the standard care group (58 vs 100 events, p = 0.009). Discrete endpoints, such as worsening HF and admission for HF were significantly reduced in the NP-guided arm (p = 0.001 and 0.002, respectively). The patient population was relatively young (mean age 63) with a low annualized mortality and only 10 cardiovascular deaths in the overall study population. However, the benefit of NP-guided therapy, unlike in other trials, was maintained in patients > 75 years of age.

The NorthStar study (NT-proBNP Stratified Follow-up in Outpatient Heart Failure Clinics)[22,23] was a large Danish study that took a subgroup of 407 clinically stable, educated, and medically optimized patients with HF and NT-proBNP levels ≥ 1,000 pg/mL to assess the benefits from long-term follow-up in a specialized HF clinic and the efficacy of NT-proBNP monitoring. Roughly, half were followed without any subsequent, routine measurement of NT-proBNP levels, while the other half had NT-proBNP measurements at every follow-up visit to the clinic. If there was a greater than 30% increase from one clinic visit to the next, the clinic staff followed a protocol for titration of HF therapy. Patients were followed for 2.5 years. The results of this study have not been published but were recently presented at a national meeting.[23] The primary endpoint, which was the combined rate of all-cause mortality or cardiovascular hospitalization, was similar in both groups. The HF patients enrolled in this study were relatively compensated and the primary purpose of the study was to determine if patients benefit from management by specialized HF clinics; thus, this study question was different from those that evaluated HF patients who were recently discharged from the hospital.

There have been two meta-analyses[24,25] done to address the issue of inadequate power by many of these small studies. These both showed a 30% reduction in mortality using NP-guided treatment compared to usual care. The first meta-analysis by Felker et al.[24] published in 2009 includes six trials with a total of 1,627 patients. Pooled analysis showed a significant mortality advantage for NP-guided therapy (HR 0.69; 95% CI: 0.55–0.86) compared to control. The second meta-analysis by Porapakkham et al.[25] published in 2010 included eight trials with a total of 1,726 patients. Again, there was an overall significantly lower risk of all-cause mortality (RR 0.76; 95% CI: 0.63–0.91, p = 0.003) with NP-guided therapy. However, in the subgroup analysis of patients < 75 years, all-cause mortality was significantly lower in the NP-guided group (RR 0.52; 95% CI: 0.33–0.82, p = 0.005), while there was no reduction in mortality in patients ≥ 75 years (RR 0.94; 95% CI: 0.71–1.25, p = 0.70). All-cause hospitalization and survival free of hospitalization were not significantly different between the two groups.

Despite the heterogeneity of trial design, including the use of different NP assays, different NP target levels, and different patient populations, there appears to be a pattern that has emerged from the NP-guided therapy trials. Patients with HF requiring admission to the hospital, who receive NP-guided therapy at the time of discharge, are more likely to achieve higher doses of evidence-based neurohormonal therapy. In addition, patients < 75 years old with reduced LVEF appear to have a significant survival benefit from NP-guided outpatient therapy. There remains a need for a well-powered, well-designed trial to confirm the efficacy of this NP-guided treatment strategy. Further studies are needed to better understand the advantage of a preset population-based cut-point for BNP or NT-proBNP versus an individualized NP level based also upon age and LVEF, to guide HF therapy.

REFERENCES

1. Maisel AS, Krishnaswamy P, Nowak RM, McCord J, Hollander JE, Duc P, et al. Rapid measurement of B-type natriuretic peptide in the emergency diagnosis of heart failure. *N Engl J Med.* 2002;347:161-7.

2. Januzzi JL Jr, Camargo CA, Anwaruddin S, Baggish AL, Chen AA, Krauser DG, et al. The N-terminal Pro-BNP Investigation of dyspnea in the emergency department (PRIDE) study. *Am J Cardiol.* 2005;95:948-54.

3. Januzzi JL, van Kimmenade R, Lainchbury J, Bayes-Genis A, Ordonez-Llanos J, Santalo-Bel M, et al. NT-proBNP testing for diagnosis and short-term prognosis in acute destabilized heart failure: an international pooled analysis of 1256 patients. The International Collaborative of NT-proBNP (ICON) Study. *Eur Heart J.* 2006;27:330-7.

4. Heart Protection Study Collaborative Group, Emberson JR, Ng LL, Armitage J, Bowman L, Parish S, Collins R. N-Terminal Pro-B-Type Natriuretic Peptide, Vascular Disease Risk, and Cholesterol Reduction Among 20,536 Patients in the MRC/BHF heart protection study. *J Am Coll Cardiol.* 2007;49:311-19.

5. Maisel A, Hollander JE, Guss D, McCullough P, Nowak R, Green G, et al. Primary results of the Rapid Emergency Department Heart Failure Outpatient (REDHOT). A multicenter study of B-type natriuretic peptide levels, emergency department decision making, and outcomes in patients presenting with shortness of breath. *J Am Coll Cardiol.* 2004;44:1328-33.

6. Kazanegra R, Cheng V, Garcia A, Krishnaswamy P, Gardetto N, Clopton P, et al. A rapid test for B-type natriuretic peptide correlates with falling wedge pressures in patients treated for decompensated heart failure: a pilot study. *J Card Fail.* 2001;7:21-9.

7. Latini R, Masson S, Anand I, Judd D, Maggioni AP, Chiang YT, et al. Effects of valsartan on circulating brain natriuretic peptide and norepinephrine in symptomatic chronic heart failure. The Valsartan Heart Failure Trial (Val-HeFT). *Circulation.* 2002;106:2454-8.

8. Masson S, Latini R, Anand IS, Barlera S, Angelici L, Vago T, et al. Prognostic value of changes in N-terminal pro-brain natriuretic peptide in Val-HeFT (Valsartan Heart Failure Trial). *J Am Coll Cardiol.* 2008;52:997-1003.

9. Murdoch DR, McDonagh TA, Byrne J, Blue L, Farmer R, Morton JJ, et al. Titration of vasodilator therapy in chronic heart failure according to plasma brain natriuretic peptide concentration: randomized comparison of the hemodynamic and neuroendocrine effects of tailored versus empirical therapy. *Am Heart J.* 1999;355:1126-32.

10. Frantz RP, Olson LJ, Grill D, Moualla SK, Nelson SM, Nobrega TP, et al. Carvedilol therapy is associated with a sustained decline in brain natriuretic peptide levels in patients with congestive heart failure. *Am Heart J.* 2005;149:541-7.

11. Troughton RW, Richards AM, Yandle TG, Frampton CM, Nicholls MG. The effects of medications on circulating levels of cardiac natriuretic peptides. *Ann Med.* 2007;39: 242-60.

12. Fruhwald FM, Fahrleitner-Pammer A, Berger R, Leyva F, Freemantle N, Erdmann E, et al. Early and sustained effects of cardiac resynchronization therapy on N-terminal pro-B-type natriuretic peptide in patients with moderate to severe heart failure and cardiac dyssynchrony. *Eur Heart J.* 2007;28:1592-7.

13. Troughton RW, Frampton CM, Yandle TG, Espiner EA, Nicholls MG, Richards AM. Treatment of heart failure guided by plasma amino-terminal brain natriuretic peptide (N-BNP) concentrations. *Lancet.* 2000;355:1126-30.

14. Jourdain P, Jondeau G, Funck F, Gueffet P, Le Helloco A, Donal E, et al. Plasma brain natriuretic peptide-guided therapy to improve outcome in heart failure: the STARS-BNP Multicenter Study. *J Am Coll Cardiol.* 2007;49:1733-9.

15. Shah MR, Califf RM, Nohria A, Bhapkar M, Bowers M, Mancini DM, et al. The STARBRITE investigators. STARBRITE: a Randomized Pilot Trial of BNP-Guided Therapy in Patients with Advanced Heart Failure. *J Card Fail.* 2011;17:613-21.

16. Pfisterer M, Buser P, Rickli H, Gutmann M, Erne P, Rickenbacher P, et al. BNP-guided vs symptom-guided heart failure therapy: The Trial of Intensified vs Standard Medical Therapy in Elderly Patients With Congestive Heart Failure (TIME-CHF) randomized trial. *JAMA.* 2009;301:383-92.

17. Lainchbury JG, Troughton RW, Strangman KM, Frampton CM, Pilbrow A, Yandle TG, et al. NTproBNP-guided Treatment for Chronic Heart Failure: results from the BATTLESCARRED trial. *J Am Coll Cardiol.* 2010;55:53-60.

18. Eurlings LW, van Pol PE, Kok WE, van Wijk S, Lodewijks-van der Bolt C, Balk AH, et al. Can Pro-Brain Natriuretic Peptide Guided Therapy of Heart Failure Improve Heart Failure Morbidity and Mortality? Main Outcome of the PRIMA-Study. *J Am Coll Cardiol.* 2010;56:2090-100. (abstract).

19. Berger R, Moertl D, Peter S, Ahmadi R, Huelsmann M, Yamuti S, et al. N-terminal pro-B-type natriuretic peptide-guided, intensive patient management in addition to multidisciplinary care in chronic heart failure a 3-arm, prospective, randomized pilot study. *J Am Coll Cardiol.* 2010;55:645-53.

20. Bhardwaj A, Rehman U, Mohammed A, Baggish AL, Moore SA, Januzzi JL Jr. Design and methods of the Pro-B Type Natriuretic Peptide Outpatient Tailored Chronic Heart Failure Therapy (PROTECT) Study. *Am Heart J.* 2010;159:532-8.

21. Januzzi JL, Rehman SU, Mohammed AA, et al. Use of amino-terminal Pro-B type natriuretic peptide to guide outpatient therapy of patients with chronic left ventricular systolic dysfunction. IN PRESS.

22. Schou M, Gustafsson F, Videbaek L, Markenvard J, Ulriksen H, Ryde H, et al. Design and methodology of the NorthStar Study: NT-proBNP stratified follow-up in outpatient heart failure clinics: a randomized Danish multicenter study. *Am Heart J.* 2008:156:649-55.

23. NorthStar Study: NT-proBNP stratified follow-up in outpatient heart failure clinics: a randomized Danish multicenter study. Data presented at late-breaking clinical trials session here at the European Society of Cardiology's Heart Failure Congress, May 21, 2011; Gothenburg, Sweden.

24. Felker GM, Hasselblad V, Hernandez AF, O'Connor CM. Biomarker-guided therapy in chronic heart failure: a meta-analysis of randomized controlled trials associated with a significant reduction in all-cause mortality compared to usual care in patients with chronic heart failure. *Am Heart J.* 2009;158:422-30.

25. Porapakkham P, Porapakkham P, Zimmet H, Billah B, Krum H. B-type natriuretic peptide-guided heart failure therapy: A meta-analysis. *Arch Intern Med.* 2010;170:507-14.

10   Cardiorenal Syndromes

Dinna N Cruz, Manish Kaushik,
Claudio Ronco, Alan S Maisel

INTRODUCTION

Various organ systems within the human body are intimately connected to each other. This so-called 'organ crosstalk' refers to the complex biological communication and feedback between organ systems, mediated via various soluble and cellular mediators. Although this crosstalk helps maintain normal homeostasis and optimal functioning of the human body, during disease states this very crosstalk can carry over the influence of the diseased organ to initiate and perpetuate structural and functional dysfunction in the other organs. Of the various organ systems in the human body, the link between heart and kidney was recognized and described as early as 60 years ago.[1]

The lack of a consensus definition and standardization of diagnostic criteria has led to the limited understanding of cardiorenal disease, and a consequent fragmentation in its clinical management. In 2008, the Acute Dialysis Quality Initiative (ADQI) proposed a consensus definition and classification of cardiorenal syndromes (CRS).[2] CRS was formally defined as 'a complex pathophysiological disorder of the heart and the kidneys whereby acute or chronic dysfunction in one organ may induce acute or chronic dysfunction in the other organ.' In addition, this definition and classification of CRS takes into account the bidirectional nature of the organ interactions and also defines the temporal relationship between the primary and secondary diseased organs. More importantly, this classification also recognizes that while the heart-kidney interactions share similarities in their pathophysiological processes, variations exist between subtypes in terms of predisposing events risk, identification, natural history, and outcomes. On the basis of the above considerations, CRS is further classified into five subtypes as shown in table 10-1.

Two important aspects of the CRS classification are worth a special mention. Firstly, the classification is not meant to label patients into fixed categories. The ADQI consensus acknowledges that many patients may move between subtypes during the course of their disease. A classic clinical situation is that of a patient with CRS type 2 who presents with acute decompensated heart failure (ADHF). The hospital

Table 10-1	Classification of Cardiorenal Syndromes		
Class	Type	Description	Clinical situation
1.	Acute cardiorenal syndrome	Abrupt worsening of cardiac function leading to AKI	Acute decompensated heart failure Cardiac surgery ACS CIN after coronary angiogram
2.	Chronic cardiorenal syndrome	Chronic abnormalities of cardiac function leading to CKD	IHD/hypertension CHD Chronic heart failure
3.	Acute renocardiac syndrome	Abrupt worsening of renal function leading to acute cardiac dysfunction	Acute pulmonary edema in AKI Arrhythmia CIN with adverse cardiac outcomes
4.	Chronic renocardiac syndrome	CKD leading to chronic cardiac dysfunction	Cardiac hypertrophy in CKD Adverse CV events in CKD ADPKD with cardiac manifestations
5.	Secondary cardiorenal syndrome	Systemic disorders causing both cardiac and renal dysfunction	Sepsis SLE DM

ACS, acute coronary syndrome; ADPKD, autosomal dominant polycystic kidney disease; AKI, acute kidney injury; CKD, chronic kidney disease; IHD, ischemic heart disease; CHD, congenital heart disease; CIN, contrast-induced nephropathy; DM, diabetes mellitus; SLE, systemic lupus erythematosus.

stay may be complicated by acute kidney injury (AKI) and the patient will then slip into CRS type 1. Treatment of the ADHF will restore the patient to his/her baseline state. The AKI in such situation is often transient, and the renal function recovers to its preexisting level and the patient moves back into CRS type 2. Another scenario often encountered clinically is that of patients with both coronary artery disease (CAD) and chronic kidney disease (CKD) at the time of disease presentation. These diseases share common pathophysiological mechanisms of disease progression. It may therefore prove difficult for the clinicians to identify whether the organ of primary insult is the heart (CRS type 2) or the kidney (CRS type 4), as CAD and CKD frequently coexist in the majority of these patients. In such cases, it has been proposed to classify these patients as having CRS type 2/4.[3] Secondly, further sub-classifications into transient or reversible dysfunction, slowly or acutely progressive versus stable disease are avoided to keep the classification parsimonious.

EPIDEMIOLOGY

CRS type 1 is characterized by an acute worsening of heart function leading to AKI and/or renal dysfunction. Examples of common clinical scenarios leading to this eventuality are ADHF, acute coronary syndrome (ACS), and cardiac surgery associated with low output state.[4] CRS type 1 secondary to ADHF and ACS are commonly seen in clinical practice with a reported incidence of 17–34% and 5–55%, respectively.[4] Most studies have found that CRS type 1, also known as 'worsening renal function' (WRF), occurs within the first seven days of admission.[5,6] Moreover, the acute deterioration in kidney function may be transient or persistent, and in either case it portends a poor prognosis.[7] There appears to be a biological gradient between AKI severity and the risk of death. In a meta-analysis of 16 studies involving 80,098 patients with heart failure (HF), there was a 15% increased risk for all-cause death for every 0.5 mg/dL increase in serum creatinine (sCr) and 7% increase in mortality risk for every 10 mL/min decrease in estimated glomerular filtration rate (eGFR).[8]

CRS types 2 and 4 are characterized by chronic cardiac or renal abnormalities causing renal or cardiac dysfunction, respectively. As alluded to earlier, chronic heart and kidney diseases commonly coexist. For example, in the ADHERE registry of 118,465 patients with ADHF admissions, 27%, 44%, and 13% of patients were found to have mild, moderate, or severe renal dysfunction at the time of hospital admission, respectively.[9] Studies like these are unable to clearly distinguish the temporal relationship between heart and kidney disease. Therefore, often this does not allow for clear discrimination between CRS types 2 and 4. In contrast, congenital heart and kidney diseases could potentially be unequivocal examples of CRS type 2 and type 4, respectively, since the temporal relationships of heart and kidney diseases in these circumstances are clearly defined. 'Cyanotic nephropathy' is a classic example of CRS type 2. In a recent series of 1,102 patients with congenital heart disease surviving into adulthood (mean age 36 years), Dimopoulos et al. observed that 41% of patients had mild CKD (eGFR 60–89 mL/min/1.73 m^2) and 9% had moderate-severe CKD (eGFR < 60 mL/min). Importantly, kidney dysfunction had a substantial impact on mortality (adjusted HR 3.25, p = 0.002 for CKD vs normal eGFR).[10] In a similar manner, autosomal dominant polycystic kidney disease (ADPKD) can be considered a prototype for CRS type 4.[11] In ADPKD, multiple cardiac conditions have been described and cardiovascular complications are the leading cause of death in this population. As with CKD in general, the prevalence of left ventricular hypertrophy (LVH) is higher in ADPKD when compared to a control population, and the frequency increases progressively as GFR decreases. However, several studies have also shown increased left ventricular (LV) mass indices, LV diastolic dysfunction, and endothelial dysfunction in young otherwise normotensive ADPKD subjects with well-preserved renal function.[12]

There were few studies on CRS type 3, which is defined as acute renal dysfunction leading to cardiac dysfunction. An example of this clinical scenario is that of radiocontrast-induced AKI (RCI-AKI) affecting cardiac outcomes negatively. In a recent study by Wi et al., transient and persistent renal dysfunction after contrast was associated with increased short- and long-term mortality and morbidity in AMI patients treated by percutaneous coronary intervention.[13]

Finally, CRS type 5 is characterized by systemic conditions leading to renal and cardiac dysfunction. AKI in sepsis is an established entity and is known to complicate sepsis in 11–64% of patients.[14] Furthermore, observational data have found that approximately 30–80% of patients with sepsis have elevated cardiac-specific troponins, which often correlate with reduced cardiac function.[15]

PATHOPHYSIOLOGY

HF with preserved left ventricular systolic function (PSF) is common and data from the ADHERE registry database has reported its incidence to be as high as 50.4% in patients with ADHF.[16] Although AKI can occur in patients with LV systolic dysfunction as a result of reduced renal blood flow, renal dysfunction has also been observed in patients with PSF. There is growing evidence that propagation of CRS involves not only changes in extracellular fluid volume, blood pressure, cardiac output and raised central venous pressure (CVP) but also accelerates atherosclerosis, cardiac remodeling and hypertrophy and results in progression of CKD. This is possible via a complex and multidimensional interplay between hemodynamic and neurohormonal factors involving the renin-angiotensin-aldosterone system (RAAS), sympathetic nervous system (SNS), nitric oxide (NO) and reactive oxygen species (ROS), and inflammatory cytokines.

As discussed, the most common precipitating factor that results in a decline in renal function during HF syndrome is decreased renal perfusion. Renal perfusion pressure is a function of mean arterial pressure and CVP. Under normal circumstances, any reduction in the renal blood flow is compensated for by an increase in filtration fraction to maintain GFR (via preferential efferent arteriolar vasoconstriction mediated by activation of the RAAS). In this aspect, studies have suggested that increased CVP has a direct, inverse relationship with GFR in patients with cardiac dysfunction.[17,18] A few mechanisms may explain this observation. Firstly, the increase in CVP pressure in patients with HF may distend the venules surrounding the distal end of the tubules, and thus, compromising the lumen of the tubules until the fluid pressure inside the tubules equates with the venous pressure. Alternately, the raised CVP may be transmitted backwards to the renal veins and increase the renal interstitial pressure. This may lead to a hypoxic state of the renal parenchyma and results in subsequent systemic and intrarenal activation of angiotensin II and SNS. Thirdly, elevated intra-abdominal pressure may be present in up to 60% of HF patients with hemodynamic derangements even in the absence of abdominal symptoms. This may further compromise renal perfusion by increasing CVP and by directly 'compressing' the kidneys.[19]

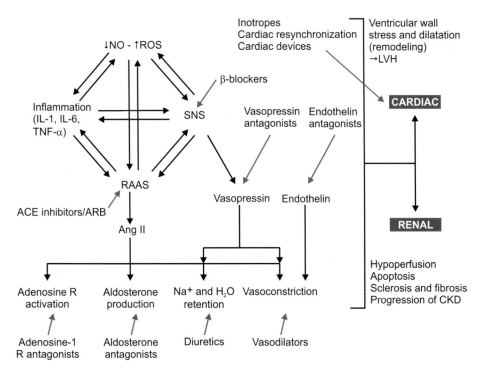

Figure 10-1 Pathophysiology of cardiorenal syndrome types 1 and 2 and sites of pharmacological interventions.

Besides renal perfusion, the neurohormonal interaction is another important aspect that is responsible for kidney injury during HF (Figure 10-1). Of note, the RAAS plays a central role in these complex neurohormonal interactions, because of its interaction with SNS, NO, and ROS and its role in inflammation. Moreover, the RAAS is a common stimulus for sympathetic overactivity in both cardiac dysfunction and renal failure. Angiotensin II-activated NADPH-oxidase results in the formation of ROS. It also induces nuclear factor-$\kappa\beta$ (NF-$\kappa\beta$) which leads to production of proinflammatory mediators, chemotactic and adhesion molecules. Increased SNS activity has been observed in both HF and kidney failure. It can cause vasoconstriction, beta-adrenoceptor insensitivity, cardiac hypertrophy, and also affect lipid metabolism. In addition, it stimulates renin release from the kidneys, generates ROS and induces inflammation. Inflammation is a common feature in both uremia and HF. C-reactive protein (CRP) and other proinflammatory markers like interleukin-6, tumor necrosis factor-α have been demonstrated in both HF and kidney disease and are predictors of atherosclerosis. NO is a potent vasodilator, natriuretic, and desensitizer of tubuloglomerular feedback. In CRS, the balance between NO and ROS is skewed towards ROS by an increase in the production of ROS, a lower antioxidant status and a lower availability of NO due to accumulation of asymmetric dimethyl arginine (ADMA), which is an endogenous nitric oxide synthase inhibitor.

Oxidative stress has been implicated in cellular dysfunction, accelerated apoptosis, and eventual cell death. Its deleterious effect, however, relies on the presence of cytosolic and extracellular labile or catalytic iron. When iron is released from injured cells and is not bound, the free iron can facilitate production of oxygen free radicals and propagation of oxidative stress and results in cellular injury across vascular tissue. It has been postulated that the loss of control over normal iron management after insults to either heart or kidneys in the form of hypoxia, chemotoxicity, or inflammation may be the fundamental pathophysiological basis of CRS.[20]

In CRS type 4, the genesis of adaptive LV remodeling is a result of two different processes.[21] First, the pressure overload state contributed by conditions, such as hypertension, arterial stiffness, arterial wall calcification, secondary hyperparathyroidism and reduced vitamin D, endothelial dysfunction and RAAS, will lead to concentric LVH. Secondly, hypervolemia, anemia, RAAS will cause lengthening of cardiac myofibers, resulting in LV dilatation and thus eccentric LVH, commonly observed in CKD patients. In a study of 432 patients, only 16% had normal LV dimensions at initiation of dialysis, while concentric LVH and LV dilatation was observed in 41% and 28%, respectively.[22] The natural history of LVH in CKD is that of progression characterized by calcification, apoptosis, and fibrosis, eventually culminating in uremic cardiomyopathy.

In addition to LV remodeling, vascular calcification is another predictor of morbidity and mortality in CKD patients. The transformation of arterial smooth muscle cells into osteoblast-like cells in the presence of increased phosphate levels, decreased calcification inhibitors and deranged mineral-bone metabolism, causes the typical arterial medial wall calcification seen in these patients.

Besides the factors highlighted above and the existing traditional and non-traditional risk factors for cardiovascular disease (CVD) in CKD (Figure 10-2), emerging postulates include increased SNS activity, cardiotonic steroids, non-osmotic sodium retention, and altered vitamin D axis.

MANAGEMENT

The multitude of pathophysiological interactions and their complexity make the management of CRS very challenging. Though there are guidelines for the treatment of HF or other cardiac disorders or CKD, respectively, there are no clear recommendations for the treatment of patients with cardiorenal or renocardiac syndromes. The approach to the management of CRS, especially for CRS types 1 and type 2, can be summarized in the following key steps—'PROTECT.' The components of management should include the following:

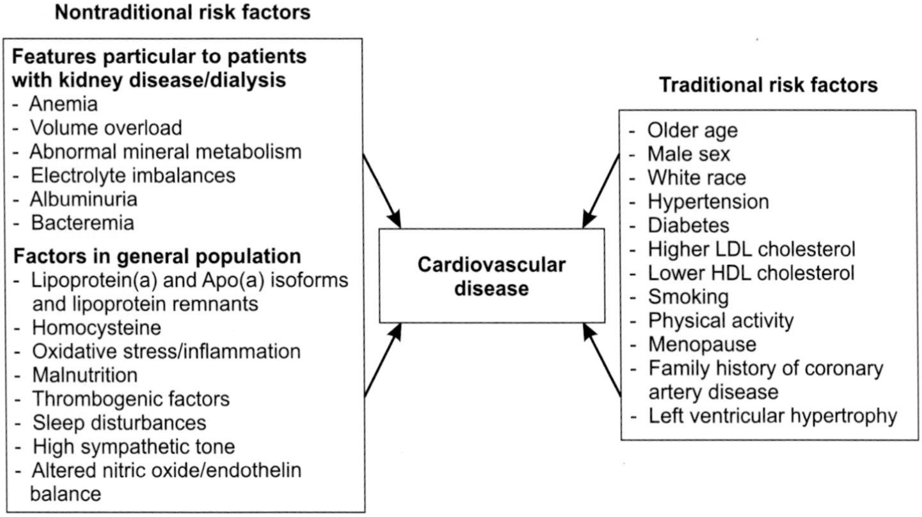

Nontraditional risk factors

Figure 10-2 Risk factors for cardiovascular disease in CKD.

Prevention: Non-pharmacological and pharmacological measures.

Recognition: Early recognition of patients at risk for CRS or developing CRS.

Optimization: Optimize outpatient therapy, titration of medication doses, and regular follow-up.

Therapy: Initiate appropriate therapy during decompensation and treat patients with CRS early and cautiously.

Education: Educate patients with regards to compliance, self-monitoring, and medications.

Cardiac devices, interventions, or transplant: Consider these options in appropriate patients.

Trial/novel therapies: Consider newer drugs or therapies.

PREVENTION

CRS are an end result of the interaction between complex pathogenic factors and once the syndromes set in, they are difficult to abort and are often not reversible in many cases. Most importantly, they are associated with adverse outcomes, including prolonged hospitalization, increased costs, need for renal replacement therapy and even death. The pathophysiology of CRS also highlights the importance of limited organ reserve to recover from insults/injury due to the chronically damaged nature of the organs in the disease process. Thus, prevention of CRS is paramount in clinical practice with an aim to identify and avoid precipitating factors, as well as employ measures to maintain optimal functioning of the diseased heart and kidney. This may involve multimodality and multidisciplinary preventive strategies, working via diverse therapeutic targets. Apart from pharmacological measures, some non-pharmacological and general preventive measures have to be reinforced across the whole spectrum of CRS. These include weight monitoring and management, smoking cessation, exercise, diet and nutrition, and compliance to pharmacological treatment.

Improving the natural history of chronic HF and avoiding decompensation are the cornerstones of prevention in CRS type 1 and type 2. Strategies for prevention in these patients should follow those recommended by the ACC/AHA for stages A and B HF.[23] These include CAD risk factor modification and avoidance of medications that may precipitate salt and water retention, including non-steroidal anti-inflammatory agents and thiozolidinediones. More importantly, medications including blockers of the RAAS and β-blockers (BB), should be used with care in selected patients.

Anemia has been closely associated with the severity and mortality of CKD and CVD. Correction of hemoglobin levels from < 10 g/dL to ~12 g/dL resulted in the reduction of LVH, improvement in ejection fraction, functional class and peak oxygen consumption with exercise testing.[24] In the FAIR-HF trial which included chronic HF patients in NYHA class II or III, significant improvement was observed after the correction of iron deficiency with intravenous carboxymaltose at week 24 (improvement to NYHA class I or II in 47% of patients on carboxymaltose vs in 30% of patients on placebo).[25] The result of RED-AHF trial, an ongoing trial that examines the impact on mortality by anemia correction with erythropoietin in HF patients, is eagerly awaited.[26]

The most common pathophysiology of acute cardiac decompensation in AKI (CRS type 3) is sodium and water retention. Hence, in AKI, a prompt aggressive avoidance of hypervolemia may avoid cardiac decompensation. Moreover, uremic changes, acid-base and electrolyte abnormalities (such as metabolic acidosis) exhibit adverse consequences on the cardiac contractility and its responsiveness to catecholamines. Electrolyte disturbances, such as hyperkalemia and hypokalemia, should be corrected to prevent arrhythmias with undesirable hemodynamic effects. Correction of the abnormal milieu in AKI with timely and appropriate interventions, including renal replacement therapy, may avert these complications.

CRS type 4 is commonly seen in clinical practice. There is a close relationship between CKD and CVD, and the risk of CVD is related to the severity of CKD. In addition, CKD has been associated with accelerated atherosclerosis, progressive LVH and development of diastolic and systolic cardiac dysfunction. It is well recognized that patients with CKD are more likely to die from CVD than progress to dialysis.[27] Despite this, major trials in the management of HF or CVD excluded patients with significant CKD. This 'therapeutic nihilism' has been well recognized in the literature. A review of medication prescription patterns for CKD patients revealed that only 24% of patients with known CAD received statins, despite their clear proven benefits in non-CKD patients.[28] Similarly, after adjustment for baseline characteristics, patients on long-term dialysis or having predialysis CKD were less likely to undergo coronary angiography as compared to patients with normal renal function (42% and 45% vs 56%, respectively). Moreover, these patients were less likely to receive revascularization or coronary intervention after diagnostic angiogram.

RECOGNITION OF PATIENTS AT RISK FOR ACUTE CRS

Patients who develop CRS type 1 are generally older, and have history of previous episodes of HF, and often demonstrate baseline renal dysfunction and hypertension. Forman et al. devised a scoring system to identify patients at risk of developing HF, which takes into account the following factors: history of HF, systolic blood pressure > 160 mmHg, diabetes (each 1 point), serum creatinine ≥ 1.5 mg/dL and < 2.5 mg/dL (2 points) and serum creatinine ≥ 2.5 mg/dL (3 points). In their cohort, patients with a score of ≥ 4 had a 53% likelihood of developing WRF.[29] Similarly, Mehran et al. devised a risk score for the development of RCI-AKI after percutaneous coronary intervention.[30] Such scoring systems can be used to recognize preemptively the patients at a high intrinsic risk of developing acute renal or cardiac complications. Prophylactic measures can then be selectively instituted in these patients with the aim of reducing the risk of acute CRS.

In addition to the clinical risk scoring systems, the use of biomarkers during the course of illness or treatment may serve to identify patients (early in the disease process) who are at risk of developing CRS, especially in the setting of acute CRS. Aghel et al. found that serum neutrophil gelatinase-associated lipocalin (NGAL) value of > 140 ng/mL on hospital admission was associated with a 7.2-fold increase in the development of WRF in patients with ADHF. Similarly, both urinary NGAL and interleukin-18 demonstrated a good performance in diagnosing RCI-AKI 24 hours earlier when compared to serum creatinine.[31] These biomarkers are discussed in further detail in other chapters of this book.

OPTIMIZATION OF OUTPATIENT THERAPY

As discussed previously, patients who are at highest risk of CRS are the ones who are receiving suboptimal therapy and experience poor control of risk factors. In patients with CKD, the aforementioned 'therapeutic nihilism' should be avoided and efforts must be made to cautiously introduce cardioprotective agents. The use of angiotensin converting enzyme inhibitor (ACEi) and angiotensin receptor blocker (ARB) deserves a special mention as they are not only cardioprotective but also have proven benefit in retarding CKD. There is no particular level of sCr above which ACEi cannot be started and they exhibit their beneficial effects even late into the disease process.[32] However, a nephrology consultation is recommended at sCr level > 2.8 mg/dL.[33] In patients with HF, digoxin has been shown to reduce hospitalization for worsening HF as compared to placebo treatment (26.8% vs 34.7%, p < 0.001) in over

6,000 HF patients with LVEF < 45%. In addition, there was a trend toward a decrease in the risk of HF death in the group who received digoxin (p = 0.06).[34]

In chronic HF especially, therapy needs to be individualized, reviewed frequently and titrated against the patient's status regularly to avoid episodes of acute decompensation. In a recent meta-analysis of 14 trials involving 4,264 patients, the use of remote telephone monitoring to ensure compliance and monitoring has shown to decrease hospitalization by 21% and all-cause mortality by 20%.[35] The use of biomarkers may further enhance telemedicine.[36] In the proposed algorithm, patients are monitored in the outpatient with regular weight monitoring. When patients report a weight gain of 3–5 lbs with HF symptoms, diuretic dose is to be adjusted and optimized via telephone advice. However, patients who report a weight gain of 3–5 lbs but without any overt signs of HF are subjected to further test with a natriuretic peptide (NP) level measurement. Accordingly, the diuretic dose can be titrated on the basis of changes in NP levels from baseline to avert further volume overload. However, in two recent studies, telemonitoring and telephone-based interactive voice response system failed to improve outcomes in HF patients as compared to high standard conventional care.[37]

THERAPY OF CRS IN ACUTE DECOMPENSATION

Patients with CRS that need inpatient management are usually those who end up in decompensation of CRS (types 1 and 3). Patients with ADHF that usually present to the hospital can be divided into two broad categories: patients with congestion and high or normal blood pressure, and patients with low blood pressure with or without congestion. Various pharmacological and interventional agents used in the treatment of these patients are represented in figure 10-1 and table 10-2.

Diuretics

Diuretics have been the cornerstone of treatment of HF for a long time despite the fact that it may be associated with AKI and increased mortality.[38] It is well-known that diuretic braking phenomenon exists and post-diuretic sodium retention may further decrease responsiveness to diuretics in CRS. Therefore, aggressive diuresis to achieve clinical goals can have undesirable consequences, such overstimulation of the RAAS and SNS, both of which may play a role in the pathogenesis of AKI/CRS type 1. The optimal regimen for diuretics remains unclear. Continuous intravenous use of diuretics has traditionally been considered more effective in severe ADHF.[39,40] In the recent randomized DOSE-AHF trial enrolling 308 patients admitted for ADHF, Felker et al. compared low-dose diuretic (equivalent to patients' oral dose) versus high-dose diuretics (equivalent to 2.5 times patients' oral dose) given either as intravenous bolus every 12 hours or continuous intravenous infusion. Comparing bolus with continuous infusion, there was no significant difference in terms of

Table 10-2	Therapeutic Options in Cardiorenal Syndromes	
Drugs	Indicated in CRS type(s)	Remarks
ACEi /ARB	1–4	Lifesaving, reduces morbidity and cardiac remodeling in type 2, in type 4 offers nephroprotection and proteinuria reduction, in type 1 continue if already on or initiate before discharge, contraindicated in renal artery stenosis
Beta-blockers	1,2,4	In type 1 use with caution in low CO state, reduce dose if already on and initiate before discharge; lifesaving and reduces cardiac remodeling in type 2; offers cardioprotection and reduces arrhythmias in type 4
Aldosterone antagonists	2,4	In type 2 is lifesaving in moderate-severe symptomatic HF, reduces morbidity and reduces myocardial and vascular fibrosis; in type 4 prevents myocardial and vascular fibrosis
Diuretics	1–4	Induces diuresis, reduces fluid overload and offers symptomatic relief; may help maintain non-oliguric AKI in type 3; helps control hypertension in type 4
Digoxin	1,2,4	In type 1 can reduce ventricular rate in AF; in types 2 and 4 reduces HF admissions, improves symptoms; mortality unchanged
Hydralazine and nitrates	2	May improve survival in patients who cannot tolerate ACEi or ARB, in African Americans reduces mortality and morbidity and improves QOL
Inotropes (dopamine, dobutamine, milrinone, levosimendan)	1	Improves CO in low output states in presence of signs of hypoperfusion or congestion despite the use of vasodilators or diuretics, some may decrease peripheral resistance
Vasopressors	1	Only indicated in cardiogenic shock when all other inotropes fail. Epinephrine is indicated only for rescue therapy in cardiac arrest
Nesiritide	1	BNP analog vasodilator, data on mortality uncertain
Vasopressin antagonists	1	Symptom relief, promotes water elimination and weight loss in short-term
Endothelin antagonists	2,4	Aimed at blocking endothelin II mediated vasoconstriction
Adenosine A-1 receptor antagonists	1,2	Block adenosine mediated glomerular vasoconstriction, may improve symptoms and improve deterioration in renal function
Erythropoiesis stimulating agents (ESA)	2,4	In type 2 may improve exercise capacity in patients with anemia, no clear impact on mortality and morbidity in HF; improves survival in CKD

Continued

Continued

Drugs	Indicated in CRS type(s)	Remarks
Parenteral iron	2,4	In type 2 improves exercise capacity and QOL in iron deficient patients; no clear impact on mortality and morbidity
Warfarin/ antiplatelets	1,4	Prevention of thromboembolism in patients with AF and reduced LVEF. Warfarin better than antiplatelets
Ultrafiltration	1,2	Removal of excess fluid in patients with diuretic resistance
Cardiac resynchronization	2	Long-term extremely low CO with right and left ventricular dys-synchrony

ACEi, angiotensin-converting enzyme inhibitor; AF, atrial fibrillation; AKI, acute kidney injury; ARB, angiotensin receptor blocker; CKD, chronic kidney disease; CO, cardiac output; HF, heart failure; QOL, quality of life.

patients' symptoms or in the mean change in the sCr level. There was a trend toward a greater improvement in patients' symptoms in the high-dose strategy as compared to the low-dose strategy, although the mean change in the sCr did not differ between the high-dose or low-dose strategies.[41]

Neurohormonal Blockade

There is abundant evidence on the role of ACEi, ARB, and BB in neurohormonal blockade via the RAAS system and SNS, respectively, in CRS.[42-46] In particular, ACEi induce favorable LV remodeling in patients with both preserved and reduced systolic function, especially after myocardial infarction. Intrinsic to ACEi, with an inherent reduction of intraglomerular pressure secondary to efferent arteriole vasodilatation, up to 30% increase in sCr and its associated drop in GFR is to be expected. BB use in HF has been shown to associate with reduced morbidity and mortality, even among patients with CKD.[47,48] However, the administration of BB in patients with CRS type 1 merits great caution and generally should be avoided until the patients have been stabilized. This is due to the fact that in such situations, maintenance of cardiac output is achieved via activation of the SNS and reflex tachycardia. Blunting of this compensatory response can thus precipitate cardiogenic shock.[49]

Use of spironolactone, an aldosterone antagonist, on top of standard medical therapy was associated with a 30% reduction in the risk of death, as well as a 35% reduction in frequency of hospitalization for HF.[50] The beneficial effect of aldosterone antagonism was reiterated in the recent EMPHASIS-HF trial wherein the addition of eplerenone to standard chronic heart failure medication significantly reduced the death from cardiovascular cause and hospitalization for heart failure.[51] It is important to note that aldosterone antagonist therapy is associated with a small, but significant, risk of severe hyperkalemia. Careful monitoring is, therefore, essential, particularly in patients with CKD.[38]

Vasodilators

Vasodilators including nitroglycerin, isosorbide dinitrate, nitroprusside, and hydralazine have been used in the management of CRS, especially in situations where ACE-i/ARB are contraindicated.[52] Nesiritide, a recombinant B-type natriuretic peptide, has been used in HF for its potent vasodilatory and modest natriuretic effects. In a recently published study by Ng et al. including 131 patients with ADHF and LVEF < 40%, nesiritide was associated with better preserved GFR and blood urea nitrogen (BUN) levels as compared to nitroglycerin, despite having lower baseline and treatment blood pressures.[53] Also, the ASCEND-HF study found nesiritide to be safe in severe HF and without an increase in risk of kidney dysfunction, but its benefits on symptoms, hospital readmissions, or mortality were unconvincing.[51]

Inotropes

Inotropes, such as dopamine, dobutamine, and milrinone are used in low cardiac output states, in presence of signs of hypoperfusion or congestion despite the use of vasodilators or diuretics, with the aim to increase cardiac output and restore perfusion. Levosimendan, a newer class of agent, called lusitropic agents or 'calcium sensitizers,' is being studied in the treatment of ADHF. In a recent study, levosimendan was compared with dobutamine, and with the combination of dobutamine and levosimendan in a cohort of 63 patients with NYHA functional class IV. Levosimendan was found to have beneficial effects with regards to the composite endpoint of death or urgent LV device implantation than dobutamine alone (p = 0.037) or the combined therapy (p = 0.009) at six months (80% vs 48% vs 43%, respectively).

EDUCATION

Two-thirds of the patients present with ADHF have established HF and the most common precipitants for decompensation are noncompliance to low sodium diet and medications. Thus, the patient education is critical in these settings to avoid repeated admissions. A study by Ekman et al. found that 20% of the patients with mild to moderate HF did not know that they had HF.[54] In addition, Ni et al. found that 40% of the patients did not understand the importance of daily weighing and one-third of the patients believed they should drink a lot of fluids.[55] In a review on the patient education in HF, cognitive and functional limitations, misconceptions, and lack of 'basic knowledge', low motivation and interest and low self-esteem have been cited as various barriers in patient education.[56] The process of patient education involves five steps including assessment, identification of barriers and learning needs, planning of education, delivery, and finally, evaluation. Patient education is a multidisciplinary process and HF nurses have a very important role to play in patient education. The venue of patient education can be at the outpatient clinic, hospital, home or a combination of these. Though the patients can be educated at any time by the health care professionals, the most appropriate time patient education should be reinforced is when the patient is stable and has started to adapt living with HF. The various educational materials that can be used are verbal information, booklets, videos, computer-based web pages or programs, and patient support groups.

CARDIAC DEVICES AND TRANSPLANTATION

In selected HF patients who have poor LVEF (< 35%) and QRS prolongation (≥ 120 ms) and who remain in NYHA functional class III–IV HF despite optimal medical management, cardiac resynchronization therapy should be considered. In the Multicenter In Sync Randomized Clinical Evaluation (MIRACLE) study, CRT was associated with improved LV function in all patients. Notably, however, there was an improvement in eGFR of patients with a baseline eGFR of < 60 mL/min and ≥ 30 mL/min.[33] Moreover, in these patients with HF and poor LVEF, implantable cardiac defibrillators (ICD) should be added, on top of CRT, in patients who have sustained ventricular arrhythmias or survived cardiac arrests.[57] This was echoed in the RAFT trial where addition of CRT to ICD therapy reduced the incidence of all-cause mortality and HF hospitalizations in patients with NYHA III–IV HF as compared to ICD alone.[37] Intra-aortic balloon pump, ventricular assist device, or artificial hearts may be beneficial, as a bridge to eventual recovery of cardiac function or heart transplant. In eligible patients who are in end-stage heart disease and have failed medical therapy, heart transplant has been shown to improve survival, exercise capacity and quality of life as compared to conventional therapy.[33] Even in patients with CKD who have CRS type 2/4, there is a documented survival benefit post-renal transplant as compared to patients on the wait list for transplant. Wali et al. have documented an improvement in the LVEF and HF functional class following renal transplant in 103 patients of end-stage kidney disease who had HF and poor LVEF (< 40%). In fact, the LVEF improved to ≥ 50% in 69.9% of patients and the mean LVEF increased from 31.6% to 52% at 12 months post-renal transplant.[58]

TRIAL OR NOVEL THERAPIES

Novel therapies, such as adenosine receptor blockers, vasopressin antagonists, and endothelin receptor antagonists are being studied. To date, the results are not yet convincing with regards to mortality and preservation of renal function. In the PROTECT study with 2,033 patients, the adenosine receptor antagonist (rolofylline) was similar to placebo in terms of changes in sCr and eGFR at day 14 of hospitalization. Moreover, the EVEREST involving 4,133 patients confirmed the efficacy of early administration of vasopressin antagonists (tolvaptan) in decreasing mean body weight and improvement in symptoms but failed to demonstrate an improvement in the long-term outcomes.

Patients with CRS type 4 represent a high-risk group for CVD and sudden cardiac death. Mineral metabolism disorders, such as hyperphosphatemia, hypocalcemia, and vitamin D deficiency, have been deeply associated not only with bone disease but also with vascular calcification and CVD. In addition, the decrease in vitamin D production stimulates the RAAS, resulting in vasoconstriction and salt and water retention, which further promotes arterial stiffening. Vitamin D receptor activators, commonly used to treat the metabolic bone disease associated with CKD, may help to reduce cardiovascular morbidity and mortality in these patients. The effect of vitamin D receptor activation using paricalcitol on LVH in patients with CKD stage 3–4 is being currently studied in the PRIMO trial.[59]

Ultrafiltration (UF) which involves the isotonic removal of water has been studied in patients with ADHF, who respond poorly to diuretics or develop diuretic resistance. The UNLOAD trial, in which 200 patients were randomized to UF or intravenous diuretics, demonstrated that in decompensated HF, UF safely produced greater weight and fluid removal than intravenous diuretics, reduced 90-day resource utilization for HF, and was an effective alternative therapy.[60] The role of UF as a rescue therapy in patients with CRS type 1, who still manifest symptoms and signs of decompensated HF, will be evaluated in the coming CARESS-HF trial.[61]

CONCLUSION

CRS is a complex and multidimensional entity that is commonly encountered in clinical practice but has significant impact on morbidity and mortality. The recently proposed consensus definition and classification will enable a better understanding of the pathophysiology of the syndromes and encourage multidisciplinary management of the syndromes. Preventive strategies in general for all patients with CKD and cardiac diseases, including HF and especially those in the high-risk patients, will help decrease the incidence of acute deterioration of organ function. Biomarkers of cardiac and renal functions have a potentially important role to play in identifying high-risk patients that will go on to develop CRS and in guiding therapy. Further studies evaluating diagnostic and therapeutic options are needed to optimize CRS management and to reduce its impact on health outcomes both clinical and economical.

REFERENCES

1. Ledoux P. Cardiorenal syndrome. *Avenir Med.* 1951;48:149-53.
2. Ronco C, McCullough P, Anker SD, Anand I, Aspromonte N, Bagshaw SM, et al. Cardiorenal syndromes: report from the consensus conference of the Acute Dialysis Quality Initiative. *Eur Heart J.* 2010;31:703-11.

3. Bagshaw SM, Cruz DN, Aspromonte N, Daliento L, Ronco F, Sheinfeld G, et al. Epidemiology of cardio-renal syndromes: workgroup statements from the 7th ADQI Consensus Conference. *Nephrol Dial Transplant.* 2010;25:1406-16.

4. Cruz DN, Gheorghiade M, Palazuolli A, Ronco C, Bagshaw SM. Epidemiology and outcome of the cardio-renal syndrome. *Heart Fail Rev.* 2010.

5. Gottlieb SS, Abraham W, Butler J, Forman DE, Loh E, Massie BM, et al. The prognostic importance of different definitions of worsening renal function in congestive heart failure. *J Cardiac Fail.* 2002;8:136-41.

6. Cowie MR, Komajda M, Murray-Thomas T, Underwood J, Ticho B. Prevalence and impact of worsening renal function in patients hospitalized with decompensated heart failure: results of the prospective outcomes study in heart failure (POSH). *Eur Heart J.* 2006;27:1216-22.

7. Aronson D, Burger AJ. The relationship between transient and persistent worsening renal function and mortality in patients with acute decompensated heart failure. *J Card Fail.* 2010;16:541-7.

8. Smith GL, Lichtman JH, Bracken MB, Shlipak MG, Phillips CO, DiCapua P, et al. Renal impairment and outcomes in heart failure: systematic review and meta-analysis. *J Am Coll Cardiol.* 2006;47:1987-96.

9. Heywood JT, Fonarow GC, Costanzo MR, Mathur VS, Wigneswaran JR, Wynne J. High prevalence of renal dysfunction and its impact on outcome in 118,465 patients hospitalized with acute decompensated heart failure: a report from the ADHERE database. *J Card Fail.* 2007;13:422-30.

10. Dimopoulos K, Diller G-P, Koltsida E, Pijuan-Domenech A, Papadopoulou SA, Babu-Narayan SV, et al. Prevalence, predictors, and prognostic value of renal dysfunction in adults with congenital heart disease. *Circulation.* 2008;117:2320-8.

11. Virzi GM, Corradi V, Panagiotou A, Gastaldon F, Cruz DN, de Cal M, et al. ADPKD: prototype of cardiorenal syndrome type 4. *Int J Nephrol.* 2010;490795:2011.

12. Cruz DN, Bagshaw SM. Heart-kidney interaction: epidemiology of cardiorenal syndromes. *Int J Nephrol.* 2010;351291:2011.

13. Wi J, Ko YG, Kim JS, Kim BK, Choi D, Ha JW, et al. Impact of contrast-induced acute kidney injury with transient or persistent renal dysfunction on long-term outcomes of patients with acute myocardial infarction undergoing percutaneous coronary intervention. *Heart.* 2011.

14. Bagshaw SM, Uchino S, Bellomo R, Morimatsu H, Morgera S, Schetz M, et al. Septic acute kidney injury in critically Ill patients: clinical characteristics and outcomes. *Clin J Am Soc Nephrol.* 2007;2:431-9.

15. Ammann P, Maggiorini M, Bertel O, Haenseler E, Joller-Jemelka HI, Oechslin E, et al. Troponin as a risk factor for mortality in critically ill patients without acute coronary syndromes. *J Am Coll Cardiol.* 2003;41:2004-9.

16. Yancy CW, Lopatin M, Stevenson LW, De Marco T, Fonarow GC. Clinical presentation, management, and in-hospital outcomes of patients admitted with acute decompensated heart failure with preserved systolic function: a report from the Acute Decompensated Heart Failure National Registry (ADHERE) database. *J Am Coll Cardiol.* 2006;47:76-84.

17. Damman K, van Deursen VM, Navis G, Voors AA, van Veldhuisen DJ, Hillege HL. Increased central venous pressure is associated with impaired renal function and mortality in a broad spectrum of patients with cardiovascular disease. *J Am Coll Cardiol.* 2009;53:582-8.

18. Mullens W, Abrahams Z, Francis GS, Sokos G, Taylor DO, Starling RC, et al. Importance of venous congestion for worsening of renal function in advanced decompensated heart failure. *J Am Coll Cardiol.* 2009;53:589-96.

19. Tang WH, Mullens W. Cardiorenal syndrome in decompensated heart failure. *Heart.* 2010;96:255-60. Epub 2009 Apr 27.

20. McCullough PA, Ahmad A. Cardiorenal syndromes. *World J Cardiol.* 2011;26:1-9.

21. Taddei S, Nami R, Bruno RM, Quatrini I, Nuti R. Hypertension, left ventricular hypertrophy and chronic kidney disease. *Heart Fail Rev.* 2010.

22. Parfrey PS, Foley RN, Harnett JD, Kent GM, Murray DC, Barre PE. Outcome and risk factors for left ventricular disorders in chronic uraemia. *Nephrol Dial Transplant.* 1996; 11:1277-85.

23. Hunt SA. ACC/AHA 2005 guideline update for the diagnosis and management of chronic heart failure in the adult: a report of the American College of Cardiology/American Heart Association Task Force on Practice Guidelines (Writing Committee to Update the 2001 Guidelines for the Evaluation and Management of Heart Failure). *J Am Coll Cardiol.* 2005;46:e1-82.

24. McCullough PA, Lepor NE. The deadly triangle of anemia, renal insufficiency, and cardiovascular disease: implications for prognosis and treatment. *Rev Cardiovasc Med.* 2005;6:1-10.

25. Anker SD, Comin Colet J, Filippatos G, Willenheimer R, Dickstein K, Drexler H, et al. Ferric carboxymaltose in patients with heart failure and iron deficiency. *N Engl J Med.* 2009;361:2436-48.

26. McMurray JJ, Anand IS, Diaz R, Maggioni AP, O'Connor C, Pfeffer MA, et al. Design of the reduction of events with darbepoetin alfa in heart failure (RED-HF): a phase III, anaemia correction, morbidity-mortality trial. *Eur J Heart Fail.* 2009;11:795-801.

27. Keith DS, Nichols GA, Gullion CM, Brown JB, Smith DH. Longitudinal follow-up and outcomes among a population with chronic kidney disease in a large managed care organization. *Arch Intern Med.* 2004;164:659-63.

28. Bailie GR, Eisele G, Liu L, Roys E, Kiser M, Finkelstein F, et al. Patterns of medication use in the RRI-CKD study: focus on medications with cardiovascular effects. *Nephrol Dial Transplant.* 2005;20:1110-15.

29. Forman DE, Butler J, Wang Y, Abraham WT, O'Connor CM, Gottlieb SS, et al. Incidence, predictors at admission, and impact of worsening renal function among patients hospitalized with heart failure. *J Am Coll Cardiol.* 2004;43:61-7.

30. Mehran R, Aymong ED, Nikolsky E, Lasic Z, Iakovou I, Fahy M, et al. A simple risk score for prediction of contrast-induced nephropathy after percutaneous coronary intervention: development and initial validation. *J Am Coll Cardiol.* 2004;44:1393-9.

31. Ling W, Zhaohui N, Ben H, Leyi G, Jianping L, Huili D, et al. NGAL as early predictive biomarkers in contrast-Induced nephropathy after coronary angiography. *Nephron Clin Pract.* 2008;108:c176-81.

32. Hou FF, Zhang X, Zhang GH, Xie D, Chen PY, Zhang WR, et al. Efficacy and safety of benazepril for advanced chronic renal insufficiency. *N Engl J Med.* 2006;354:131-40.

33. Dickstein K, Cohen-Solal A, Filippatos G, McMurray JJ, Ponikowski P, Poole-Wilson PA, et al. ESC guidelines for the diagnosis and treatment of acute and chronic heart failure 2008: the Task Force for the Diagnosis and Treatment of Acute and Chronic Heart Failure 2008 of the European Society of Cardiology. Developed in collaboration with the Heart Failure Association of the ESC (HFA) and endorsed by the European Society of Intensive Care Medicine (ESICM). *Eur Heart J.* 2008;29:2388-442.

34. The effect of digoxin on mortality and morbidity in patients with heart failure. The Digitalis Investigation Group. *N Engl J Med.* 1997;336:525-33.

35. Clark RA, Inglis SC, McAlister FA, Cleland JG, Stewart S. Telemonitoring or structured telephone support programmes for patients with chronic heart failure: systematic review and meta-analysis. *BMJ.* 2007;334:942.

36. Maisel A, Mueller C, Adams K, Anker SD, Aspromonte N, Cleland JGF, et al. State of the art: using natriuretic peptide levels in clinical practice. *Eur J Heart Fail.* 2008;10:824-39.

37. Cleland JG, Coletta AP, Buga L, Antony R, Pellicori P, Freemantle N, et al. Clinical trials update from the American Heart Association meeting 2010: EMPHASIS-HF, RAFT, TIM-HF, Tele-HF, ASCEND-HF, ROCKET-AF, and PROTECT. *Eur J Heart Fail.* 2011;13: 460-5.

38. Aspromonte N, Cruz DN, Valle R, Bonello M, Tubaro M, Gambaro G, et al. Metabolic and toxicological considerations for diuretic therapy in patients with acute heart failure. *Expert Opin Drug Metab Toxicol.* 2011.

39. Howard PA, Dunn MI. Aggressive diuresis for severe heart failure in the elderly. *Chest.* 2001;119:807-10.

40. Salvador DR, Rey NR, Ramos GC, Punzalan FE. Continuous infusion versus bolus injection of loop diuretics in congestive heart failure. *Cochrane Database Syst Rev.* 2005;CD003178.

41. Felker GM, Lee KL, Bull DA, Redfield MM, Stevenson LW, Goldsmith SR, et al. Diuretic strategies in patients with acute decompensated heart failure. *N Engl J Med.* 2011;364:797-805.

42. Effects of enalapril on mortality in severe congestive heart failure. Results of the Co-operative North Scandinavian Enalapril Survival Study (CONSENSUS). The CONSENSUS Trial Study Group. *N Engl J Med.* 1987;316:1429-35.

43. Effect of enalapril on survival in patients with reduced left ventricular ejection fractions and congestive heart failure. The SOLVD Investigators. *N Engl J Med.* 1991;325:293-302.

44. Weir RA, McMurray JJ, Puu M, Solomon SD, Olofsson B, Granger CB, et al. Efficacy and tolerability of adding an angiotensin receptor blocker in patients with heart failure already receiving an angiotensin-converting inhibitor plus aldosterone antagonist, with or without a beta blocker. Findings from the Candesartan in Heart failure: Assessment of Reduction in Mortality and morbidity (CHARM)-added trial. *Eur J Heart Fail.* 2008;10: 157-63.

45. Cohn JN, Tognoni G. A randomized trial of the angiotensin-receptor blocker valsartan in chronic heart failure. *N Engl J Med.* 2001;345:1667-75.

46. Pfeffer MA, Braunwald E, Moye LA, Basta L, Brown EJ Jr, Cuddy TE, et al. Effect of captopril on mortality and morbidity in patients with left ventricular dysfunction after myocardial infarction. Results of the survival and ventricular enlargement trial. The SAVE Investigators. *N Engl J Med.* 1992;327:669-77.

47. Packer M, Coats AJ, Fowler MB, Katus HA, Krum H, Mohacsi P, et al. Effect of carvedilol on survival in severe chronic heart failure. *N Engl J Med.* 2001;344:1651-8.

48. Effect of metoprolol CR/XL in chronic heart failure: Metoprolol CR/XL Randomised Intervention Trial in Congestive Heart Failure (MERIT-HF). *Lancet.* 1999;353:2001-7.

49. Chen ZM, Pan HC, Chen YP, Peto R, Collins R, Jiang LX, et al. Early intravenous then oral metoprolol in 45,852 patients with acute myocardial infarction: randomised placebo-controlled trial. *Lancet.* 2005;366:1622-32.

50. Pitt B, Zannad F, Remme WJ, Cody R, Castaigne A, Perez A, et al. The effect of spirono-lactone on morbidity and mortality in patients with severe heart failure. Randomized Aldactone Evaluation Study Investigators. *N Engl J Med.* 1999;341:709-17.

51. Gensch C, Hoppe U, Bohm M, Laufs U. Late-breaking clinical trials presented at the American Heart Association Congress in Chicago 2010. *Clin Res Cardiol.* 2011;100:1-9.

52. Taylor AL, Ziesche S, Yancy C, Carson P, D'Agostino R Jr, Ferdinand K, et al. Combination of isosorbide dinitrate and hydralazine in blacks with heart failure. *N Engl J Med.* 2004;351:2049-57.

53. Ng TM, Ackerbauer KA, Hyderi AF, Hshieh S, Elkayam U. Comparative effects of nesiritide and nitroglycerin on renal function, and incidence of renal injury by traditional and RIFLE criteria in acute heart failure. *J Cardiovasc Pharmacol Ther.* 2011.

54. Ekman I, Norberg A, Lundman B. An intervention aimed at reducing uncertainty in elderly patients with chronic heart failure. *Int J Hum Caring.* 2000;4:7-13.

55. Ni H, Nauman D, Burgess D, Wise K, Crispell K, Hershberger RE. Factors influencing knowledge of and adherence to self-care among patients with heart failure. *Arch Intern Med.* 1999;159:1613-9.

56. Strömberg A. The crucial role of patient education in heart failure. *Eur J Heart Fail.* 2005; 7:363-9.

57. Vardas PE, Auricchio A, Blanc JJ, Daubert JC, Drexler H, Ector H, et al. Guidelines for cardiac pacing and cardiac resynchronization therapy: The Task Force for Cardiac Pacing and Cardiac Resynchronization Therapy of the European Society of Cardiology. Developed in collaboration with the European Heart Rhythm Association. *Eur Heart J.* 2007;28:2256-95.

58. Wali RK, Wang GS, Gottlieb SS, Bellumkonda L, Hansalia R, Ramos E, et al. Effect of kidney transplantation on left ventricular systolic dysfunction and congestive heart failure in patients with end-stage renal disease. *J Am Coll Cardiol.* 2005;45:1051-60.

59. Thadhani R, Appelbaum E, Chang Y, Pritchett Y, Bhan I, Agarwal R, et al. Vitamin D receptor activation and left ventricular hypertrophy in advanced kidney disease. *Am J Nephrol.* 2011;33:139-49.

60. Costanzo MR, Guglin ME, Saltzberg MT, Jessup ML, Bart BA, Teerlink JR, et al. Ultrafiltration versus intravenous diuretics for patients hospitalized for acute decompensated heart failure. *J Am Coll Cardiol.* 2007;49:675-83.

61. Costanzo MR. Cardiorenal Rescue Study in Acute Decompensated Heart Failure (CARESS-HF Clinical Trial). www.hfnetwork.org (21 June 2011).

CHAPTER 11

Assessing Kidney Injury in Heart Failure: The Role of Biomarkers

Arrash Fard, Navaid Iqbal,
Ravindra L Mehta, Yang Xue, Alan S Maisel

INTRODUCTION

In modern medicine it is quite difficult and arguably irresponsible to discuss cardiovascular disease and not mention the kidneys. The proper function of the heart and kidney are intricately linked through organ cross talk via neurohumoral feedback mechanisms, and, therefore, damage and ensuing dysfunction of one system can often cause concomitant dysfunction of the other. Consequently, during the assessment and treatment of those with cardiovascular disease, a clinician must always be aware of the patient's renal function and carefully manage the many insults (such as drugs and contrast) that can lead to acute kidney injury.

Acute kidney injury (AKI) is generally defined as a sudden and continuous decline in renal function leading to a steady accumulation of nitrogenous and non-nitrogenous products and toxins, with rapid development of fluid, electrolyte, and acid-base disorders. Unfortunately, AKI is often unrecognized as criteria for the disease vary from quantitative and qualitative changes in serum creatinine to changes in urine output and need for dialysis. Recognizing this dilemma, the Acute Dialysis Quality Initiative (ADQI) group proposed consensus recommendations of the RIFLE criteria for the definition and staging of AKI.[1] Subsequently, the Acute Kidney Injury Network (AKIN) revised these standards to necessitate a 0.3 mg/dL or $\geq$ 50% increase in serum creatinine from baseline or a decreased urine output of < 0.5 mL/kg/hour over 6 hours, within a 48-hour period, following sufficient volume repletion. These criteria were based on mounting evidence that even minor changes in serum creatinine are linked to severe clinical consequences[1-7] and the RIFLE stage correlated with unfavorable events.[8] In addition, the AKIN criteria distinguish the severity of kidney dysfunction at diagnosis and several time points along the course of the disease.[9] AKI is found in 5% of all hospitalized patients and in up to half of ICU patients.[10-14] With about 172 cases per million adults annually, the amount of AKI diagnoses is continuing to grow.[12] Nowhere is it more of an issue as in the ICU, where there are large cohorts of cardiovascular and cardiorenal patients. In fact, a study done by Cruz et al. in 2009 on 301 ICU patients reported that

44% of them had AKI during their stay, and almost 30% were diagnosed within 24 hours of admission.[10] Another study, this time by Kolhe et al. revealed that 6.3% of 276,731 patients admitted to 170 ICUs in a 10-year period had indications of severe AKI (serum creatinine $\geq$ 300 µmol/L and/or urea $\geq$ 40 mmol/L) during the first 24 hours, requiring intense and expensive interventions.[14]

The availability of the RIFLE and AKIN criteria (Table 11-1) have facilitated the recognition and reporting of AKI in various clinical settings and provided a framework for assessing cardiac and renal interactions. Ronco et al. have proposed a new definition for cardiorenal syndromes based on whether the heart or the kidney are the primary organ that is involved and the acuity of the situation.[15] As these new definitions of cardiorenal interactions are being evaluated further it is apparent that there is a great need clinically to ascertain the extent of kidney involvement in heart failure and define whether the increase in serum creatinine represents structural damage or a reversible functional change. The available clinical data, information on the timing and format of the event, rapidity, and duration of the changes and the response to improved hemodynamics and hydration all contribute to the differential diagnosis. However, the lack of any standardized criteria for "prerenal failure" and the absence of any specific markers for structural damage have contributed to a gap in our knowledge and led to variation in the management of AKI. Furthermore, it is particularly challenging to distinguish the coexistence of structural damage and a

Table 11-1	RIFLE and AKIN Criteria for Kidney Injury
RIFLE	*Definition*
Risk	x1.5 serum creatinine or urine production of < 0.5 mL/kg for 6 hours
Injury	x2.0 serum creatinine or urine production of < 0.5 mL/kg for 12 hours
Failure	x3.0 serum creatinine or creatinine > 355 µmol/L or urine output below 0.3 mL/kg for 24 hours
Loss	Persistent AKI or complete loss of kidney function for more than 4 weeks
End-stage renal disease	Complete loss of kidney function for more than 3 months
AKIN (Acute kidney injury network)	*Definition*
AKI (Acute kidney injury)	1. Kidney damage within a 48-hour window 2. Increase in serum creatinine of ≥ 0.3 mg/dL (≥ 26.4 µmol/L) 3. Increase in serum creatinine of ≥ 50% 4. Reduction in urine output of < 0.5 mL/kg/hr for more than 6 hours

Bellomo R, Ronco C, Kellum JA, Mehta RL, Palevsky P. Acute renal failure–definition, outcome measures, animal models, fluid therapy and information technology needs: the Second International Consensus Conference of the Acute Dialysis Quality Initiative (ADQI) Group. *Crit Care.* 2004;8:R204-12.

Lameire N, Van Biesen W, Vanholder R. Acute renal failure. *Lancet.* 2005;365:417-30.

Mehta RL, Kellum JA, Shah SV, Molitoris BA, Ronco C, Warnock DG, et al. Acute Kidney Injury Network: report of an initiative to improve outcomes in actue kidney injury. *Crit Care.* 2007;11:R31.

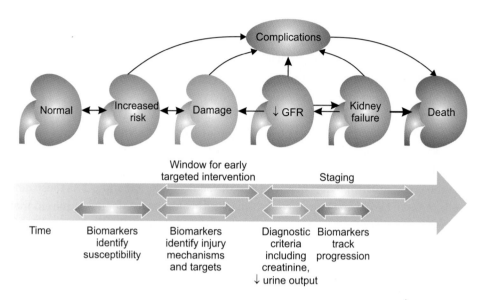

Figure 11-1 Varying time points for the use of biomarkers in acute kidney injury. Different biomarkers may have different capabilities of defining prerenal states depending on the nature and timing of the biomarker and the status of renal structure and function. Biomarkers of kidney injury could allow clinicians act early to limit renal damage. This is in contrast to markers of renal function, such as creatinine, which only rise when the damage is enough to significantly reduce kidney function. *From* Mehta RL. Timed and targeted therapy for acute kidney injury: a glimpse of the future. *Kidney Int.* 2010;77:947-9.

prerenal condition when there is chronic kidney disease (CKD). In both the past and present, blood urea nitrogen (BUN) and creatinine levels have been used as markers of kidney injury.[7,16] Unfortunately, creatinine is an inadequate marker of early renal injury. Therefore, there is a great need for kidney specific biomarkers that can help clinician in managing patients with cardiorenal syndromes much as the availability of cardiac troponins and BNP have enhanced the management of patients with cardiac ischemia and heart failure (Figure 11-1).[17]

In this chapter, we examine several prominent novel markers of kidney injury that have emerged and are being readied for clinical application. These biomarkers may potentially help identify those with renal injuries sooner than conventional markers, differentiate the etiology of renal injury, suggest the optimal timing of treatment initiation, and ultimately lead to improved patient management and outcomes.[10]

TRADITIONAL MARKERS: BUN, CREATININE, AND URINE OUTPUT

Blood urea nitrogen (BUN) is a serum byproduct of protein metabolism and is probably one of the oldest prognostic biomarkers in AKI. Urea is formed in the liver and carried to the kidneys for excretion. Diseased or damaged kidneys cause BUN to accumulate in the blood as the GFR goes down. Conditions, such as hypovolemic shock, congestive heart failure, high protein diet and bleeding into the gastrointestinal tract will also cause BUN elevations. Similarly, creatinine also accumulates in the blood when GFR decreases in the setting of renal dysfunction. Creatinine, a catabolic product of creatine phosphate in muscle tissue, is generated at a reasonably steady rate and is cleared by the kidneys with little-to-no tubular resorption. As a result, serum creatinine levels are commonly utilized to calculate the creatinine clearance (CrCl), which is a surrogate for GFR and renal function. Both traditionally and currently, BUN and creatinine are routinely used as standard biomarkers for AKI diagnosis and risk stratification.[18]

Despite their widespread use, these older biomarkers are far from ideal and can lead to inaccuracies. Bouchard et al.[19] compared the three major methods for estimation of renal function (Cockcroft-gault estimated CrCl, modification of diet in renal disease, and modified Jelliffe estimated CrCl) with urine CrCl and elevation in serum creatinine level in nondialyzed, critically ill subjects. They found that these methods overestimated urinary CrCl by 80%, 33%, and 10%, respectively, and the Jelliffe method underestimated GFR by 2%. While these equations serve as a widely available, noninvasive and cost effective method for approximating GFR, their principle fallacy is that they rely on a creatinine level presumed to be in "steady state." Unfortunately, the marker has been revealed to be a nonspecific, fairly insensitive marker for AKI.[20-22] Because it is an indicator of kidney function rather than structural damage, a person's glomerular filtration rate (GFR) must decline substantially before a rise in creatinine is detectable. Therefore, it is generally undependable with acute fluctuations in renal function.[23] To make matters worse, its concentration is influenced by several extrarenal factors, such as race, weight, gender, age, drugs, total body volume, protein intake, and muscle metabolism.[17]

Although urine output has been suggested as criterion for AKI diagnosis, there have been limited studies validating it utility. Macedo et al. have recently shown that reductions in urine output < 0.5 mL/kg/hr over 6 hours are early predictors of adverse outcomes and the number of episodes and duration of oliguria magnify the risk.[24] A follow-up study in ICU patients further validates these findings even when diuretics are used highlighting the utility of urine output as a physiological biomarker of interest.[25] Certainly oliguria is commonly encountered in heart failure and prompts the aggressive use of diuretics, an approach that may not always be beneficial to the patient.

Over the last decade, numerous new biomarkers, measured in blood and urine have emerged for diagnosing AKI. A model biomarker for renal dysfunction would be kidney specific, sensitive to small alterations in kidney function, correlate with gravity of injury, distinguish functional changes from structural damage and reveal the progression of damage.[17] We will now consider several novel biomarkers in this field and discuss the merits and limitations of each.

NEUTROPHIL GELATINASE-ASSOCIATED LIPOCALIN (NGAL)

Arguably the most analyzed and promising novel biomarker for AKI is neutrophil gelatinase-associated lipocalin (NGAL). It is a 25 kDa protein primarily used to transport substances of low molecular weight and is expressed by neutrophils and various epithelial cells, such as those in the proximal convoluted tubule (PCT).[26] While NGAL is found in a variety of tissues, it has been demonstrated as one of the most up-regulated proteins in the kidney following acute damage.[27-29] In fact, it is detectable in human blood and urine at the earliest stages of AKI, 48–72 hours before the rise in creatinine.[17] Both serum and urinary levels of NGAL have been studied as possible early structural markers of AKI in a variety of clinical locales and subject cohorts.

A landmark NGAL study in the emergency department (ED) has gathered a large amount of attention recently. Nikolas et al. calculated urine NGAL on 635 ED patients and demonstrated that uNGAL (corrected for urinary creatinine in this study) had a sensitivity of 90% and specificity of 99% (at a 130 mcg/g Cr cut-off) as well as the power to differentiate between AKI and other causes of elevated creatinine such as CKD and prerenal azotemia.[30] A study by Singer et al.[31] provides support for NGAL as a marker of kidney damage to discriminate 'prerenal' from 'intrinsic' AKI. These investigators measured urine NGAL in 145 hospitalized patients with elevated serum creatinine values meeting the RIFLE criteria for AKI (either a > 50% elevation in serum creatinine concentration or a > 25% decrease in GFR compared to a baseline measurement). Patients were followed through their hospital course to ascertain if they met a composite outcome of death, dialysis, or progression of RIFLE class. Two clinicians reviewed the clinical data and determined whether the patients had "prerenal" (22.1%), intrinsic AKI (51.7%), or were unclassifiable (26.2%). Urine NGAL levels were evaluated in context of this stratification for its diagnostic accuracy and prognostic ability. Urine NGAL levels at thresholds > 104 µg/L and < 47 µg/L identified patients who had intrinsic and prerenal AKI, respectively, with an AUC of 0.87 and a high specificity and predictive value for meeting a composite outcome when the levels were higher than 104 µg/L. Higher NGAL levels were related with a greater probability of reaching the composite outcome. However, it is necessary to understand that prerenal states can occur independently of structural changes or concurrent with structural changes. Thus threshold values for NGAL to distinguish prerenal from intrinsic AKI maybe very different in a patients with prior normal kidney function versus patients with CKD. Consequently, a combination of biomarkers may be more valuable than a single biomarker alone.[31,32]

NGAL has been studied specifically in the ICU as well as the ED. Cruz et al. found similar results as the studies above while analyzing the plasma NGAL of 301 ICU patients. Incredibly, plasma NGAL permitted the diagnosis of AKI earlier than the RIFLE criteria by up to 48 hours. It possessed an AUC of 0.78 in this scenario to go along with an AUC of 0.82 to anticipate the need for dialysis.[10] Constantin et al. performed a ICU study as well: they measured a single plasma NGAL measurement for 88 patients upon ICU admission. They reported NGAL to also elevate up to 48 hours before the RIFLE criteria were fulfilled while earning an AUC of 0.92, sensitivity and sensitivity of 82% and 97%, respectively, for a cut-off of 155 nmol/L.[33] It must be noted that the researchers in this study excluded those with a prior history of CKD. Removing this key demographic is most likely not a completely accurate portrayal of an ICU cohort.

A meta-analysis of NGAL's diagnostic and prognostic qualities in AKI had favorable results for the marker. The authors analyzed both plasma/serum and urine studies with measurements within 6 hours of kidney injury (if known) or from 24 to 48 hours prior to AKI diagnosis by traditional means. NGAL's diagnostic odds ratio (DOR) for predicting AKI in this analysis was 18.6 with sensitivity and specificity of 76.4% and 85.1%, respectively, and an AUC of 0.815. The utility of NGAL was better in children than in adults and was superior when standard NGAL assays were used. In cases of cardiac surgery, NGAL had a DOR of 13.1 with an AUC of 0.775, a sensitivity of 75.5%, and specificity of 75.1%. Urine NGAL was better than blood levels in the analysis with an AUC of 0.837 compared to 0.775 for plasma or serum. NGAL also appeared to predict the need for RRT well with an AUC of 0.782 but did not correlate as well with in-hospital mortality.[34]

NGAL research has also been done in relation to heart failure and early results are very promising in regard to both the kidneys of these patients as well as the myocardium. Various cohorts of chronic HF patients have been found to possess significantly higher levels of both serum and urine NGAL when compared with control subjects despite having only modest reductions in estimated glomerular filtration rates (eGFR).[35-38] The elevated urine NGAL in these cases was felt to represent tubular damage.[35] Furthermore, both serum and urine NGAL levels correlated with various indices of renal function[35-38] such as creatinine, eGFR, cystatin C, and urinary albumin excretion.[35] Investigators have therefore speculated that both serum and urine NGAL may be a sensitive and early marker of renal injury in chronic HF patients. Regarding acute HF, NGAL has demonstrated the ability to predict worsening renal function similarly to the chronic HF cohort mentioned above. One study showed that patients with an admission NGAL level of ≥ 140 ng/mL had a risk 7.4 times greater to develop worsening renal function with a sensitivity and specificity of 86% and 54%, respectively.[39]

Interestingly, NGAL's role is not confined to the kidney. The lipocalin is expressed within the failing myocardium as well as systemically. In fact, it has been demonstrated that patients with chronic HF have significantly elevated levels of NGAL compared with controls, with NYHA class III and IV patients possessing the highest levels.[38] The NGAL level also appears to be correlated with the NT-proBNP level, which is a cleavage product of proBNP.[38] These results indicate that NGAL can be an useful biomarker for cardiorenal syndrome, but clinically the addition of other biomarkers may be needed to improve diagnostic and prognostic accuracy.

Of the novel renal biomarkers being researched today, NGAL seems to have the strongest body of evidence thus far and has the greatest potential to be a stand-alone biomarker for kidney injury. It has been shown to increase significantly up to 48 hours before traditional markers and accurately detect kidney injury. This would give the physician time to adjust treatments to shield their patients from further renal injury and decrease morbidity in addition to the financial strain on healthcare systems. However, the lipocalin is not without its limitations.[40,41] These limitations can be assigned to imperfect time restraints on AKI diagnostic criteria or erroneously adding transient prerenal azotemia patients to AKI groups.[42] Additionally, the overall evidence for NGAL is stronger in children. This could perhaps be explained by the increased bypass times and various comorbidities in adult and elderly patients. Further research is needed to fully understand and possibly even rectify these limitations.

CYSTATIN C

Cystatin C (CysC) is protein produced by all nucleated cells. It is a cationic non-glycosylated low molecular weight cysteine protease (13 kD) that is not tubularly secreted and is filtered freely at the glomerulus, although it can be reabsorbed and catabolized.[43-44] As opposed to NGAL which is a structural marker of cell damage, CysC is a functional marker of GFR along the lines of creatinine. CysC does not appear to be influenced by race, gender, or muscle mass as creatinine is which makes it a better marker for glomerular function. Unfortunately, there is evidence connecting variations in CysC levels in patients with glucocorticoid abnormalities, aortic aneurysm, and thyroid dysfunction.[44] A variety of studies have been performed with CysC and several of them have focused on specific cohorts such as those in the ICU.

In 85 ICU patients with normal creatinine at baseline, CysC was able to detect AKI 24–48 hours earlier than creatinine with a sensitivity of 82% and specificity of 95%.[44] The same study had an AUC of 0.76 for predicting the severity of AKI, suggesting that CysC may have some value in gauging the degree of kidney injury as well as detecting renal damage earlier than current markers such as creatinine.

Another recent ICU study looked at 442 heterogeneous patients and found that those with elevations in both plasma CysC and creatinine > 50% of their baselines, a plasma CysC elevation preceded Cr elevation by 5.8 ± 13 hours. This was substantially less time than in the study mentioned above that had a disparity of 1.5 ± 0.6 days between the two.[44] Nejat et al. attribute their reduced time to the bigger patient cohort and heterogeneous qualities of their cohort which included some with recognized AKI and even CKD.[45] Plasma CysC was prognostic of AKI with an AUC of 0.87 [95% CI: 0.84–0.91] across the entire group of patients. This value was better than creatinine's AUC of 0.78 [95% CI: 0.73–0.83]. With regard to those patients that did not possess AKI on admission to the ICU, CysC predicted sustained AKI with an AUC of 0.80 (p < 0.0001) while pCr was not significantly prognostic. However, CysC was less than preferable in prognosticating AKI within seven days or at predicting death and RRT with AUC's of 0.65 [95% CI: 0.58–0.71] and 0.63 [95% CI: 0.56–0.71], respectively, in that cohort without established AKI. The authors did, interestingly, find a significant association between plasma CysC values and age. This could perhaps reverberate the understood age related decreases in GFR in elderly patients.[45] Several preceding studies had not found such a connection between CysC levels and age.

CysC performed favorably in the diagnosis of established AKI according to a recent systematic review, with an AUC of 0.88–0.97.[46] Based on earlier results for CysC as a dependable functional marker of GFR, these are not surprising findings. The review went on to point out that CysC had very good accuracy for the early diagnosis of AKI at one to two days prior to traditional clinical means.

Despite favorable experimental evidence for CysC, a reasonable critique is that it is not a direct marker of tissue injury, rather a functional GFR marker such as creatinine.[47] Thus it has the potential to be plagued by the same fallacies that have hindered creatinine as a marker; including the postponement in its rise due to its dependency on a substantial fall in GFR. Additionally, the effects of several comorbidities such as adrenal disorders or thyroid disease on CysC's levels are another limitation of the marker. Therefore, in order to obtain more widespread credibility, CysC needs further assessment in these and other clinical circumstances. If it can hold up to this scrutiny, CysC has promised to be a reliable marker of GFR over serum creatinine clinically. Studies have shown that it can identify a decrease in kidney function earlier than we are presently able to with BUN and creatinine. However, a direct marker of kidney injury would be vastly preferred to a functional marker of kidney decline such as cystatin C when faced the difficult early diagnosis of AKI.

INTERLEUKIN-18

Interleukin-18 (IL-18) holds an essential role in the pathophysiology of sepsis as an 18-kDa pro-inflammatory cytokine.[48] IL-18 in the urine arises from tubular epithelial cells and has the potential to be an early marker of AKI as it has been demonstrated in mice to mediate ischemic acute tubular necrosis.[49,50] The interleukin has also been analyzed within several clinical settings in a variety of patient cohorts.

ROC-AUCs for IL-18's ability to diagnose early AKI have varied according to a recent systematic review. In this review AUC values ranged anywhere from a paltry 0.54 to an impressive 0.90.[46] Furthermore, they found a faint correlation to AKI duration or severity and demonstrated that as a whole IL-18 had high specificity but low sensitivity to diagnose AKI. Additionally, Parikh et al. conducted a nested case-control study within the Acute Respiratory Distress Syndrome (ARDS) Network trial to identify if urine IL-18 is an early diagnostic marker of AKI. They showed that IL-18 levels were elevated significantly in AKI patients at one and two days prior to diagnosis by creatinine; nevertheless the AUC's were a measly 0.73 at 24 hours and 0.65 at 48 hours.[51] This group also found IL-18 to be an independent predictor of mortality, but it is essential to take this results in the context of the criteria of the primary ARDS study.

In the arena of novel biomarkers of AKI, IL-18 has shown some signs of early promise, but the overall evidence has been somewhat inconsistent. In the majority of the trials, IL-18 received poorer marks than the other novel biomarkers being studied. Another issue with IL-18 is that a handful of trials have connected its up-regulation to sepsis, heart failure and systemic inflammation.[52,53] Importantly, these are all pathological conditions that can result in or often coexist with AKI. For now it seems that IL-18 could become most serviceable as a part of a renal biomarker panel due to its utility in to predicting adult and pediatric mortality in[51,54] critically ill cohorts, but it needs further research to determine if it possesses any stand-alone value.

KIDNEY INJURY MOLECULE-1

Kidney injury molecule-1 (KIM-1) is a type 1 transmembrane protein that is not detectable in normal tissue. It is highly up-regulated in dedifferentiated epithelial cells of the proximal tubule after a toxic or ischemic renal insult.[55] It is thus a structural marker of tubular injury and better suited to be used as a biomarker of AKI than creatinine. This marker has in fact shown the ability to provide information regarding the nature of the renal insult. Urinary KIM-1 has showed effectiveness in differentiating actual acute tubular necrosis from and other forms of kidney injury such as CKD and prerenal azotemia.[56]

KIM-1 was shown to be a useful biomarker in the diagnosis of established AKI but not as serviceable in predicting future AKI according to a recent review.[46] Additionally, Han et al. conducted a trial involving 44 patients with an assortment of acute and chronic kidney diseases and 30 control subjects. They showed that urinary KIM-1 levels were significantly higher in patients with AKI when compared to those with UTI or control subjects. The biomarker possessed an AUC of 0.90 to diagnose AKI in this cohort.[57]

Several KIM-1 studies have been performed in cardiac surgery patients as well. In a trial featuring 103 cardiopulmonary bypass patients devoid of preoperative renal impairment, KIM-1 outperformed other urinary biomarkers for AKI detection at two hours post bypass (AUC of 0.78).[58] At this time point, KIM-1 possessed a sensitivity of 92% and specificity of 58%. Disappointingly, significant increases in KIM-1 levels did not persist at one- and two-day time points when comparing in AKI subjects versus non-AKI subjects.[58]

KIM-1 has had some promising results in trials to date with regards to being a good structural marker of kidney injury. It has shown utility in detecting injury prior to serum creatinine and this evidence has been especially of note in cardiac surgery cohorts. Despite this results, the data for KIM-1's utility as an individual marker for AKI prediction and diagnosis is currently inadequate due to vastly different cohorts within current studies as well as an inadequate number of studies overall. Differing cohorts is a key concern: some patient groups have much greater risks of renal damage than others and this can make comparative evaluations challenging. At this point, KIM-1 appears best served as a member of kidney biomarker panel. A pairing of KIM-1 with other novel markers may be able to provide reliable results than the markers individually. In fact, Liang et al. found that combining it with IL-18 in diagnosing and gauging the advancement of AKI after CPB yielded favorable results.[59]

THE FUTURE OF RENAL BIOMARKERS IN HEART FAILURE

It is now well recognized that the development of AKI portends a poor prognosis and that there is a great clinical need to develop new methods for recognizing renal dysfunction early and intervene early in the course. While traditional markers BUN, serum creatinine, and urine output have inherent limitations we need to recognize that we do not use them optimally and they can add significantly to our management strategies. While we have reviewed some of the most studied kidney biomarkers it is apparent that there are several candidate including liver fatty acid binding protein, alpha and pi GST, NAG, and urine albumin that are being studied further and will likely add to our tool kit.[60] However, it is worth considering that none of these biomarkers will by themselves be the sole winners in this area. In fact, a recent review of all kidney biomarkers suggests that they have not added much incremental value for clinical decision making.[61] Given the rapid advances in this field it is helpful to reflect on the need for kidney biomarkers in cardiac failure. As shown in table 11-2, biomarkers can help resolve several different questions to optimize treatment of patients with renal dysfunction in the setting of heart failure. There is limited data

Table 11-2	Clinical Need for Kidney Biomarkers in Cardiorenal Syndromes			
Risk assessment	*Surveillance*	*Diagnosis*	*Interventions*	*Prognosis*
Is patient at risk for kidney dysfunction? Genomic CKD?	Change in renal function during course of heart failure	Is there evidence of renal damage or is there functional change (prerenal that is reversible)?	*When the diagnosis is uncertain to define the type and nature of initial therapy* CRS 1: a. Whether patient has "prerenal" state or has suffered structural damage b. Is the dysfunction due to the underlying disease or to the therapy? CRS 2: a. Is the decline in kidney function chronic and stable or is new injury occurring? b. What will be effect of choice of therapy on kidney function? *When the therapy is in place to define success* Has renal function decline resolved? Has a new steady state been achieved that is acceptable? Is progression occurring?	Will the patient need dialysis? Will renal function improve with improvement in heart condition?

CRS, cardiorenal syndromes.

for the utilization of biomarkers together. The combination of KIM-1 and IL-18 levels aids in the judicious evaluation of the advancement of AKI after CPB.[59] Additionally, IL-18 and urine NGAL levels, when corrected for urine creatinine, can be utilized together to identify AKI in subjects post cardiac surgery.[62] A similar combination was effective for contrast based injuries as Ling W et al. demonstrated that urinary IL-18 and NGAL are potential early markers for contrast induced nephropathy (CIN).[63] Essentially, the use of these biomarkers in conjunction with each other could result in earlier and more dependable AKI diagnosis and prognosis evaluations than traditional markers.[64] The establishment and analysis of such a kidney would be difficult in its infancy, however, succinct classifications and limitations must be thoroughly examined and recognized before the markers could be confidently used together. Our comprehension of novel urinary markers currently is somewhat incomplete. However, the studies illuminating their mechanisms of function, specificities, sensitivities, time courses of action, and utilities in clinical prognosis have shown great potential. Further investigation into the world of novel biomarkers can equip clinicians with the necessary equipment to quickly and reliably appraise their patients' renal function so that appropriate management can be utilized; for example, determining if intermittent or permanent hemodialysis must be employed.[65]

We propose that now as we have a fair amount of information on individual biomarkers, we move rapidly towards evaluating combinations of biomarkers encompassing clinical, physiological, and structural changes in the kidney in the setting of heart failure. We believe that these approaches will enhance risk assessment, surveillance, and diagnosis and will facilitate primary and secondary prevention, targeted intervention and appropriate timely interventions to improve outcomes in these patients. We look forward to an era where the specter of kidney involvement in heart failure does not evoke anxiety but leads to biomarker-guided specific targeted interventions with beneficial effects.

REFERENCES

1. Bellomo R, Ronco C, Kellum JA, Mehta RL, Palevsky P. Acute renal failure–definition, outcome measures, animal models, fluid therapy and information technology needs: the Second International Consensus Conference of the Acute Dialysis Quality Initiative (ADQI) Group. *Crit Care.* 2004;8:R204-12.
2. Chertow GM, Burdick E, Honour M, Bonventre JV, Bates DW. Acute kidney injury, mortality, length of stay, and costs in hospitalized patients. *J Am Soc Nephrol.* 2005;16: 3365-70.
3. Gruberg L, Mintz GS, Mehran R, Gangas G, Lansky AJ, Kent KM, et al. The prognostic implications of further renal function deterioration within 48 h of interventional coronary procedures in patients with pre-existent chronic renal insufficiency. *J Am Coll Cardiol.* 2000;36:1542-8.
4. Lassnigg A, Schmidlin D, Mouhieddine M, Bachmann LM, Druml W, Bauer P, et al. Minimal changes of serum creatinine predict prognosis in patients after cardiothoracic surgery: a prospective cohort study. *J Am Soc Nephrol.* 2004;15:1597-605.
5. Levy MM, Macias WL, Vincent JL, Russell JA, Silva E, Trzaskoma B, et al. Early changes in organ function predict eventual survival in severe sepsis. *Crit Care Med.* 2005;33:2194-201.
6. McCullough PA, Soman SS. Contrast-induced nephropathy. *Crit Care Clin.* 2005;21:261-80.
7. Praught ML, Shlipak MG. Are small changes in serum creatinine an important risk factor? *Curr Opin Nephrol Hypertens.* 2005;14:265-70.
8. Ricci Z, Cruz D, Ronco C. The RIFLE criteria and mortality in acute kidney injury: A systematic review. *Kidney Int.* 2008;73:538-46.
9. Mehta RL, Kellum JA, Shah SV, Molitoris BA, Ronco C, Warnock DG, et al. Acute Kidney Injury Network (AKIN): report of an initiative to improve outcomes in acute kidney injury. *Crit Care.* 2007;11:R31.

10. Cruz DN, de Cal M, Garzotto F, Perazella MA, Lentini P, Corradi V, et al. Plasma neutrophil gelatinase-associated lipocalin is an early biomarker for acute kidney injury in an adult ICU population. *Intensive Care Med.* 2010;36:444-51.

11. Liu KD, Chertow GM. Acute renal failure. In: Anthony SF, Eugene B, Dennis LK, Stephen LH, Dan LL, Larry JJ, et al., editors. Harrison's Principles of Internal Medicine. 17th ed. New York: McGraw-Hill Medical. 2008. Vol. II. p. 1752-61.

12. Feest TG, Round A, Hamad S. Incidence of severe acute renal failure in adults: results of a community-based study. *BMJ.* 1993;306:481-3.

13. Hsu CY, McCulloch CE, Fan D, Ordonez JD, Chertow GM, Go AS. Community-based incidence of acute renal failure. *Kidney Int.* 2007;72:208-12.

14. Kolhe NV, Stevens PE, Crowe AV, Lipkin GW, Harrison DA. Case mix, outcome and activity for patients with severe acute kidney injury during the first 24 hours after admission to an adult general critical care unit: application of predictive models from a secondary analysis of the ICNARC Case Mix Programme Database. *Crit Care.* 2008;12 Suppl 1:S2.

15. Ronco C, Haapio M, House AA, Anavekar N, Bellomo R. Cardiorenal syndrome. *J Am Coll Cardiol.* 2008;52:1527-39.

16. Macedo E, Mehta R. Prerenal azotemia in congestive heart failure. *Contrib Nephrol.* 2010;164:79-87.

17. Mehta RL. Timed and targeted therapy for acute kidney injury: a glimpse of the future. *Kidney Int.* 2010;77:947-9.

18. Bjornsson TD. Use of serum creatinine concentrations to determine renal function. *Clin Pharmacokinet.* 1979;4:200-22.

19. Bouchard M, Macedo C, Soroko S, Chertow GM, Himmelfarb J, Ikizler TA, et al. Comparison of methods for estimating glomerular filtration rate in critically ill patients with acute kidney injury. *Nephrol Dial Transplant.* 2010;25:102-7.

20. Lattanzio M, Kopyt N. Acute kidney injury: new concepts in definition, diagnosis, pathophysiology, and treatment. *J Am Osteopath Assoc.* 2009;109:13-9.

21. Awdishu L. Drug dosing in acute kidney injury—do we underdeliver? Paper presented at: International Conference on Continuous Renal Replacement Therapies; February 2010: San Diego, CA.

22. Ostermann M, Chang RW. Acute kidney injury in the intensive care unit according to RIFLE. *Crit Care Med.* 2007;35:1837-43.

23. Bellomo R, Kellum JA, Ronco C. Defining acute renal failure: physiological principles. *Intensive Care Med.* 2004;30:33-7.

24. Macedo E, Malhotra R, Claure-Del Granado R, Fedullo P, Mehta RL. Defining urine output criterion for acute kidney injury in critically ill patients. *Nephrol Dial Transplant.* 2011;26:509-15.

25. Macedo E, Malhotra R, Bouchard J, Wynn SK, Mehta RL. Oliguria is an early predictor of higher mortality in critically ill patients. *Kidney Int.* 2011

26. Uttenthal O. NGAL: a marker molecule for the distressed kidney? *Clin Lab Int.* 2005;29: 39-41.

27. Supavekin S, Zhang W, Kucherlapati R, Kaskel FJ, Moore LC, Devarajan P. Differential gene expression following early renal ischemia-reperfusion. *Kidney Int.* 2003;63:1714-24.

28. Keiran NE, Doran PP, Connolly SB, Greenan MC, Higgins DF, Leonard M, et al. Modification of the transcriptome response to renal ischemia/reperfusion injury by lipoxin analog. *Kidney Int.* 2003;64:480-92.

29. Yuen PST, Jo SK, Holly MK, Hu X, Star RA. Ischemic and nephrotoxic acute renal failure are distinguished by their broad transcriptomic responses. *Physiol Genomics.* 2006;25:375-86.

30. Nickolas TL, O'Rourke MJ, Yang J, Sise ME, Canetta PA, Barasch N, et al. Sensitivity and specificity of a single emergency department measurement of urinary neutrophil gelatinase-associated lipocalin for diagnosing acute kidney injury. *Ann Intern Med.* 2008;148:810-9.

31. Singer E, Elger A, Elitok S, Kettritz R, Nickolas TL, Barasch J, et al. Urinary neutrophil gelatinase-associated lipocalin distinguishes pre-renal from intrinsic renal failure and predicts outcomes. *Kidney Int.* 2011;80:405-14.

32. Mehta RL. Biomarker explorations in acute kidney injury: the journey continues. *Kidney Int.* 2011;80:332-4.

33. Constantin JM, Futier E, Perbet S, Roszyk L, Lautrette A, Gillart T, et al. Plasma neutrophil gelatinase-associated lipocalin is an early marker of acute kidney injury in adult critically ill patients: a prospective study. *J Crit Care.* 2010;25:176.e1-6.

34. Haase M, Bellomo R, Devarajan P, Schlattmann P, Haase-Fielitz A. Accuracy of neutrophil gelatinase-associated lipocalin (NGAL) in diagnosis and prognosis in acute kidney injury: a systematic review and meta-analysis. *Am J Kidney Dis.* 2009;54:1012-24.

35. Damman K, van Veldhuisen DJ, Navis G, Voors AA, Hillege HL. Urinary neutrophil gelatinase associated lipocalin (NGAL), a marker of tubular damage, is increased in patients with chronic heart failure. *Eur J Heart Fail.* 2008;10:997-1000.

36. Poniatowski B, Malyszko J, Bachorzewska-Gajewska H, Malyszko JS, Dobrzycki S. Serum neutrophil gelatinase-associated lipocalin as a marker of renal function in patients with chronic heart failure and coronary artery disease. *Kidney Blood Press Res.* 2009;32:77-80.

37. Bolignano D, Basile G, Parisi P, Coppolino G, Nicocia G, Buemi M. Increased plasma neutrophil gelatinase-associated lipocalin levels predict mortality in elderly patients with chronic heart failure. *Rejuvenation Res.* 2009;12:7-14.

38. Yndestad A, Landro L, Ueland T, et al. Increased systemic and myocardial expression of neutrophil gelatinase-associated lipocalin in clinical and experimental heart failure. *Eur Heart J.* 2009;30:1229-36.

39. Aghel A, Shrestha K, Mullens W, Borowski A, Tang WH. Serum neutrophil gelatinase-associated lipocalin (NGAL) in predicting worsening renal function in acute decompensated heart failure. *J Card Fail.* 2010;16:49-54.

40. Koyner JL, Bennett MR, Worcester EM, Ma Q, Raman J, Jeevanandam V, et al. Urinary cystatin C as an early biomarker of acute kidney injury following adult cardiothoracic surgery. *Kidney Int.* 2008;74:1059-69.

41. Wagener G, Gubitosa G, Wang S, Borregaard N, Kim M, Lee HT. Urinary neutrophil gelatinase-associated lipocalin and acute kidney injury after cardiac surgery. *Am J Kidney Dis.* 2008;52:425-33.

42. Devarajan P. NGAL in acute kidney injury: from serendipity to utility. *Am J Kidney Dis.* 2008;52:395-9.

43. Dharnidharka VR, Kwon C, Stevens G. Serum cystatin C is superior to serum creatinine as a marker of kidney function: a meta-analysis. *Am J Kidney Dis.* 2002;40:221-6.

44. Herget-Rosenthal S, Marggraf G, Hüsing J, Göring F, Pietruck F, Janssen O, et al. Early detection of acute renal failure by serum cystatin C. *Kidney Int.* 2004;66:1115–22.

45. Nejat M, Pickering JW, Walker RJ, Endre ZH. Rapid detection of acute kidney injury by plasma cystatin C in the intensive care unit. *Nephrol Dial Transplant.* 2010;25:3283-9.

46. Coca SG, Yalavarthy R, Concato J, Parikh CR. Biomarkers for the diagnosis and risk stratification of acute kidney injury: a systematic review. *Kidney Int.* 2008;73:1008-16.

47. Mishra J, Dent C, Tarabishi R, et al. Neutrophil gelatinase-associated lipocalin (NGAL) as a biomarker for acute renal injury after cardiac surgery. *Lancet.* 2005;365:1231-8.

48. Tschoeke SK, Oberholzer A, Moldawer LL. Interleukin-18: a novel prognostic cytokine in bacteria-induced sepsis. *Crit Care Med.* 2006;34:1225-33.

49. Melnikov VY, Faubel S, Siegmund B, Lucia MS, Ljubanovic D, Edelstein CL. Neutrophil-independent mechanisms of caspase-1- and IL-18-mediated ischemic acute tubular necrosis in mice. *J Clin Invest.* 2002;110:1083-91.

50. Melnikov VY, Ecder T, Fantuzzi G, Siegmund B, Lucia MS, Dinarello CA, et al. Impaired IL-18 processing protects caspase-1-deficient mice from ischemic acute renal failure. *J Clin Invest.* 2001;107:1145-52.

51. Parikh CR, Abraham E, Ancukiewicz M, Edelstein CL. Urine IL-18 is an early diagnostic marker for acute kidney injury and predicts mortality in the intensive care unit. *J Am Soc Nephrol.* 2005;16:3046-52.

52. Haase M, Bellomo R, Story D, Davenport P, Haase-Fielitz A. Urinary interleukin-18 does not predict acute kidney injury after adult cardiac surgery: a prospective observational cohort study. *Crit Care.* 2008;12:R96.

53. Grobmyer SR, Lin E, Lowry SF, Rivadeneira DE, Potter S, Barie PS, et al. Elevation of IL-18 in human sepsis. *J Clin Immunol.* 2000;20:212-5.

54. Washburn KK, Zappitelli M, Arikan AA, Loftis L, Yalavarthy R, Parikh CR, et al. Urinary interleukin-18 is an acute kidney injury biomarker in critically Ill children. *Nephrol Dial Transplant.* 2008;23:566-72.

55. Vaidya VS, Ramirez V, Ichimura T, Bobadilla NA, Bonventre JV. Urinary kidney injury molecule-1: a sensitive quantitative biomarker for early detection of kidney tubular injury. *Am J Physiol Renal Physiol.* 2006;290:F517-29.

56. Han WK, Bailly V, Abichandani R, Thadhani R, Bonventre JV. Kidney Injury molecule-1 (KIM-1): a novel biomarker for human renal proximal tubule injury. *Kidney Int.* 2002;62:237-44.

57. Han WK, Waikar SS, Johnson A, Betensky RA, Dent CL, Devarajan P, et al. Urinary biomarkers in the early diagnosis of acute kidney injury. *Kidney Int.* 2008;73:863-9.

58. Liangos O, Tighiouart H, Perianayagam MC, Kolyada A, Han WK, Wald R, et al. Comparative analysis of urinary biomarkers for early detection of acute kidney injury following cardiopulmonary bypass. *Biomarkers.* 2009;14:423-31.

59. Liang XL, Liu SX, Chen YH, Yan LJ, Li H, Xuan HJ, et al. Combination of urinary kidney injury molecule-1 and interleukin-18 as early biomarker for the diagnosis and progressive assessment of acute kidney injury following cardiopulmonary bypass surgery: a prospective nested case-control study. *Biomarkers.* 2010;15:332-9.

60. Devarajan P. Biomarkers for the early detection of acute kidney injury. *Curr Opin Pediatr.* 2011;23:194-200.

61. Lameire NH, Vanholder RC, Van Biesen WA. How to use biomarkers efficiently in acute kidney injury. *Kidney Int.* 2011;79:1047-50.

62. Xin C, Yulong X, Yu C, Changchun C, Feng Z, Xinwei M. Urine neutrophil gelatinase-associated lipocalin and interleukin-18 predict acute kidney injury after cardiac surgery. *Ren Fail.* 2008;30:904-13.

63. Ling W, Zhaohui N, Ben H, Leyi G, Jianping L, Huili D, et al. Urinary IL-18 and NGAL as early predictive biomarkers in contrast-induced nephropathy after coronary angiography. *Nephron Clin Pract.* 2008;108:c176-81.

64. Parikh CR, Mishra J, Thiessen-Philbrook H, Dursun B, Ma Q, Kelly C, et al. Urinary IL-18 is an early predictive biomarker of acute kidney injury after cardiac surgery. *Kidney Int.* 2006;70:199-203.

65. Desai AA, Baras J, Berk BB, Nakajima A, Garber AM, Owens D, et al. Management of acute kidney injury in the intensive: a cost-effectiveness analysis of daily vs alternate-day hemodialysis. *Arch Intern Med.* 2008;168:1761-7.

Adrenomedullin

John T Parissis, Alan S Maisel, Gerasimos S Filippatos

INTRODUCTION

Adrenomedullin (ADM) is a novel 52 amino acid vasoactive peptide that was discovered for the first time in 1993 in human pheochromocytoma.[1,2] This molecule has structural homology with calcitonin-gene-related peptide and is synthesized by many human tissues, including adrenal medulla, vascular endothelium, myocardium, and central nervous system.[1,2] It is well known that ADM can act as a potent vasodilator promoting also diuresis and natriuresis. Moreover, recent data suggest that ADM is a multifunctional mediator involved in processes so diverse as embryogenesis, normal and malignant growth, inflammation and immunity. Plasma ADM levels are increased in various pathological conditions, such as arterial hypertension, acute and chronic heart failure, acute coronary syndromes, renal insufficiency, and sepsis.[3,4] ADM may play important role in the pathophysiology of many of these syndromes; and in some of them, evaluation of ADM concentration may provide important prognostic information. This chapter summarizes the current knowledge regarding the biologic role of ADM in cardiovascular system as well as the utility of this molecule as a novel biomarker for risk stratification of patients with cardiovascular disease.

BIOLOGIC EFFECTS ON CARDIOVASCULAR SYSTEM

Vasodilatory Effects

ADM is a vasoactive agent, in that when administered into systemic circulation, it lowers arterial blood pressure by decreasing peripheral vascular resistance.[5] This effect can lead to a substantial increase in cardiac output due to reduction of afterload. A potential mechanism of vasodilatory action of ADM is the agent-induced endothelium-independent relaxation through the increase of cAMP level in vascular smooth muscle cells. Because ADM is secreted by endothelial cells, it may act as one of endothelium-derived relaxing factors. In addition, ADM binds to specific receptors in endothelial cells and elicits endothelium-dependent vasorelaxation, mediated by nitric oxide and/or vasoactive prostanoids. The effects of ADM on vascular endothelial cells as well as its antiproliferative action on vascular smooth muscle cells may play an important role in vascular remodeling in arterial hypertension or during the development of post-PTCA restenosis.

Inotropic Effects

Although systemic infusion of ADM increases cardiac output, this is secondary to peripheral vasodilatory action. The direct effect of ADM on myocardial contractility still remains controversial. ADM reduces contractility of isolated rabbit ventricular myocytes by stimulating NO production, which decreases intracellular calcium concentration through cGMP-dependent mechanism.[6] In contrast, ADM has positive inotropic effect on isolated perfused rat heart and isolated rat papillary muscles. Several studies have demonstrated that ADM inhibits protein synthesis and hypertrophy of cardiomyocytes, as well as proliferation of cardiac fibroblasts and production of extracellular matrix.[7,8] Since ADM is synthesized and secreted by isolated cardiomyocytes and cardiac fibroblasts, this molecule may be an important regulator of myocardial hypertrophy and remodeling in arterial hypertension and heart failure in a paracrine/autocrine manner.

Diuretic/Natriuretic Effects

ADM administration can lead to increased urine output and urinary sodium excretion.[3,4] The drug mainly causes renal vasodilation that lead to increased renal blood flow and glomerular filtration rate. Additionally, ADM inhibits tubular sodium reabsorption leading to natriuresis. Finally, experimental data suggest that ADM inhibits angiotensin II-induced migration and proliferation of mesangial cells and the generation of reactive oxygen species by these cells. These antioxidative effects may attenuate the progression of chronic nephropathies and suggest a renoprotective role of this substance in cardiorenal syndromes.

ADRENOMEDULLIN/PROADRENOMEDULLIN AS BIOMARKERS OF CARDIOVASCULAR DISEASE

Arterial Hypertension

Experimental pressure overload induced by the infusion of angiotensin II, arginine vasopressin, or by surgical aortic banding increases myocardial ADM gene expression. In addition, mechanical stretch promotes ADM secretion from cultured cardiomyocytes. Thus, ADM gene is up-regulated by myocardial pressure overload and myocardial hypertrophy.[9] It is suggested that up-regulation of cardiac ADM system in arterial hypertension is a protective mechanism decreasing myocardial overload due to vasodilatory and natriuretic properties of ADM, as well as limiting further myocardial hypertrophy and remodeling. Furthermore, plasma ADM concentrations are elevated in patients with idiopathic arterial hypertension and are associated with complications of the disease, such as left ventricular hypertrophy and nephrosclerosis.[10]

Heart Failure

There are several reports, which have shown that plasma ADM levels are increased in heart failure in proportion to the disease severity. In 1995,[11] Nishikimi et al. demonstrated a significant and proportionate increase in plasma levels of ADM in patients with moderate to severe heart failure (Figure 12-1). In addition, they observed a significant correlation between plasma levels of ADM, norepinephrine, atrial natriuretic peptide (ANP), and BNP. Plasma levels of ADM in patients with severe heart failure decreased after treatment including beta-blockade, with a concomitant decrease in ANP and BNP levels. These results suggest that the increased plasma volume and an activated sympathetic nervous system may be involved in the increased levels of circulating ADM. Given that ADM exerts potent cardiovascular effects in animal models and that vascular endothelial cells and

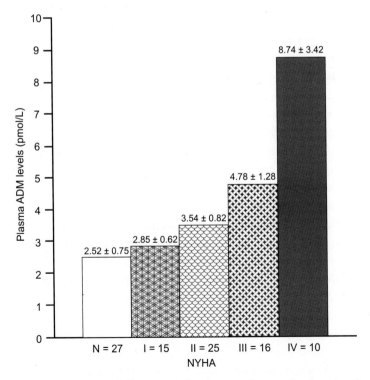

Figure 12-1 Plasma adrenomedullin (ADM) levels according to the functional severity of chronic heart failure. *Data from* Nishikimi T, Saito Y, Kitamura K, Ishimitsu T, Eto T, Kangawa K, et al. Increased plasma levels of adrenomedullin in patients with heart failure. *J Am Coll Cardiol.* 1995;26:1424-31.

vascular smooth muscle cells synthesize and secrete ADM, increased levels of this substance in heart failure may be involved in the defence mechanism against further elevation in peripheral vascular resistance.

In another prospective study,[12] plasma levels of ADM were measured by radioimmunoassay in 117 chronic heart failure patients with idiopathic or ischemic cardiomyopathy who treated with ACE inhibitors and diuretics. Plasma levels of ADM were significantly increased in chronic heart failure patients by comparison to controls (p = 0·01). During the follow-up period, fourteen cardiovascular deaths and four urgent cardiac transplantations occurred. In the univariate Cox model, ADM plasma levels were related to prognosis (p = 0·004). A multivariate analysis, including heart rate, systolic blood pressure, NYHA class, left ventricular ejection fraction, left ventricular echocardiographic end-diastolic diameter, plasma levels of ADM, endothelin-1, norepinephrine, and ANP was performed: plasma levels of ADM (p = 0·03), of endothelin-1 (p = 0·0001), and systolic blood pressure (p = 0·003) were significantly associated with outcome. These findings suggest that elevated plasma concentrations of ADM are an independent predictor of prognosis in predominantly mild to moderate chronic heart failure treated by conventional therapy and provide additional prognostic information.

Moreover, it has been reported that plasma NT-proBNP and ADM levels in patients with established ischemic left ventricular dysfunction receiving standard therapy with ACE inhibitors and loop diuretics (with or without digoxin) are independently predictive of mortality and heart failure. Elevated plasma levels of both of these peptides predict a long-term benefit from initiation of carvedilol use.[13]

It is known that ADM is synthesized as part of a larger precursor molecule, termed preproADM (Figure 12-2). In humans, this precursor consists of 185 amino acids. ADM is difficult to measure in plasma because it is partially complexed with complement factor H and is rapidly cleared from the circulation. The more stable midregional fragment of proADM (MR-proADM), comprising amino acids 45–92 of preproADM, has been identified, and is more stable than the active molecule being secreted in equimolar amounts to ADM.[14] Recently, it has been reported[15] that in patients with acute dyspnea, MR-proADM levels are elevated in nonsurvivors compared with survivors, regardless of the underlying disease. MR-proADM on admission predicted 30-day and one-year mortality and seemed to be even better than the natriuretic peptides regarding short-term mortality. Finally, MR-proADM used in addition to natriuretic peptides helped to better risk stratify dyspneic patients.

Recently, MR-proADM were assessed by von Haehling et al.[16] in 501 chronic heart failure patients with impaired left ventricular systolic function. MR-proADM levels increased according to the severity of NYHA class (p < 0.0001). During 1 year follow-up, 70 patients (14%) died. Elevated plasma MR-proADM concentration was

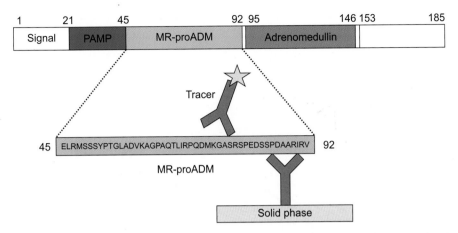

Figure 12-2 Schematic representation of preproadrenomedullin (preproADM) molecule. Signal: signal peptide; PAMP: Pro-adrenomedullin N-terminal 20 peptide; MR-proADM: Mid regional proadrenomedullin. *From* Khan S, O'Brien R, Struck J, Quinn P, Morgenthaler N, Squire I, et al. Prognostic value of midregional proadrenomedullin in patients with acute myocardial infarction: the LAMP (Leicester Acute Myocardial Infarction Peptide) study. *J Am Coll Cardiol.* 2007;49:1525-32, with permission.

a predictor of poor survival at 12 months (p < 0.002) after multivariable adjustment. In receiver-operating characteristic curve analysis of 12-month survival, the areas under the curve for MR-proADM and NT-proBNP did not significantly differ (p < 0.3). Comparing Cox proportional hazard models using the likelihood ratio x2 statistic, authors found that both NT-proBNP and MR-proADM added prognostic value to a base model of left ventricular ejection fraction, age, creatinine, and NYHA class. Adding MR-proADM to the base model offered stronger prognostic power than adding NT-proBNP. Thus, MR-proADM is a predictor of mortality in patients with CHF, independent of established clinical and biochemical markers. The assessment of MR-proADM seems to add prognostic information to classical natriuretic peptides.

Finally, in the prognostic arm of the BACH (Biomarkers in Acute Heart Failure) trial,[17] investigators found that MR-proADM was superior to traditional natriuretic peptides for predicting 90-day mortality in patients with dyspnea due to acute heart failure. This finding was especially true in an exploratory analysis of the important first 30 days after baseline evaluation, for which MR-proADM clearly outperformed BNP and NT-proBNP. Troponin, which was recently shown to have prognostic value in patients with heart failure, was also added to a multivariable model with the other three markers. In this model, MR-proADM still remained an independent prognostic factor. In the 568 BACH patients with a confirmed diagnosis of acute heart failure, the prognostic accuracy of MR-proADM levels evaluated in blood samples taken on admission to the emergency department was 73%. Prognostic accuracy was found

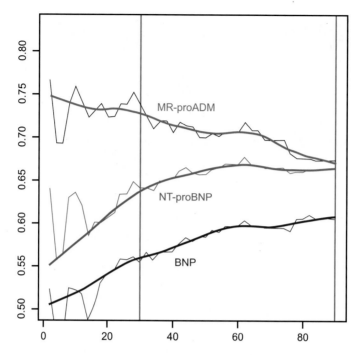

Figure 12-3 Area under the receiver-operating characteristic curve for survival to 90 days for MR-proADM (red line), BNP (blue line), and NT-proBNP (green line) in patients with acute heart failure included in BACH trial. *From* Maisel A, Mueller C, Nowak R, Peacock WF, Landsberg JW, Ponikowski P, et al. Mid-region pro-hormone markers for the diagnosis and prognosis in acute dyspnea: results from the BACH (Biomarkers in Acute Heart Failure) trial. *J Am Coll Cardiol.* 2010;55:2062-76, with permission.

to be lower for BNP and NT-proBNP (62% and 64%, respectively) (Figure 12-3). This remained also in the same way when investigating all 1,641 enrolled patients, regardless of final diagnosis. Consequently, these findings highlight the prognostic importance of MR-proADM levels in patients with acute heart failure that may help clinicians optimize therapeutic interventions, especially in patients at high risk.

Acute Coronary Syndromes

Plasma ADM has been initially investigated in small studies as a prognostic marker compared with B type natriuretic peptides. One study identified plasma ADM as an independent predictor of cardiogenic shock and short-term mortality in patients with an acute coronary syndrome.[18] Other investigators found that ADM had no independent additional prognostic value to NT-proBNP in patients with acute coronary syndromes.[19] The potential role of the more stable prohormone MR-proADM in prognostication after AMI has been investigated in patient population of the LAMP (Leicester Acute Myocardial Infarction Peptide) study.[20] Plasma MR-proADM and NTproBNP were assessed in 983 consecutive post-AMI patients 3–5 days after chest pain onset. There were 101 deaths and 49 readmissions with heart failure during follow-up. The MR-proADM was increased in patients with death or HF compared with survivors ($p < 0.0001$). Using a sophisticated multivariate logistic model, log MR-proADM (odds ratio 4.22) and log NT-proBNP (odds ratio 3.20) were significant independent predictors of death or heart failure (with creatinine, age, gender, and history of AMI). The areas under the receiver operating characteristic curve for MR-proADM, NT-proBNP, and the logistic model with both markers were 0.77, 0.79, and 0.84, respectively. Cox models for the predictors of death or heart failure showed the same variables (including log MR-proADM, hazard ratio 3.63; log NT-proBNP, hazard ratio 2.67). The MR-proADM provided further risk stratification in those patients who had NT-proBNP levels above the median ($p < 0.0001$) (Figure 12-4). Findings were similar for death and heart failure as individual end-points.

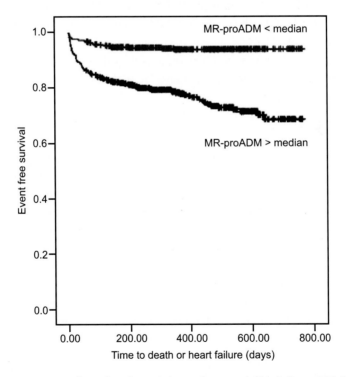

Figure 12-4 Prognostic value of midregional proadrenomedullin (MR-proADM) in patients with acute myocardial infarction. Kaplan-Meier analysis on death or heart failure as individual end-points showed a significantly better clinical outcome in patients with MR-proADM below the median compared with those with MR-proADM above the median (log rank chi-square test 42.4 and 28.65, respectively, $p < 0.0001$). *From* Khan S, O'Brien R, Struck J, Quinn P, Morgenthaler N, Squire I, et al. Prognostic value of midregional pro-adrenomedullin in patients with acute myocardial infarction: the LAMP (Leicester Acute Myocardial Infarction Peptide) study. *J Am Coll Cardiol.* 2007;49:1525-32, with permission.

These observations suggest that the ADM system is activated after AMI, and MR-proADM is a powerful predictor of adverse outcome, especially in post-MI patients with elevated NT-proBNP concentrations. In this context, MR-proADM may represent a clinically valuable marker of prognosis after AMI.

Dhillon et al. also[21] measured plasma MR-proADM on admission and discharge in 745 non-ST-elevation MI patients. The primary end-point was a composite of death, heart failure, hospitalization, and recurrent acute MI over mean follow-up of 760 days, with each event assessed individually as secondary end-points. Both admission and discharge MR-proADM levels were increased compared with established normal ranges. Multivariate adjusted Cox regression models revealed that both were associated with the primary end-point (both $p < 0.001$). Admission MR-proADM was particularly associated with early (< 30 days) mortality ($p < 0.001$), and when compared with NT-proBNP and GRACE clinical score, it was the only independent predictor of this end-point. Admission ADM > 1.11 nmol/L identified those at highest risk of death ($p < 0.001$). Additionally, patients with above-median admission MR-proADM may benefit from revascularization. Consequently, MR-proADM seems to have independent prognostic value in patients with non-ST-elevation MI, identifying also the patients at highest risk that need aggressive therapeutic interventions.

CONCLUSIONS

Current literature confirms that there is an activation of the ADM system in various abnormal cardiovascular conditions, especially in heart failure and after MI. MR-proADM as a more stable molecule in comparison to ADM seems to be a powerful and accurate new prognostic marker of adverse outcomes in patients with AMI and heart failure, having independent and/or additive value to established conventional risk factors and traditional plasma biomarkers such as natriuretic peptides. A multimarker approach with MR-proADM and natriuretic peptides may be more informative than either marker alone and may be useful for risk stratification in patients with cardiovascular disease. This multimarker strategy may also help clinicians optimize therapeutic interventions in various stages of cardiovascular disease.

REFERENCES

1. Eto T. A review of the biological properties and clinical implications of adrenomedullin and proadrenomedullin N-terminal 20 peptide (PAMP), hypotensive and vasodilating peptides. *Peptides.* 2001;22:1693-711.
2. Beltowski J, Jamroz A. Adrenomedullin – what do we know 10 years since its discovery? *Pol J Pharmacol.* 2004;56:5-27.
3. Hinson JP, Kapas S, Smith DM. Adrenomedullin, a multifunctional regulatory peptide. *Endocr Rev.* 2000;21:138-67.

4. Israel A, Diaz E. Diuretic and natriuretic action of adrenomedullin administered intracerebroventricularly in conscious rats. *Regul Pept.* 2000;89:13-8.

5. Kitamura K, Kangawa K, Kawamoto M, Ichiki Y, Nakamura S, Matsuo H, et al. Adrenomedullin: a novel hypotensive peptide isolated from human pheochromocytoma. *Biochem Biophys Res Commun.* 1993;192:553-60.

6. Szokodi I, Kinnunen P, Tavi P, Weckstrom M, Toth M, Ruskoaho H. Evidence for cAMP-independent mechanisms mediating the effects of adrenomedullin, a new inotropic peptide. *Circulation.* 1998;97:1062-70.

7. Tsuruda T, Kato J, Kitamura K, Kuwasako K, Imamura T, Koiway Y, et al. Adrenomedullin: a possible autocrine or paracrine inhibitor of hypertrophy of cardiomyocytes. *Hypertension.* 1998;31:505-10.

8. Jougasaki M, Rodeheffer RJ, Redfield MM, Yamamoto K, Wei CM, McKinley LJ, et al. Cardiac secretion of adrenomedullin in human heart failure. *J Clin Invest.* 1996;97: 2370-6.

9. Kato J, Tsuruda T, Kitamura K, Eto T. Adrenomedullin: a possible autocrine or paracrine hormone in the cardiac ventricles. *Hypertens Res.* 2003;26:S113-9.

10. Kuwasako K, Kitamura K, Kangawa K, Ishiyama Y, Kato J, Eto T. Increased plasma proadrenomedullin N-terminal 20 peptide in patients with essential hypertension. *Ann Clin Biochem.* 1999;36:622-8.

11. Nishikimi T, Saito Y, Kitamura K, Ishimitsu T, Eto T, Kangawa K, et al. Increased plasma levels of adrenomedullin in patients with heart failure. *J Am Coll Cardiol.* 1995;26: 1424-31.

12. Pousset F, Masson F, Chavirovskaia O, Isnard R, Carayon A, Golmard JL, et al. Plasma adrenomedullin, a new independent predictor of prognosis in patients with chronic heart failure. *Eur Heart J.* 2000;21:1009-14.

13. Richards M, Doughty R, Nicholls G, MacMohan S, Sharpe N, Murphy J, et al. Plasma N-terminal pro-brain natriuretic peptide and adrenomedullin prognostic utility and prediction of benefit from carvedilol in chronic ischemic left ventricular dysfunction. *J Am Coll Cardiol.* 2001;37:1781-7.

14. Morgenthaler NG, Struck J, Alonso C, Bergmann A. Measurement of midregional proadrenomedullin in plasma with an immunoluminometric assay. *Clin Chem.* 2005;51: 1823-9.

15. Potocki M, Breidthardt T, Reichlin T, Morgenthaler NG, Bergmann A, Noveanu M, et al. Midregional pro-adrenomedullin in addition to b-type natriuretic peptides in the risk stratification of patients with acute dyspnea: an observational study. *Crit Care.* 2009;13:R122-33.

16. von Heahling S, Filippatos GS, Papassotiriou J, Cicoira M, Jankowska EA, Doehner W, et al. Mid-regional pro-adrenomedullin as a novel predictor of mortality in patients with chronic heart failure. *Eur J Heart Fail.* 2010;12:484-91.

17. Maisel A, Mueller C, Nowak R, Peacock WF, Landsberg JW, Ponikowski P, et al. Mid-region pro-hormone markers for the diagnosis and prognosis in acute dyspnea: results from the BACH (Biomarkers in Acute Heart Failure) trial. *J Am Coll Cardiol.* 2010;55: 2062-76.

18. Richards AM, Nicholls MG, Yandle TG, Frampton C, Espiner EA, Turner JG, et al. Plasma N-terminal pro-brain natriuretic peptide and adrenomedullin: new neurohormonal predictors of left ventricular function and prognosis after myocardial infarction. *Circulation.* 1998;97:1921-9.

19. Katayama T, Nakashima H, Furudono S, Honda Y, Suzuki S, Yano K. Evaluation of neurohumoral activation (adrenomedullin, BNP, catecholamines, etc.) in patients with acute myocardial infarction. *Intern Med.* 2004;43:1015-22.

20. Khan S, O'Brien R, Struck J, Quinn P, Morgenthaler N, Squire I, et al. Prognostic value of midregional pro-adrenomedullin in patients with acute myocardial infarction: the LAMP (Leicester Acute Myocardial Infarction Peptide) study. *J Am Coll Cardiol.* 2007;49:1525-32.

21. Dhillon OS, Khan SQ, Narayan HK, Ng KH, Struck J, Quinn PA, et al. Prognostic value of mid-regional pro-adrenomedullin levels taken on admission and discharge in non-ST-elevation myocardial infarction: the LAMP (Leicester Acute Myocardial Infarction Peptide) II study. *J Am Coll Cardiol.* 2010;56:125-33.

Galectin-3

Rudolf A de Boer, Maxi Meissner, Dirk J van Veldhuisen

INTRODUCTION

Despite recent treatment advances, heart failure (HF) remains a progressive disorder. Its associated high mortality and morbidity indicates that key pathological morbidity mechanisms are not targeted and modified by current therapies, and that diagnostic and prognostic strategies are not optimal.

The leading biomarkers being utilized currently for heart failure diagnosis and prognosis are natriuretic peptides [brain natriuretic peptide (BNP), amino-terminal-pro-brain natriuretic peptide (NT-proBNP), and atrial natriuretic peptide, (ANP)]. These markers respond predominantly to mechanical stretch imposed on the myocardium (cardiac loading) and hence are referred to as so-called loading markers. However, they are not specific for inflammation and fibrosis. An ever growing body of evidence confirms the prominent role of fibrosis and changes in the intracellular matrix in the pathogenesis of HF.[1,2] These matricellular changes are evoked by damaging events like tissue ischemia, necrosis, and inflammation. The utilization of a biomarker that is directly linked to inflammation and fibrosis could potentially improve the diagnostic and/or prognostic yield in HF patients. Simultaneously, the development of anti-inflammatory and antifibrotic agents may offer improved therapy and outcome in HF patients by directly targeting a key pathophysiological event contributing to the progression of this condition.

Herein, galectin-3 appears to be a promising candidate, as it has recently gained attention as a biomarker.[3] Galectin-3 not only showed to be involved in inflammatory and fibrotic processes[1,4-7] but moreover plasma galectin-3 levels have repeatedly been shown to be increased in patients with acute[8] and chronic heart failure.[5,9,10] Additionally, galectin-3 has strong prognostic value for adverse outcome, and this prognostic value of galectin-3 is independent of NT-proBNP.[8] Thus, including galectin-3 in combination with the traditional biomarker NT-proBNP may improve the prediction of long-term prognosis.

Importantly, galectin-3 appears to have particular prognostic value in predicting the transition of compensated HF to decompensated HF, a suggestion that was supported by observations that plasma galectin-3 correlates with diastolic measures of HF, and seems of particular value in patients with HF with preserved ejection fraction (HFPEF).[11,12]

Finally, the utility of measuring galectin-3 in the clinical assessment of HF has recently gained acceptance, as an easy-to-perform galectin-3 ELISA[13] has been cleared by the FDA for this purpose (http://www.galectin-3.com/?p=2102). This altogether prompts stimulating discussion on the applicability of galectin-3 as a novel biomarker in HF.

Galectin-3: Biology

Galectin-3 belongs to a family of galectins that bind β-galactosides,[14,15] and it is expressed in a wide range of species and tissues.[16] Contrary to other galectins, galectin-3 displays an extended nonlectin N-terminal region constituted of tandem repeats of short amino acid segments (about 120 amino acids) connected to a single C-terminal carbohydrate recognition domain (CRD) of about 130 amino acids; which is why, it is often referred to as a "chimera-like" galectin. Thus, galectin-3 is comprised of a carbohydrate recognition domain and collagen-like domains enabling communication with a variety of carbohydrates, e.g., extracellular matricellular proteins, such as laminin, fibronectin and tenascin, and unglyscosylated matrix proteins, e.g., cell surface receptors (macrophage CD11b/CD18) and extracellular receptors (collagen IV). In fact, galectin-3 exerts a high binding with lactose and N-acetyllactosamine and affinity for N-acetyllactosamine is five times stronger than for lactose.[17-19]

Galectin-3 is primarily found in the cytoplasm. However, by an endoplasmic reticulum and Golgi complex-independent pathway, galectin-3 can be secreted into the extracellular space,[20] herein the plasma membrane plays a central role.[21] Although galectin-3 lacks specific signal peptides, it can cross the plasma membrane by interacting with extracellular matrix (ECM) proteins. In addition to being expressed in the cytosol, galectin-3 can also be expressed in the nucleus where it is associated with proliferative effects, while loss of nuclear galectin-3 is implicated in the malignant phenotype of cancers.

Galectin-3: Expression

Galectin-3 expression is observed in cells mediating inflammatory response, such as mast cells, macrophages, fibroblasts, eosinophils, and neutrophils.[22] Herein, galectin-3 is required for normal phagocytotic activity and is localized in the phagocytic cups and phagosomes of macrophages.[7] Moreover, upon macrophage, galectin-3 expression is upregulated by sixfold in granulocyte-macrophage colony-stimulating factor transgenic mice.[23] Further, co-localization of galectin-3 with macrophages was found in hypertrophied hearts[1] and during active myocarditis,[6] which both coincided with significant infiltration of macrophages. Abundant galectin-3 was also reported within the cytoplasm and nucleus of macrophages, which were found to secrete considerable amounts of galectin-3 into the supernatant in cell culture, indicating localization of galectin-3 to the extracellular space.[24]

Further, co-localization of galectin-3 with proliferating fibroblasts was observed in a murine model of hepatic fibrosis.[4] Moreover, a study of hypertrophied hearts revealed that galectin-3 binding sites are predominatly present around the nucleus of proliferating fibroblasts, while resting cells only displayed little binding sites in cytoplasm.[6]

In tissues, galectin-3 expression is predominant in lung, spleen, stomach, colon, adrenal gland, uterus, and ovary; its expression levels are lower in the kidney, heart, cerebrum, pancreas, and liver.[25] However, a low constitutive expression level cannot be translated to function (e.g., in liver and heart), because the level of galectin-3 expression may change substantially under pathological conditions.

ROLE OF GALECTIN-3 IN HEART FAILURE

A hallmark of chronic heart failure is the development of cardiac remodeling and interstitial fibrosis, prompting changes in the extracellular matrix. Cardiac remodeling is an important player in the clinical outcome of heart failure, because it is associated with disease progression and poor prognosis.[26] Cardiac remodeling manifests clinically as structural and functional modulations of the heart; while histopathological characterization involves structural derangement, specifically cardiomyocytes hypertrophy, cardiac fibroblast proliferation, fibrosis, and cell death. Slowing or reversing the progression of remodeling has only recently become a therapeutic goal of heart failure therapy. Galectin-3 is importantly involved in cardiac remodeling and the fibrotic process as demonstrated by animal and clinical studies.

Animal Studies

The initial observation indicating a role of galectin-3 in the onset of HF came from a study of hypertensive Ren-2 rats that overexpresses the murine *Ren-2d* renin gene.[1] While some of the homozygous Ren-2 rats displayed overt failure after about 15 weeks, indicated by signs of HF, such as dyspnea, lethargy as well as severely compromised hemodynamics, other rats remained compensated at the same age. Galectin-3 showed to be the strongest regulated gene as analyzed by comparing compensated and decompensated Ren-2 rats utilizing a complementary DNA array with whole RNA from rat hearts. Galectin-3 was more than fivefold upregulated in decompensated hearts compared with compensated hearts.[1] Subsequently, an increased galectin-3 expression was observed in another murine model of left ventricular remodeling (the angiotensin II-infused mice),[27] confirming implication of galectin-3 in left-ventricular remodeling.

Further, rather than loading-dependent factors, e.g., natriuretic peptides, the genes that were most differentially regulated in Ren-2 rats pertained to matricellular proteins, such as collagens, osteoactivin, and fibronectin.[1] The co-expression of galectin-3 with these factors furthermore suggests a role for galectin-3 in fibrosis. This was corroborated by infusion of recombinant galectin-3 in the pericardial sac of Sprague Dawley rats prompted left ventricular dysfunction and extensive myocardial fibrosis.[1] Specifically, infusion of galectin-3 increased infiltration of macrophage and mast cells, all processes associated with the development of fibrosis and left ventricular dysfunction.

Several studies suggest a potential role for *N*-acetyl-Ser-Asp-Lys-Pro (ac-SDKP), a tetrapeptide hydrolyzed by angiotensin-converting enzyme, in modulating the negative effects of galectin-3. It was first demonstrated that ac-SDKP decreased fibrosis and expression of galectin-3 in left ventricular tissue of mice treated with angiotensin II.[27] Then, it was reported that the galectin-3-induced fibrosis and inflammation were inhibited and cardiac dysfunction was alleviated upon co-infusion of galectin-3 with ac-SDKP in the pericardial sac of Sprague-Dawley rats.[28] Although the role of ac-SDKP in alleviating the adverse effects of galectin-3 needs further clarification, it is attractive to speculate that targeted treatment against galectin-3 may benefit cardiac remodeling and HF.

Fibrosis is central in the maladaptive cardiac response to injury. Fibroblasts, myofibroblasts and macrophages are key players in the initiation and progression of tissue scarring.[29,30] While galectin-3 co-localized with macrophages and fibroblasts but not with cardiomyocytes, it is thus present at the immediate sites of fibrosis. Importantly, galectin-3 binding sites are localized to fibrotic areas[1] and recombinant galectin-3 causes collagen production *in vivo*[27,28] as well as proliferation and collagen production of cardiac fibroblasts cultures *in vitro*.

The discussed experimental results pertaining to cardiac tissue complement an array of studies associating galectin-3 with fibrosis in general: liver cirrhosis,[4,31] idiopathic lung fibrosis;[32] as well as hepatic[4] and renal[24,33] fibrosis animal models. Herein, it was also recently suggested that galectin-3 actually limits renal tubular apoptosis and extracellular matrix remodeling in murine model of progressive renal fibrosis.[34] Moreover, Henderson and colleagues reported temporal and spatial association of galectin-3 with fibrosis, which was found to be minimal in normal rat liver, maximal at peak fibrosis but absent after recovery from fibrosis.[24]

Cardiac remodeling and fibrosis are mediated by the inflammatory response, and galectin-3 has been successfully linked to inflammatory processes leading to fibrosis and damage, especially in renal models of inflammation.[24,33,35] For example, in a model of murine renal fibrosis, specific macrophage depletion caused significantly decreased activation of myofibroblast and also reduced fibrosis, shown by decreased α-SMA and collagen expression.[24] The authors stated that renal galectin-3 expression and secretion by macrophages was the key player in renal fibrosis, as galectin-3 deficiency (galectin-3 knockout) did not show any effects on proinflammatory cytokine profiles nor macrophage recruitment after stimulation with interferon-gamma/LPS.[24] In contrast, complete depletion of macrophage in the Ren-2 rat model appeared to accelerate cardiac remodeling, complementing the idea that (temporary) macrophage influx is instrumental in adaptive remodeling.[36] Additionally, it has been found that TGF-β activates myofibroblasts in a galectin-3-mediated manner.[4]

No direct evidence has yet been observed for inflammatory effects *via* galectin-3 in the heart; however, it has been found that besides galectin-3 other genes encoding for immune factors are differentially regulated between hypertensive Ren-2 rats developing overt heart failure or remaining compensated.[1,27] Moreover, a recent clinical study found a significant positive correlation between galectin-3 levels at admission for acute heart failure and inflammatory cytokines linked to the outcome of heart failure, such as VEGF, IL-6, and CRP.[12] Additionally, an increased infiltration of galectin-3 macrophages as well as mRNA expression of proinflammatory cytokines has been observed in myocardial tissue in interferon-gamma-induced chronic active myocarditis and cardiomyopathy.[6]

Although more research is warranted, the previous research clearly indicates that myofibroblast activation and accumulation by mechanisms related to galectin-3 expression and macrophage secretion leads to cardiac and renal fibrosis. Altogether these animal studies strongly indicate a pathophysiological role for galectin-3 in the development and progression of fibrogenesis and HF. Importantly, clinical data supports this notion.

Clinical Studies

Thus far, three studies addressed the predictive value of galectin-3 in HF. These studies collectively show that serum/plasma galectin-3 levels were elevated in patients with acute as well as chronic HF, that they were prognostic of adverse outcome,[5,8,11,12] and that galectin-3 may be a promising prognostic biomarker in patients with HFPEF.[12]

The first evidence for a role of galectin-3 in human heart failure came from Sharma et al.[1] who found that galectin-3 was up-regulated in tissues from ventricular biopsies of patients with aortic stenosis. Galectin-3 levels were up-regulated, specifically in patients with depressed versus preserved ejection fraction.

The first report on the prognostic value of plasma galectin-3 in human *acute* heart failure was published by van Kimmenade et al. In the ProBNP Investigation of Dyspnea in the Emergency Department (PRIDE) cohort, 599 acutely dyspneic patients were studied, of whom 209 patients were diagnosed with heart failure. Plasma galectin-3 levels offered relative poor diagnostic value in acute heart failure, but strong prognostic value in predicting heart failure outcome.[8] The analysis of biomarkers for the diagnosis of acute heart failure revealed that NT-proBNP was superior in diagnosis compared to galectin-3 and apelin: the area under the curve for NT-proBNP was 0.94 (p < 0.0001) vs 0.72 (p < 0.0001) for galectin-3 and 0.52 (p = 0.23) for apelin. However, plasma galectin-3 was found to be the most powerful predictor for 60-day mortality: the area under the curve for plasma galectin-3 was 0.74 (P = 0.0001) vs 0.67 (P = 0.009) and 0.54 (P = 0.33) for NT-proBNP and apelin, respectively (Figure 13-1).[8] Multivariate logistic regression analysis furthermore uncovered elevated plasma galectin-3 to be the strongest predictor for death and the combination of death and recurrent heart failure within 60 days.[8] Recently, a long term follow-up of the same cohort was published.[11] In this subanalysis, echographic indices were correlated with plasma galectin-3 levels in a small subset of the PRIDE patients (N = 106). It was shown that galectin-3 levels were not related to markers of left ventricular structure or systolic function but that higher galectin-3 levels

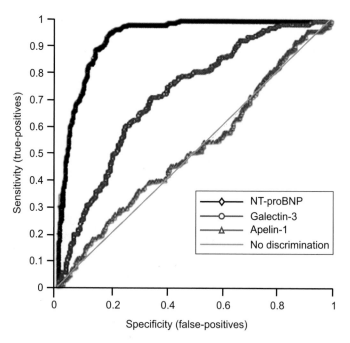

Figure 13-1 Combined receiver-operating characteristic (ROC) curves for amino-terminal pro-brain natriuretic peptide (NT-proBNP), galectin (gal)-3 and apelin for the diagnosis of heart failure in dyspneic patients. The ROC analysis for NT-proBNP showed an area under the curve (AUC) for NT-proBNP of 0.94 (p < 0.0001). The ROC analysis for gal-3 showed an AUC of 0.72 (p < 0.0001). The AUC for apelin for diagnosis of acute heart failure was 0.52 (p = 0.23). *From* van Kimmenade RR, Januzzi JL Jr, Ellinor PT, Sharma UC, Bakker JA, Low AF, et al. Utility of amino-terminal pro-brain natriuretic peptide, galectin-3, and apelin for the evaluation of patients with acute heart failure. *J Am Coll Cardiol*. 2006;48:1217-24, with permission.

were specifically correlated to incidences of diastolic function: Doppler indices of higher filling pressure and more extensive diastolic relaxation abnormalities.[11] This supports a role for galectin-3 in fibrosis, a condition where the diastolic properties of the myocardium are impaired due to its progressive stiffening. Moreover, the highest levels of plasma galectin-3 were the most strongly associated with a higher risk of 4-year mortality, independent of left ventricular dimensions, function, or right ventricular pressures as analyzed in a smaller subset of this study (n = 53).[11]

Subsequently, plasma galectin-3 levels were reported to be strongly correlated to long-term outcome in a larger cohort of 240 patients with stable *chronic* heart failure (mean follow-up 3.4 years; HR 1.95; 95% CI: 1.24–3.09, P = 0.004).[9] This study also analyzed the incremental risk of the combination of galectin-3 (below/above median) with NT-proBNP (above/below median) (Figure 13-2). Patients with high baseline values of both galectin-3 and NT-proBNP were found to have a 1.5- to 2-fold higher mortality rate compared to patients in other groups (low galectin-3

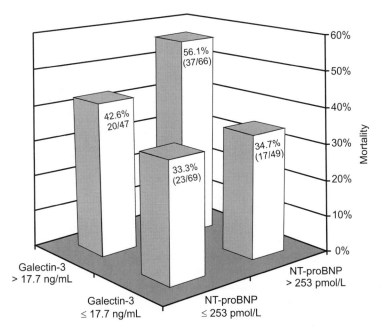

Figure 13-2 Mortality as a function of baseline galectin-3 and NT-proBNP categories. The median value of NT-proBNP (253 pmol/L) was used to define two levels of NT-proBNP concentration. Of the 232 subjects, 231 had both a galectin-3 and NT-proBNP measurement. The number of patients in the each category is as follows: high galectin-3 and high NT-proBNP (n = 66); low galectin-3 and low NT-proBNP (n = 69); low galectin-3 and high NT-proBNP (n = 49); high galectin-3 and low NT-proBNP (n = 47). *From* Lok DJ, van Der Meer P, de la Porte PW, Lipsic E, van Wijngaarden J, Hillege HL, et al. Prognostic value of galectin-3, a novel marker of fibrosis, in patients with chronic heart failure: data from the DEAL-HF study. *Clin Res Cardiol.* 2010;99:323-8, with permission.

and low NT-proBNP; low galectin-3 and high NT-proBNP; high galectin-3 and low NT-proBNP).[9] Given that NT-proBNP and galectin-3 are markers for different pathophysiological processes in heart failure, as explained later, such a combination of traditional (NT-proBNP) with a novel biomarker (here: galectin-3) in a multi-biomarker score may thus provide better prognostic prediction compared to using either single biomarker. This should be given more attention in future studies.

Prognostic value of galectin-3 was further explored in patients enrolled in the Coordinating Study Evaluating Outcomes of Advising and Counseling in Heart failure (COACH).[12] Plasma samples were collected from 592 patients at discharge after patients were stabilized after an acute heart failure admission, and mean follow-up was 18 months. Two hundred and ninety-one patients were sampled again after six months in an outpatient setting. Galectin-3 levels were divided into quartiles and the patients in the lowest quartile were used as a reference group (HR for the primary outcome set to 1.00) (Figure 13-3). Compared to the reference group patients in the second quartile had a HR of 1.98 (95% CI: 1.29–3.02; P = 0.0016) for rehospitalization for heart failure or death, patients in the third quartile a HR of 2.66 (95% CI: 1.76–

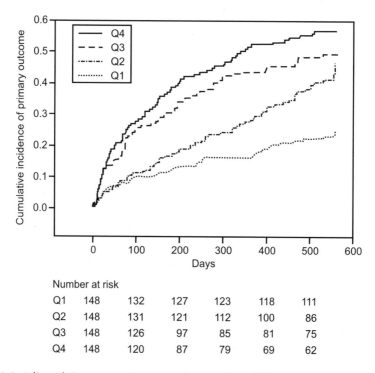

Number at risk

Q1	148	132	127	123	118	111
Q2	148	131	121	112	100	86
Q3	148	126	97	85	81	75
Q4	148	120	87	79	69	62

Figure 13-3 Adjusted Cox regression curves for quartiles of plasma galectin-3 showing the cumulative risk for the combined end-point all-cause mortality and hospitalization for HF. *From* de Boer RA, Lok DJ, Jaarsma T, van Der Meer P, Voors AA, Hillege HL, et al. Predictive value of plasma galectin-3 levels in heart failure with reduced and preserved ejection fraction. *Ann Med.* 2011;43:60-8, with permission.

4.03; P < 0.001) and patients in the fourth quartile a HR of 3.34 (95% CI: 2.23–5.01; P < 0.001). Baseline galectin-3 had independent prognostic value even after correction for established risk factors for poor outcome of heart failure like age, sex, BNP, renal function, and diabetes mellitus: HR 1.38 (1.07–1.78; P = 0.015). Furthermore, serial sampling did not seem to add substantially to the prognostic value of galectin-3, thus, baseline galectin-3 levels appears to be sufficient to predict outcome. Combining plasma galectin-3 and BNP levels increased prognostic value over either biomarker alone (ROC analysis, P < 0.05). In a subanalysis, it appeared that the predictive value of galectin-3 may be stronger in patients with preserved LVEF (HFPEF, N = 114) compared to the patients with reduced LVEF (HFREF, N = 478). Importantly, while absolute galectin-3 levels did not differ between patients with HFPEF and HFREF, a significant interaction between depressed LVEF (≤ 40%) and preserved LVF (> 40%) and a predictive value of plasma galectin-3 was found. Specifically, the predictive power of plasma galectin-3 appeared to be stronger in HFPEF compared to HFREF (P < 0.001). Thus, an identical increase in plasma galectin-3 levels represents a much stronger incremental risk for experiencing rehospitalization or death in patients with HFPEF in comparison to patients with HFREF (Figure 13-4). Although exploratory, this finding should be explored as HF with preserved ejection fraction is common and we lack biomarkers for this disease.

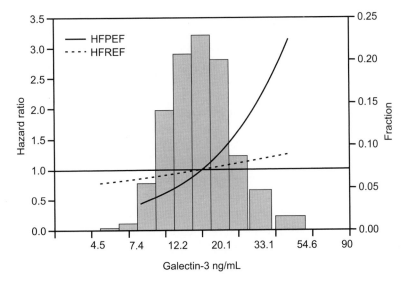

Figure 13-4 Graphical depiction of the risk estimates for experiencing the primary outcome in patients with HFPEF and HFREF with increasing levels of plasma galectin-3. The distribution of (log-transformed) galectin-3 is depicted in the background in brown bars. A similar increase in galectin-3 causes a much more pronounced increase in risk in patients with HFPEF compared to patients with HFREF. *From* de Boer RA, Lok DJ, Jaarsma T, van Der Meer P, Voors AA, Hillege HL, et al. Predictive value of plasma galectin-3 levels in heart failure with reduced and preserved ejection fraction. *Ann Med.* 2011;43:60-8, with permission.

Importantly, the prognostic value of galectin-3 was repeatedly found to be independent from NT-proBNP levels,[8,9,12] which is currently considered the most commonly used biomarker in heart failure. This suggests that galectin-3 and NT-proBNP characterize different pathophysiological events involved in the etiology of heart failure. Specifically, NT-proBNP is a loading marker corresponding to ventricular stretch or overload.[37] Contrarily, galectin-3 is less responsive to (un-) loading and rather viewed as a marker of interstitial fibrosis. Underscoring that galectin-3 marks specific pathological events in the development of heart failure are observations from Milting et al.[5] who show that fibrosis-related biomarkers, including galectin-3 were increased in 55 patients with end-stage heart failure compared to controls. Interestingly, mechanical circulatory support only reduced the loading-related biomarker BNP but not tissue inhibitor of metalloproteinase-1 (TIMP-1), tenascin, osteopontin, nor galectin-3; all fibrosis-related biomarkers.[5]

An essential process of interstitial fibrosis is ECM turnover[38] and markers of ECM turnover have proven prognostic value in heart failure.[38-40] Lin et al.[10] recently described the relationship between serum galectin-3 and ECM turnover in 106 patients with chronic heart failure (NYHA II-III; mean left ventricular ejection fraction (LVEF) 35 ± 9%). Serum galectin-3 was significantly correlated with serum type III amino-terminal propeptide of procollagen (PIIINP), tissue inhibitor of metalloproteinase-1 (TIMP-1) and matrix metalloproteinase-2 (MMP-2), all markers of EMC turnover. However, serum galectin-3 was not correlated with LVEF, age, and sex. The correlation between galectin-3 and PIINP and MMP-2 remained significant after correction, implying a link between galectin-3 and cardiac ECM turnover in heart failure patients[10] further undermining a role for galectin-3 in fibrosis.

GALECTIN-3: FUTURE PERSPECTIVES

Recent data suggest that galectin-3 may be utilized in clinical practice for predicting prognosis, possibly diagnosis, and may even guide therapy. Since many biomarkers have emerged, we should ask ourselves what advantage galectin-3 may have over other biomarkers.

First, galectin-3 is produced by activated macrophages and fibroblasts, and thus seems to be associated with so-called remodeling heart failure (Figure 13-5). Thus, galectin-3 is involved clearly in a specific pathway of the pathophysiology of heart failure. In contrast, the currently well-used biomarkers in diagnosis and prognosis of heart failure (BNP, NT-proBNP, and ANP) are loading markers and hence not sensitive for other processes underlying heart failure etiology, such as fibrosis. In line with this, galectin-3 has demonstrated predictive value of adverse outcome by itself but also in combination with the loading biomarker NT-proBNP. Thus, its prognostic utilization of galectin-3 within the clinic, alone or in combination with other biomarkers (multimarker approach), is supported by the pathophysiology.

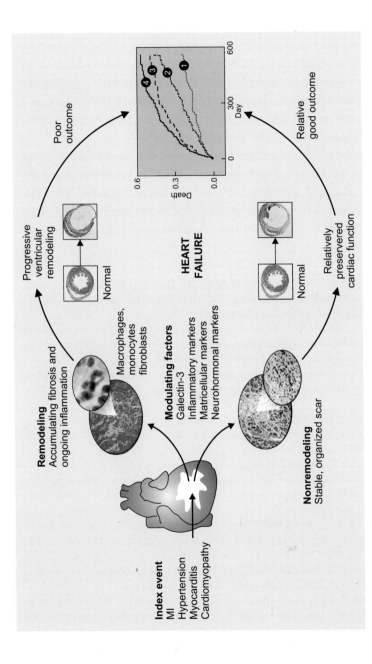

Figure 13-5 Working scheme representing the sequence of events following an index event (such as myocardial infarction (MI), hypertension, myocarditis and cardiomyopathy) leading to remodeling and nonremodeling. The graph within this graphic is taken *from* de Boer RA, Lok DJ, Jaarsma T, van Der Meer P, Voors AA, Hillege HL, et al. Predictive value of plasma galectin-3 levels in heart failure with reduced and preserved ejection fraction. *Ann Med.* 2011;43:60-8; and represents the adjusted Cox regression curves for quartiles of plasma galectin-3 showing the cumulative risk for the combined end-point, death. The black circles with the white numbers represent quartile 1 through 4, respectively. Galectin-3 is displayed as a central modulating factor involved in the remodeling process which leads to ongoing damage and eventually poor heart failure outcome. Therapeutically, galectin-3 inhibition could favor nonremodeling, thereby improving heart failure outcome by relatively preserved cardiac function.

Second, the observation that galectin-3 may be a specifically strong predictor of adverse outcome in HFPEF is clinically important.[5] HFPEF is a very common condition[41] distinct to HFREF and characterized by fibrosis-related features, such as hypertrophy, matrix apposition and myocardial stiffening.[42,43] Approximately 50% of heart failure patients have normal left ventricular ejection fraction. Currently, prognosis is poor; a 5-year survival rate of 43% was recently reported in patients with HFPEF after first hospitalization for heart failure.[41] Besides natriuretic peptides, we have no biomarkers in our arsenal that have proven usefulness in HFPEF. Galectin-3 may have additive value in this important subgroup of patients. Future studies exploring the value of galectin-3 in HFPEF are highly desirable.

Lastly, galectin-3 appears a promising target for many diseases given the broad biological functionality of galectin-3 and its involvement in processes spanning apoptosis, chemoattraction, cell adhesion, cell growth, cell differentiation, cell cycle, inflammation, and fibrosis. To date, its potential as anticancer therapy appears to be the most widely researched,[44-47] but studies in the cardiovascular field are underway.

REFERENCES

1. Sharma UC, Pokharel S, van Brakel TJ, van Berlo JH, Cleutjens JP, Schroen B, et al. Galectin-3 marks activated macrophages in failure-prone hypertrophied hearts and contributes to cardiac dysfunction. *Circulation.* 2004;110:3121-8.
2. Weber KT, Gerling IC, Kiani MF, Guntaka RV, Sun Y, Ahokas RA, et al. Aldosteronism in heart failure: a proinflammatory/fibrogenic cardiac phenotype. Search for biomarkers and potential drug targets. *Curr Drug Targets.* 2003;4:505-16.
3. de Boer RA, Voors AA, Muntendam P, van Gilst WH, van Veldhuisen DJ. Galectin-3: a novel mediator of heart failure development and progression. *Eur J Heart Fail.* 2009; 11:811-7.
4. Henderson NC, Mackinnon AC, Farnworth SL, Poirier F, Russo FP, Iredale JP, et al. Galectin-3 regulates myofibroblast activation and hepatic fibrosis. *Proc Natl Acad Sci U S A.* 2006;103:5060-5.
5. Milting H, Ellinghaus P, Seewald M, Cakar H, Bohms B, Kassner A, et al. Plasma biomarkers of myocardial fibrosis and remodeling in terminal heart failure patients supported by mechanical circulatory support devices. *J Heart Lung Transplant.* 2008; 27:589-96.
6. Reifenberg K, Lehr HA, Torzewski M, Steige G, Wiese E, Kupper I, et al. Interferon-gamma induces chronic active myocarditis and cardiomyopathy in transgenic mice. *Am J Pathol.* 2007;171:463-72.
7. Sano H, Hsu DK, Apgar JR, Yu L, Sharma BB, Kuwabara I, et al. Critical role of galectin-3 in phagocytosis by macrophages. *J Clin Invest.* 2003;112:389-97.
8. van Kimmenade RR, Januzzi JL Jr, Ellinor PT, Sharma UC, Bakker JA, Low AF, et al. Utility of amino-terminal pro-brain natriuretic peptide, galectin-3, and apelin for the evaluation of patients with acute heart failure. *J Am Coll Cardiol.* 2006;48:1217-24.
9. Lok DJ, van Der Meer P, de la Porte PW, Lipsic E, van Wijngaarden J, Hillege HL, et al. Prognostic value of galectin-3, a novel marker of fibrosis, in patients with chronic heart failure: data from the DEAL-HF study. *Clin Res Cardiol.* 2010;99:323-8.

10. Lin YH, Lin LY, Wu YW, Chien KL, Lee CM, Hsu RB, et al. The relationship between serum galectin-3 and serum markers of cardiac extracellular matrix turnover in heart failure patients. *Clin Chim Acta.* 2009;409:96-9.

11. Shah RV, Chen-Tournoux AA, Picard MH, van Kimmenade RR, Januzzi JL. Galectin-3, cardiac structure and function, and long-term mortality in patients with acutely decompensated heart failure. *Eur J Heart Fail.* 2010;12:826-32.

12. de Boer RA, Lok DJ, Jaarsma T, van Der Meer P, Voors AA, Hillege HL, et al. Predictive value of plasma galectin-3 levels in heart failure with reduced and preserved ejection fraction. *Ann Med.* 2011;43:60-8.

13. Christenson RH, Duh SH, Wu AH, Smith A, Abel G, deFilippi CR, et al. Multi-center determination of galectin-3 assay performance characteristics: anatomy of a novel assay for use in heart failure. *Clin Biochem.* 2010;43:683-90.

14. Barondes SH, Cooper DN, Gitt MA, Leffler H. Galectins. Structure and function of a large family of animal lectins. *J Biol Chem.* 1994;269:20807-10.

15. Cooper DN. Galectinomics: finding themes in complexity. *Biochim Biophys Acta.* 2002; 1572:209-31.

16. Dumic J, Dabelic S, Flogel M. Galectin-3: an open-ended story. *Biochim Biophys Acta.* 2006;1760:616-35.

17. Seetharaman J, Kanigsberg A, Slaaby R, Leffler H, Barondes SH, Rini JM. X-ray crystal structure of the human galectin-3 carbohydrate recognition domain at 2.1-A resolution. *J Biol Chem.* 1998;273:13047-52.

18. Rosenberg I, Cherayil BJ, Isselbacher KJ, Pillai S. Mac-2-binding glycoproteins. Putative ligands for a cytosolic beta-galactoside lectin. *J Biol Chem.* 1991;266:18731-6.

19. Sato S, Hughes RC. Binding specificity of a baby hamster kidney lectin for H type I and II chains, polylactosamine glycans, and appropriately glycosylated forms of laminin and fibronectin. *J Biol Chem.* 1992;267:6983-90.

20. Menon RP, Hughes RC. Determinants in the N-terminal domains of galectin-3 for secretion by a novel pathway circumventing the endoplasmic reticulum-Golgi complex. *Eur J Biochem.* 1999;264:569-76.

21. Mehul B, Hughes RC. Plasma membrane targetting, vesicular budding and release of galectin 3 from the cytoplasm of mammalian cells during secretion. *J Cell Sci.* 1997; 110:1169-78.

22. Hughes RC. Secretion of the galectin family of mammalian carbohydrate-binding proteins. *Biochim Biophys Acta.* 1999;1473:172-85.

23. Elliott MJ, Strasser A, Metcalf D. Selective up-regulation of macrophage function in granulocyte-macrophage colony-stimulating factor transgenic mice. *J Immunol.* 1991; 147:2957-63.

24. Henderson NC, Mackinnon AC, Farnworth SL, Kipari T, Haslett C, Iredale JP, et al. Galectin-3 expression and secretion links macrophages to the promotion of renal fibrosis. *Am J Pathol.* 2008;172:288-98.

25. Kim H, Lee J, Hyun JW, Park JW, Joo HG, Shin T. Expression and immunohistochemical localization of galectin-3 in various mouse tissues. *Cell Biol Int.* 2007;31:655-62.

26. Task Force for Diagnosis and Treatment of Acute and Chronic Heart Failure 2008 of European Society of Cardiology, Dickstein K, Cohen-Solal A, Filippatos G, McMurray JJ, Ponikowski P, et al. ESC Guidelines for the diagnosis and treatment of acute and chronic heart failure 2008: the Task Force for the Diagnosis and Treatment of Acute and Chronic Heart Failure 2008 of the European Society of Cardiology. Developed in collaboration

with the Heart Failure Association of the ESC (HFA) and endorsed by the European Society of Intensive Care Medicine (ESICM). *Eur Heart J.* 2008;29:2388-442.

27. Sharma U, Rhaleb NE, Pokharel S, Harding P, Rasoul S, Peng H, et al. Novel anti-inflammatory mechanisms of N-Acetyl-Ser-Asp-Lys-Pro in hypertension-induced target organ damage. *Am J Physiol Heart Circ Physiol.* 2008;294:H1226-32.

28. Liu YH, D'Ambrosio M, Liao TD, Peng H, Rhaleb NE, Sharma U, et al. N-acetyl-seryl-aspartyl-lysyl-proline prevents cardiac remodeling and dysfunction induced by galectin-3, a mammalian adhesion/growth-regulatory lectin. *Am J Physiol Heart Circ Physiol.* 2009;296:H404-12.

29. Duffield JS, Forbes SJ, Constandinou CM, Clay S, Partolina M, Vuthoori S, et al. Selective depletion of macrophages reveals distinct, opposing roles during liver injury and repair. *J Clin Invest.* 2005;115:56-65.

30. Friedman SL. Molecular regulation of hepatic fibrosis, an integrated cellular response to tissue injury. *J Biol Chem.* 2000;275:2247-50.

31. Hsu DK, Dowling CA, Jeng KC, Chen JT, Yang RY, Liu FT. Galectin-3 expression is induced in cirrhotic liver and hepatocellular carcinoma. *Int J Cancer.* 1999;81:519-26.

32. Nishi Y, Sano H, Kawashima T, Okada T, Kuroda T, Kikkawa K, et al. Role of galectin-3 in human pulmonary fibrosis. *Allergol Int.* 2007;56:57-65.

33. Sasaki S, Bao Q, Hughes RC. Galectin-3 modulates rat mesangial cell proliferation and matrix synthesis during experimental glomerulonephritis induced by anti-Thy1.1 antibodies. *J Pathol.* 1999;187:481-9.

34. Okamura DM, Pasichnyk K, Lopez-Guisa JM, Collins S, Hsu DK, Liu FT, et al. Galectin-3 preserves renal tubules and modulates extracellular matrix remodeling in progressive fibrosis. *Am J Physiol Renal Physiol.* 2011;300:F245-53.

35. Eis V, Luckow B, Vielhauer V, Siveke JT, Linde Y, Segerer S, et al. Chemokine receptor CCR1 but not CCR5 mediates leukocyte recruitment and subsequent renal fibrosis after unilateral ureteral obstruction. *J Am Soc Nephrol.* 2004;15:337-47.

36. Zandbergen HR, Sharma UC, Gupta S, Verjans JW, van den Borne S, Pokharel S, et al. Macrophage depletion in hypertensive rats accelerates development of cardiomyopathy. *J Cardiovasc Pharmacol Ther.* 2009;14:68-75.

37. Tjeerdsma G, de Boer RA, Boomsma F, van den Berg MP, Pinto YM, van Veldhuisen DJ. Rapid bedside measurement of brain natriuretic peptide in patients with chronic heart failure. *Int J Cardiol.* 2002;86:143-9; discussion 149-52.

38. Graham HK, Horn M, Trafford AW. Extracellular matrix profiles in the progression to heart failure. European Young Physiologists Symposium Keynote Lecture-Bratislava 2007. *Acta Physiol (Oxf).* 2008;194:3-21.

39. George J, Patal S, Wexler D, Roth A, Sheps D, Keren G. Circulating matrix metalloproteinase-2 but not matrix metalloproteinase-3, matrix metalloproteinase-9, or tissue inhibitor of metalloproteinase-1 predicts outcome in patients with congestive heart failure. *Am Heart J.* 2005;150:484-7.

40. Cicoira M, Rossi A, Bonapace S, Zanolla L, Golia G, Franceschini L, et al. Independent and additional prognostic value of aminoterminal propeptide of type III procollagen circulating levels in patients with chronic heart failure. *J Card Fail.* 2004;10:403-11.

41. Tribouilloy C, Rusinaru D, Mahjoub H, Souliere V, Levy F, Peltier M, et al. Prognosis of heart failure with preserved ejection fraction: a 5 year prospective population-based study. *Eur Heart J.* 2008;29:339-47. Epub 2007 Dec 22.

42. Kindermann M, Reil JC, Pieske B, van Veldhuisen DJ, Bohm M. Heart failure with normal left ventricular ejection fraction: what is the evidence? *Trends Cardiovasc Med.* 2008;18:280-92.

43. Paulus WJ, Tschope C, Sanderson JE, Rusconi C, Flachskampf FA, Rademakers FE, et al. How to diagnose diastolic heart failure: a consensus statement on the diagnosis of heart failure with normal left ventricular ejection fraction by the Heart Failure and Echocardiography Associations of the European Society of Cardiology. *Eur Heart J.* 2007;28:2539-50.

44. Sethi K, Sarkar S, Das S, Mohanty B, Mandal M. Biomarkers for the diagnosis of thyroid cancer. *J Exp Ther Oncol.* 2010;8:341-52.

45. Glinsky VV, Raz A. Modified citrus pectin anti-metastatic properties: one bullet, multiple targets. *Carbohydr Res.* 2009;344:1788-91.

46. Nakahara S, Raz A. Regulation of cancer-related gene expression by galectin-3 and the molecular mechanism of its nuclear import pathway. *Cancer Metastasis Rev.* 2007; 26:605-10.

47. Nakahara S, Oka N, Raz A. On the role of galectin-3 in cancer apoptosis. *Apoptosis.* 2005;10:267-75.

Hanna Kim Gaggin, James L Januzzi Jr

INTRODUCTION

More than two decades ago, ST2 was originally isolated and later described in the context of cell proliferation, inflammatory states, and autoimmune diseases.[1-3] Since then, a multiplicity of intriguing information regarding ST2 is now available, including an intriguing role in the development and progression of heart failure (HF) and myocardial remodeling.

NOMENCLATURE AND BIOLOGY OF ST2

The official approved symbol for ST2 gene from the human gene nomenclature database is interleukin-1 receptor-like-1 (IL1RL1) located on human chromosome 2;[4] however, commonly used names are ST2 or T1. The homologous gene in rats is Fos-induced transcript-1(Fit-1) and in mice is delayed early response gene 4 (DER4).[5]

Four protein isoforms of ST2 have been identified to date and are produced by alternative promoter splicing and 3' post-transcription processing of ST2 mRNA. The two main forms of ST2 are a secreted soluble form ST2 (sST2), and a relatively larger transmembrane form, ST2 ligand (ST2L), which has three extracellular IgG domains. ST2L is believed to have immunomodulatory function as a cell-surface marker of T helper type 2 (Th2) lymphocytes, and is also thought to play a role in T-cell mediated inflammation.[6] Importantly, the induction of both sST2 and ST2L in the setting of mechanical strain of either cardiac fibroblasts or cardiomyocytes is well-documented. Although both soluble and membrane forms of ST2 are induced when these cells are strained, in this setting, the soluble form predominates.[7]

The two variant forms (of undetermined significance to date) are ST2 (ST2v) and ST2Lv.[8-10] ST2v appears to be a transmembrane protein while ST2Lv appears to be a soluble secreted and N-glycosylated variant of the ST2 gene product.[9]

HISTORY

While searching for genes that are activated in response to oncogenes and serum growth factors, Werenskiold and colleagues isolated ST2 gene.[1] The same year,

Tominaga and colleagues also identified that ST2 gene is induced in the course of the initiation of cell proliferation.[11] The ST2 gene sequence encodes a protein that has extensive similarities to members of the immunoglobulin gene superfamily (especially to the interleukin [IL]-1 receptor).[12] The ST2 gene was subsequently found to be transiently activated in response to stimulation with a number of inflammatory and cell growth factors, including lysophosphatidic acid, several growth factors (platelet-derived growth factor, acidic fibroblast growth factor, and basic fibroblast growth factor), tissue plasminogen activator, and the proinflammatory cytokines tumor necrosis factor and IL-1.[12,13]

As noted above, despite a putative role in the immune response, it is well established at this point that the ST2 gene is potently induced in the context of cellular stretch, including cardiac fibroblasts and myocytes. This link between ST2 and biomechanical strain in the heart was found by Weinberg and colleagues who found that among 7,000 genes up-regulated in stretched cardiac cells, transcripts for ST2 were very heavily expressed.[7]

CARDIAC REMODELING AND sST2 IN HF

Significant pathologic cardiac abnormalities, no matter what the etiology, have an end-result of biomechanical strain (volume or pressure overload) on the heart. Teleologically, the heart responds with a series of biomechanical changes in an attempt to reduce this increased tension. Initially adaptive, cardiac remodeling including myocyte hypertrophy, interstitial fibrosis, inflammation and apoptosis, may paradoxically result in progression of HF, and often it does so in a prognostically meaningful way.[14] ST2 appears to play a pivotal role in the process of ventricular remodeling and fibrosis, which reflects its value as a biomarker of HF prognosis.

ST2 IN EXPERIMENTAL HF MODELS

As noted above, ST2 gene expression increases in the context of cellular stretch, as well as following ischemic insult, such as in acute myocardial infarction. In this context, both ST2L and sST2 are expressed and secreted. The primary ligand for ST2 is IL-33 (itself a cellular stretch product), the discovery of which opened a crucial window into the role of ST2 in cardiomyocyte hypertrophy and cardiac fibrosis.

Although participant in the process of inflammation and tolerance (as with ST2), IL-33 clearly has a crucial role in cardiovascular disease. IL-33/ST2 signaling is best thought of as a biomechanically activated, cardioprotective fibroblast-cardiomyocyte paracrine system (Figure 14-1). This signaling system appears to control a critical pathway in the maladaptive remodeling of the heart.

The favorable biological effects of IL-33 in experimental HF are numerous: IL-33 antagonizes the development of cardiomyocyte hypertrophy following infusion of angiotensin II and phenylephrine, a benefit that may be blocked by infusion of

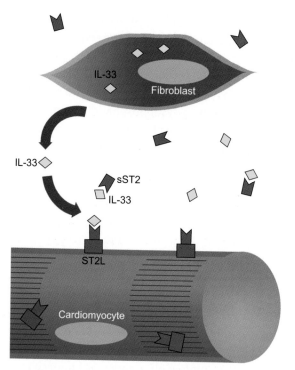

Figure 14-1 ST2 and IL-33 paracrine system.

sST2, consistent with the proposed role of sST2 as the decoy receptor for IL-33.[15] In animal models of thoracic aortic constriction, administration of IL-33 prevented the left ventricle from excessive hypertrophy, fibrosis and dysfunction. In contrast, administration of IL-33 to ST2$^{-/-}$ mice (which lack the ability of IL-33 to bind to ST2L) did not benefit the mice from ventricular overload, remodeling, and death.[15] In models of myocardial ischemia and MI, infusion of IL-33 reduced the infarct volume and limited the extent of the subsequent myocardial fibrosis; this benefit was also abrogated in ST2$^{-/-}$ animals. The antihypertrophic and antifibrotic benefits of IL-33 appear to be mitigated through up-regulation of genes that prolong cell life, resisting proapoptotic pathways; these benefits seem to be reversed by exposure to sST2.

Thus, in summary, IL-33 binds to ST2L exerting a cardioprotective, antiremodeling benefit in the context of volume or pressure overload. This benefit may be lost when sST2 competes for IL-33's binding. Thus, excessive elevation of sST2 may be viewed as a maladaptive response to myocardial stretch/strain.

ASSAYS FOR THE MEASUREMENT OF sST2

The first sST2 assay was relatively insensitive and highly imprecise at low concentrations of protein. Subsequently, a highly sensitive enzyme-linked immunosorbent assay has been described, which has exceptional sensitivity at very low concentrations of sST2 and has excellent analytical precision across the range of expected sST2 values.[16] This novel sST2 assay is able to measure the marker in various matrices, and no interaction is present with commonly encountered interferents, such as bilirubin. A moderate positive correlation between males is present in normal subjects, but sST2 is not affected by fasting state, age, renal function, or body mass index. Serum sST2 concentrations are stable through multiple freeze thaw cycles with an estimated mean recovery > 95%. The day-to-day biological variability of sST2 is currently not well-established, but thought to be approximately 30%.[16]

ST2 IN CARDIOVASCULAR DISORDERS

Acutely Decompensated Heart Failure

Although initially examined in a small cohort of subjects with chronic HF,[17] discussed below, the first compelling data to support the prognostic value of sST2 came from the ProBNP investigation of dyspnea in the emergency department (PRIDE) study, which examined sST2 values in 593 patients presenting to an emergency department with acute dyspnea.[18-20] Concentrations of sST2 in patients with acute HF were increased compared with those from patients whose dyspnea was due to other causes (0.50 ng/mL vs 0.15 ng/mL, p < 0.001). However, the area under the receiver operator characteristic (ROC) curve for sST2 as a diagnostic tool for acutely decompensated heart failure (ADHF) was lower than that of NT-proBNP.

A number of important observations have been made from the PRIDE experience. Among patients with HF, sST2 was higher in ADHF with decreased systolic left ventricular function compared with HF with preserved ejection fraction (HFpEF) (0.67 ng/mL vs 0.42 ng/mL, p = 0.012) and sST2 concentrations correlated with that of NT-proBNP, HF severity (NYHA functional classification), LVEF and creatinine clearance.[19] Although sST2 was not as useful for ADHF diagnosis as NT-proBNP, sST2 was shown in PRIDE to be exceptionally powerful for prognosis, superseding the information provided even by highly refined natriuretic peptide assays; for example, presenting sST2 concentrations in the PRIDE study strongly predicted death at 1 year in ADHF patients (Hazard ratio [HR] = 9.3, p = 003) and in all-cause dyspnea patients (HR = 5.6, p < 0.001). This risk associated with an elevated sST2 in dyspneic patients appeared early and was sustained at least to 4 years (log-rank p < 0.001); ROC analyses for 1-year mortality demonstrated an AUC of 0.80 (p < 0.001) for sST2.[19]

Mueller and colleagues also confirmed the above results in a smaller cohort of 137 patients who presented with ADHF; in this analysis presenting serum sST2 was elevated in those who had died at one year vs those who survived. sST2 was also predictive of death at 1 year independent of other traditional predictors of clinical outcomes such as age, vital signs, renal function, low LVEF, and HF severity by NYHA classes.[21]

While sST2 in these prior studies (as well as in a pooled analysis from both trials[20]) demonstrated the marker to be superior to NT-proBNP for predicting death or future HF events, both markers remained significant predictors of outcome, implying that NT-proBNP may be more indicative of wall stress and sST2 appears to be indicative of the cardiac response to injury and maladaptive remodeling. Lending credence to this concept is the fact that sST2 concentrations identified dyspneic patients with echocardiographic evidence for more adversely remodeled left ventricle, elevated filling pressures, and an overall deleterious cardiac phenotype.[22] Given that NT-proBNP and sST2 appear to reflect interrelated but independent processes, and both are uniquely prognostic, it is therefore of note that the two biomarkers provide additive information regarding prognosis in ADHF (Figure 14-2); while patients with elevation of both peptides are at highest risk, and those with low values for both are at lowest risk, those with elevation of either are reclassified to a risk category that is more intermediate. In addition to NT-proBNP, a recent study indicates that among patients with ADHF, sST2 appears independently predictive of prognosis even in the context of highly sensitive troponin measurement as well.[23]

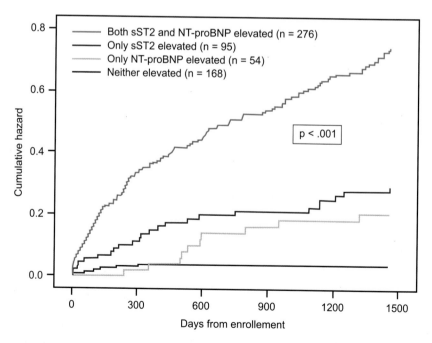

Figure 14-2 sST2 adds incremental predictive power to NT-proBNP for long-term mortality. Unpublished graph *from* Januzzi JL Jr, Rehman S, Mueller T, et al. Importance of biomarkers for long-term mortality prediction in acutely dyspneic patients. *Clin Chem.* 2010;56:1814-21.

While a single sST2 measurement at presentation with ADHF provides powerful prognostic information, the change in sST2 values over the treatment course of HF seems to inform even more robust prognostic value. Boisot and colleagues measured serial sST2 concentrations in 150 patients hospitalized with ADHF, and found that the percent change in sST2 during treatment for ADHF was strongly predictive of 90-day mortality (AUC 0.783, p < 0.001). Those patients whose sST2 values decreased by 15.5% or more during the study period had a 7% chance of death while patients whose sST2 values failed to decrease by 15.5% had a 33% chance of dying.[24] This prognostic value was actually superior to BNP, and additive to renal function and NT-proBNP, both themselves well-established gold standards for outcomes in ADHF.

Chronic HF

The first clinical analysis of sST2 in chronic HF came from the efforts of Richard Lee's group at the Brigham and Women's Hospital. In one of the first clinical studies of sST2, 139 blood samples from subjects with chronic systolic HF (LVEF < 30%) and NYHA functional classes III and IV were analyzed with an early phase assay for sST2; despite the limitations of the method, sST2 levels found to be significantly higher in patients with HF compared with control subjects without HF (median of 0.24 ng/mL vs 0.14 ng/mL; p < 0.0001),[17] and in subsequent measurements, the relative change in sST2 rather than the baseline measurement was predictive of mortality of transplantation in univariate analysis with an odds ratio of 1.32 (p = 0.048). Further analysis also showed that changes in sST2 levels were predictors of mortality or transplantation independent of established markers, such as NT-proBNP. Subsequent data in chronic HF was provided by Bayes-Genis and colleagues who demonstrated that serial measures of sST2 in an ambulatory population of subjects with chronic HF provided exceptional prognostic value for outcomes; in this analysis, an sST2 reduction of approximately 15% or more after therapy change was associated with more favorable outcome compared to those who did not show this reduction in the marker.[25]

In general, negative ventricular remodeling is thought to result in progressive HF and death due to pump failure, but an important association between myocardial fibrosis and risk for malignant ventricular arrhythmia exists.[26] Thus, it is not unreasonable to expect sST2 not only to predict pump failure death but also death from ventricular tachycardia or fibrillation; and indeed, in a cohort of patients with previously implanted cardioverter-defibrillators, data reveal a compelling association between sST2 values and the risk for sudden cardiac death.[27]

These important studies not withstanding, by far the most compelling analysis of sST2 in chronic HF thus far has come from the Penn heart failure study, an analysis of more than 1100 subjects.[28] In this study, a clearly graded association between the concentration of sST2 and adverse outcome was found; compared to those in

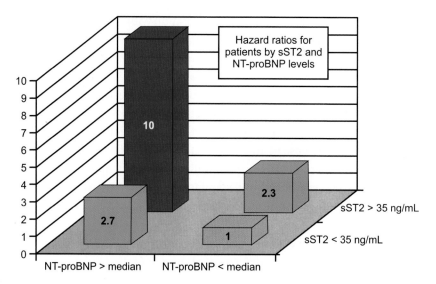

Figure 14-3 Hazard ratios for patients by sST2 and NT-proBNP levels. *Data From* Ky B, French B, McCloskey K, et al. High-sensitivity ST2 for prediction of adverse outcomes in chronic heart failure. *Circ Heart Fail.* 2011;4:180-7.

lower categories, those in the highest sST2 decile had a hazard ratio in excess of 5.0 (P < 0.0001). This risk was strikingly additive to that of NT-proBNP; those with an sST2 ≥ 35 ng/mL (using the highly-sensitive assay) and an elevated NT-proBNP had a hazard ratio of 10 (Figure 14-3). In addition, sST2 added to the prognostic value of the Seattle heart failure model, reclassifying 15% of subjects into more appropriate risk categories.

Acute MI

In 69 human subjects, Weinberg and colleagues showed that sST2 was increased 1 day after MI (3.8 ± 0.4 ng/mL) compared with 14 days (0.98 ± 0.06 ng/mL) and 90 days (0.79 ± 0.07 ng/mL) after MI. Furthermore, circulating sST2 levels correlated with the extent of myocardial injury or biomechanical load; it correlated positively with peak creatine kinase and negatively with left ventricular ejection fraction.[7]

Several large-scale studies have measured sST2 levels in patients with acute MI.[29,30] Shimpo and colleagues looked at 810 patients with acute myocardial infarction in the thrombolysis in myocardial infarction (TIMI) 14 and enoxaparin and TNK-tPA with or without GPIIb/IIIa inhibitor as reperfusion strategy in ST segment elevation MI (STEMI) (ENTIRE)-TIMI 23 clinical trials and found that baseline sST2 levels were predictive of 30-day mortality and new congestive HF.[29] In the clopidogrel as adjunctive reperfusion therapy (CLARITY)-TIMI 28 trial, Sabatine and colleagues found in 1,239 patients that even after adjusting for traditional predictors of clinical outcomes, including age, sex, comorbidities, renal function, extent of infarct and NT-proBNP, sST2 concentrations continued to be an independent predictor of 30-day cardiovascular death or HF.[30] The predictive power of sST2 for 1-year mortality in 403 patients with non-STEMI (NSTEMI) was also demonstrated in the global use of strategies to open occluded coronary arteries (GUSTO) IV study.[31]

Mechanistically, the correlation between sST2 and post-MI outcomes appears to be similarly mediated by the ability of the biomarker to predict adverse ventricular remodeling. In an analysis using cardiac magnetic resonance imaging, 100 subjects with acute MI were scanned at baseline and at 12 and 24 weeks. Concentrations of sST2 correlated with LVEF at baseline ($r = -0.30$, $P = 0.002$) and at 24 weeks ($r = -0.23$, $P = 0.026$). The change in sST2 correlated with change in LV end-diastolic volume index ($r = -0.24$, $p = 0.023$). An elevated sST2 level at baseline was associated with higher infarct volumes at baseline ($r = 0.26$, $p = 0.005$) and at 24 weeks ($r = 0.22$, $p = 0.037$) and the change in infarct volume index ($r = -0.28$, $p = 0.001$),[32] implying that sST2 values are associated with a higher risk for adverse remodeling at presentation, and predict this process prospectively. In addition, an intriguing treatment interaction was found in this analysis: not only did elevated sST2 values identify those patients most likely to have maladaptive remodeling, randomized treatment with an aldosterone blocker (with favorable anti-remodeling benefits) appeared to mainly benefit those patients following MI with elevated sST2 concentrations.[32] Thus, there may be a specific therapeutic response associated with elevated sST2 values in acute MI.

UNRESOLVED ISSUES AND FUTURE DIRECTIONS

In a relatively short period, sST2 has moved from being a poorly understood, scientific curiosity to being a strong contender for clinical application. Across a wide spectrum of cardiovascular disease, this novel biomarker has shown utility for prognostication in a manner additive to, and frequently above that of other prognostic biomarkers.

Although compellingly associated with ventricular fibrosis and remodeling in patients with cardiovascular disease, a number of questions remain about the biological role played by sST2. Indeed, as mentioned above, ST2 is an important mediator of inflammatory process and sST2 concentrations are markedly elevated in such conditions as sepsis and trauma.[33,34] ST2 also specifically mediates interactions of T helper (Th) cell type 2 responses to an insult, thus playing a pivotal role in tolerance. Dysregulation of this process has been shown to be associated with elevated sST2 and present in allergic and autoimmune disease, such as asthma,[35] systemic lupus erythematosus,[3] rheumatoid arthritis,[3] and in idiopathic pulmonary fibrosis.[36] Furthermore, it is reasonable to expect that any process leading to tissue injury and fibrosis may cause elevated sST2 values; indeed, elevation of the marker has been described in hepatic fibrosis[37] and acute respiratory distress syndrome,[38] as well as severe pulmonary syndromes, such as pneumonia.[39] Importantly, in all of these cases, prognostic value of sST2 is seen.

CONCLUSION

In conclusion, sST2 concentrations appear to be prognostically meaningful in a wide range of cardiovascular disease states; it remains unclear if the marker may be useful in other patient types with more subtle forms of cardiac dysfunction. Indeed, as ventricular remodeling associated with common but more subtle cardiovascular disease states, such as hypertension—a leading cause of HF—it is reasonable to consider sST2 measurement for prediction of HF in "apparently well" subjects. With the development of highly sensitive methods for sST2 measurement (allowing detection and resolution of low sST2 concentrations in normal patients), this is now possible, and preliminary data would indicate sST2 may be in fact predictive of future HF in apparently normal subjects (Januzzi JL, personal communication). Whether therapeutic intervention in this context can be brought to bear with the ultimate goal to prevent such fibrosis and organ dysfunction remains speculative, but it is an area ripe for future research.

REFERENCES

1. Werenskiold AK, Hoffmann S, Klemenz R. Induction of a mitogen-responsive gene after expression of the Ha-ras oncogene in NIH 3T3 fibroblasts. *Mol Cell Biol*. 1989;9: 5207-14.
2. Kumar S, Tzimas MN, Griswold DE, et al. Expression of ST2, an interleukin-1 receptor homologue, is induced by proinflammatory stimuli. *Biochem Biophys Res Commun*. 1997;235:474-8.
3. Kuroiwa K, Arai T, Okazaki H, et al. Identification of human ST2 protein in the sera of patients with autoimmune diseases. *Biochem Biophys Res Commun*. 2001;284:1104-8.
4. Tominaga S, Inazawa J, Tsuji S. Assignment of the human ST2 gene to chromosome 2 at q11.2. *Hum Genet*. 1996;97:561-3.
5. Lanahan A, Williams JB, Sanders LK, et al. Growth factor-induced delayed early response genes. *Mol Cell Biol*. 1992;12:3919-29.
6. Xu D, Chan WL, Leung BP, et al. Selective expression of a stable cell surface molecule on type 2 but not type 1 helper T cells. *J Exp Med*. 1998;187:787-94.
7. Weinberg EO, Shimpo M, De Keulenaer GW, et al. Expression and regulation of ST2, an interleukin-1 receptor family member, in cardiomyocytes and myocardial infarction. *Circulation*. 2002;106:2961-6.
8. Tominaga S, Kuroiwa K, Tago K, et al. Presence and expression of a novel variant form of ST2 gene product in human leukemic cell line UT-7/GM. *Biochem Biophys Res Commun*. 1999;264:14-8.
9. Iwahana H, Hayakawa M, Kuroiwa K, et al. Molecular cloning of the chicken ST2 gene and a novel variant form of the ST2 gene product, ST2LV. *Biochim Biophy Acta (BBA) - Gene Structure and Expression*. 2004;1681:1-14.

10. Tago K, Noda T, Hayakawa M, et al. Tissue distribution and subcellular localization of a variant form of the human ST2 gene product, ST2V. *Biochem Biophys Res Commun.* 2001;285:1377-83.

11. Tominaga S. A putative protein of a growth specific cDNA from BALB/c-3T3 cells is highly similar to the extracellular portion of mouse interleukin 1 receptor. *FEBS Lett.* 1989;258:301-4.

12. Klemenz R, Hoffmann S, Werenskiold AK. Serum- and oncoprotein-mediated induction of a gene with sequence similarity to the gene encoding carcinoembryonic antigen. *Proc Natl Acad Sci U S A.* 1989;86:5708-12.

13. Laursen NB, Kessler R, Frohli E, et al. Effects of ras transformation on the induction of the IL-1 receptor related T1 gene in response to mitogens, anisomycin, IL-1 and TNFalpha. *Oncogene.* 1998;16:575-86.

14. Manabe I, Shindo T, Nagai R. Gene expression in fibroblasts and fibrosis: involvement in cardiac hypertrophy. *Circ Res.* 2002;91:1103-13.

15. Sanada S, Hakuno D, Higgins LJ, et al. IL-33 and ST2 comprise a critical biomechanically induced and cardioprotective signaling system. *J Clin Invest.* 2007;117:538-49.

16. Dieplinger B, Januzzi JL Jr, Steinmair M, et al. Analytical and clinical evaluation of a novel high-sensitivity assay for measurement of soluble ST2 in human plasma—the Presage ST2 assay. *Clin Chim Acta.* 2009;409:33-40.

17. Weinberg EO, Shimpo M, Hurwitz S, et al. Identification of serum soluble ST2 receptor as a novel heart failure biomarker. *Circulation.* 2003;107:721-6.

18. Januzzi JL Jr, Camargo CA, Anwaruddin S, et al. The N-terminal Pro-BNP investigation of dyspnea in the emergency department (PRIDE) study. *Am J Cardiol.* 2005;95:948-54.

19. Januzzi JL Jr, Peacock WF, Maisel AS, et al. Measurement of the interleukin family member ST2 in patients with acute dyspnea: results from the PRIDE (Pro-Brain Natriuretic Peptide Investigation of Dyspnea in the Emergency Department) study. *J Am Coll Cardiol.* 2007;50:607-13.

20. Rehman SU, Mueller T, Januzzi JL Jr, Characteristics of the novel interleukin family biomarker ST2 in patients with acute heart failure. *J Am Coll Cardiol.* 2008;52:1458-65.

21. Mueller T, Dieplinger B, Gegenhuber A, et al. Increased plasma concentrations of soluble ST2 are predictive for 1-year mortality in patients with acute destabilized heart failure. *Clin Chem.* 2008;54:752-6.

22. Shah RV, Chen-Tournoux AA, Picard MH, et al. Serum levels of the interleukin-1 receptor family member ST2, cardiac structure and function, and long-term mortality in patients with acute dyspnea. *Circ Heart Fail.* 2009;2:311-9.

23. Pascual-Figal DA, Manzano-Fernandez S, Boronat M, et al. Soluble ST2, high sensitivity troponin T and N-terminal pro-B-type natriuretic peptide: complementary role for risk stratification in acutely decompensated heart failure patients. *Eur J Heart Fail.* 2011 May 6. (Epub ahead of print).

24. Boisot S, Beede J, Isakson S, et al. Serial sampling of ST2 predicts 90-day mortality following destabilized heart failure. *J Card Fail.* 2008;14:732-8.

25. Bayes-Genis A, Pascual-Figal D, Januzzi JL, et al. Soluble ST2 monitoring provides additional risk stratification for outpatients with decompensated heart failure. *Rev Esp Cardiol.* 2010;63:1171-8.

26. Iles L, Pfluger H, Lefkovits L, et al. Myocardial fibrosis predicts appropriate device therapy in patients with implantable cardioverter-defibrillators for primary prevention of sudden cardiac death. *J Am Coll Cardiol.* 2011;57:821-8.

27. Pascual-Figal DA, Ordonez-Llanos J, Tornel PL, et al. Soluble ST2 for predicting sudden cardiac death in patients with chronic heart failure and left ventricular systolic dysfunction. *J Am Coll Cardiol.* 2009;54:2174-9.

28. Ky B, French B, McCloskey K, et al. High-sensitivity ST2 for prediction of adverse outcomes in chronic heart failure. *Circ Heart Fail.* 2011;4:180-7. Epub 2010 Dec 22.

29. Shimpo M, Morrow DA, Weinberg EO, et al. Serum levels of the interleukin-1 receptor family member ST2 predict mortality and clinical outcome in acute myocardial infarction. *Circulation.* 2004;109:2186-90.

30. Sabatine MS, Morrow DA, Higgins LJ, et al. Complementary roles for biomarkers of biomechanical strain ST2 and N-terminal prohormone B-type natriuretic peptide in patients with ST-elevation myocardial infarction. *Circulation.* 2008;117:1936-44.

31. Eggers KM, Armstrong PW, Califf RM, et al. ST2 and mortality in non-ST-segment elevation acute coronary syndrome. *Am Heart J.* 2010;159:788-94.

32. Weir RA, Miller AM, Murphy GE, et al. Serum soluble ST2: a potential novel mediator in left ventricular and infarct remodeling after acute myocardial infarction. *J Am Coll Cardiol.* 2010;55:243-50.

33. Trajkovic V, Sweet MJ, Xu D. T1/ST2—an IL-1 receptor-like modulator of immune responses. *Cytokine Growth Factor Rev.* 2004;15:87-95.

34. Brunner M, Krenn C, Roth G, et al. Increased levels of soluble ST2 protein and IgG1 production in patients with sepsis and trauma. *Intensive Care Med.* 2004;30:1468-73. Epub 2004 Feb 28.

35. Oshikawa K, Kuroiwa K, Tago K, et al. Elevated soluble ST2 protein levels in sera of patients with asthma with an acute exacerbation. *Am J Respir Crit Care Med.* 2001;164:277-81.

36. Tajima S, Oshikawa K, Tominaga S, et al. The increase in serum soluble ST2 protein upon acute exacerbation of idiopathic pulmonary fibrosis. *Chest.* 2003;124:1206-14.

37. Amatucci A, Novobrantseva T, Gilbride K, et al. Recombinant ST2 boosts hepatic Th2 response *in vivo*. *J Leukoc Biol.* 2007;82:124-32. Epub 2007 Apr 5.

38. Januzzi J, Bajwa EK, Gong MN, et al. Abstract P118: Plasma levels of interleukin receptor soluble ST2 predict disease severity and mortality in patients with acute respiratory distress syndrome (ARDS). *Circulation.* 2009;120(18_MeetingAbstracts):S1466-c-1467.

39. Martinez-Rumayor A, Camargo CA, Green SM, et al. Soluble ST2 plasma concentrations predict 1-year mortality in acutely dyspneic emergency department patients with pulmonary disease. *Am J Clin Pathol.* 2008;130:578-84.

Copeptin

Nils G Morgenthaler

INTRODUCTION

Arginine vasopressin (AVP or antidiuretic hormone) is one of the key hormones in the human body responsible for a variety of cardiovascular functions. Despite its pivotal role in cardiovascular disease, the measurement and diagnostic use of AVP have so far escaped introduction into the routine clinical laboratory due to technical difficulties and preanalytical errors. Copeptin, the C-terminal part of the AVP precursor peptide, was found to be a stable and sensitive surrogate marker for AVP release. Copeptin behaves in a similar manner to mature AVP in the circulation, with respect to osmotic stimuli and hypotension. Copeptin is a relatively new biomarker. Till September 2011, there are only 150 publications in Medline if the search term "copeptin" is used. About 100 of those were written in the last few years as a result of the development of the copeptin assay.[1] For comparison, there are more than 38,000 papers under the search term "vasopressin". Despite its young age, copeptin has been shown to be of interest in a variety of clinical indications,[2] including cardiovascular diseases, such as heart failure, myocardial infarction, and stroke.[3]

Copeptin is a glycosylated, 39 amino acid long peptide with a leucine-rich core segment, and was described for the first time by Holwerda in 1972.[4] AVP and copeptin share the same precursor peptide, the 164 amino acid long preprovasopressin, which consists of a signal peptide, AVP, neurophysin II, and copeptin (Figure 15-1).[5] Thus, copeptin is the C-terminal part of pro-AVP (CT-proAVP) and is released together with

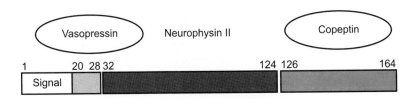

Figure 15-1 Arginine vasopressin (AVP) precursor peptide. Numbers indicate the amino acid positions of the preprohormone.

AVP, during precursor processing. In contrast to AVP, copeptin is very stable in the serum or plasma at room temperature, and is easy and robust to measure.[1,6]

RELEASE MECHANISM OF COPEPTIN AS PART OF THE AVP PRECURSOR PEPTIDE

Pro-AVP, the precursor peptide of AVP and copeptin, is produced and released by two endocrine mechanisms. In the first mechanism, the precursor peptide pro-AVP is produced in the magnocellular neurons of the supraoptic and paraventricular hypothalamic nuclei. During axonal transport through the infundibulum to the posterior lobe of the pituitary gland, AVP, neurophysin II, and copeptin are processed from the precursor peptide (Figure 15-2). Pro-AVP is subjected to a four-enzyme cascade to reach the bioactive conformation of mature AVP.[7] During this process, copeptin and neurophysin II seem to help in the correct folding of AVP.[8] Processing is usually complete at the level of the neurohypophysis.[7] All three peptides are subsequently secreted from the neurohypophysis upon hemodynamic or osmotic stimuli.

The second release mechanism is part of the endocrine stress response, involving two hormones from the hypothalamus for the release of adrenocorticotropic

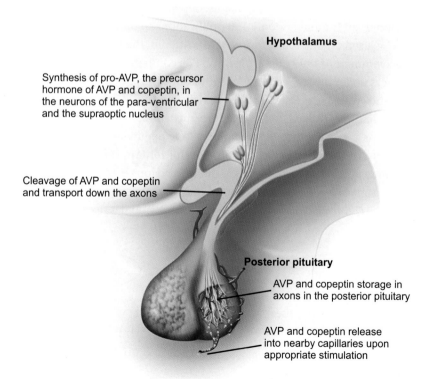

Figure 15-2 AVP and copeptin release from the hypothalamus (mechanism 1).

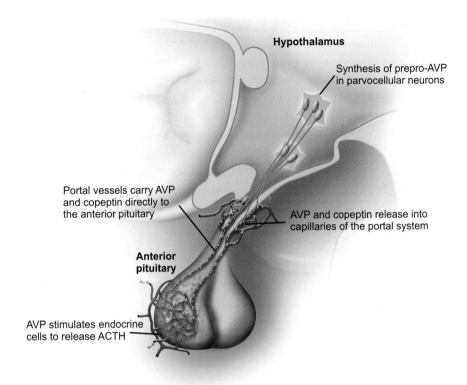

Hypothalamus

Synthesis of prepro-AVP
in parvocellular neurons

Portal vessels carry AVP
and copeptin directly to
the anterior pituitary

AVP and copeptin release into
capillaries of the portal system

**Anterior
pituitary**

AVP stimulates endocrine
cells to release ACTH

Figure 15-3 AVP and copeptin release from the hypothalamus (mechanism 2).

hormone (ACTH). For this mechanism, the precursor peptide is synthesized and processed in the parvocellular neurons of the hypothalamus, the same part of the brain that produces also corticotropin-releasing hormone (CRH). AVP produced by this mechanism is subsequently released into the pituitary portal system at the eminentia mediana and acts immediately on the endocrine cells of the adenohypophysis (Figure 15-3). The synergistic effect of CRH and AVP stimulates the release of ACTH, and through ACTH eventually to cortisol.[9-12]

AVP RECEPTORS AND FUNCTION

The function of AVP is well understood, but the physiologic relevance of copeptin is still unsolved. AVP exerts its peripheral effects in the circulation by binding to tissue-specific G-protein-coupled receptors (GPCR).[13,14] Two predominant receptor types are known: the V_1-receptor, which mediates arteriolar vasoconstriction, and the V_2-receptor, which is responsible for the antidiuretic effect in the kidneys. V_1-receptors are found in high density on vascular smooth muscle cells and cause vasoconstriction by an increase in intracellular calcium via G-protein-induced inositol triphosphate and diacylglycerol. V_1-receptors are also present on cardiac myocytes, but the vasoconstrictive effect on these cells is still under debate.[14,15]

V_2-receptors are located on the cells of the renal collecting tubules, where they increase intracellular cyclic adenosine monophosphate (cAMP)[13] that has two effects on water homeostasis: first, it stimulates the synthesis of mRNA encoding aquaporin-2; and second, it increases the traffic of aquaporin-2 vesicles to the apical plasma membrane of the collecting duct, where aquaporin-2 allows the absorption of most of the water present in the urine. A third AVP receptor, the V_3-receptor (or V_{1b}-receptor), is restricted to certain cells of the adenohypophysis, and is involved in the secretion of ACTH.[16] AVP also binds to the oxytocin receptor with a similar affinity to oxytocin[17] and to certain purinergic receptors, also members of the GPCR superfamily. These binding effects are not yet completely understood and subject to ongoing research.

MEASUREMENT OF AVP AND COPEPTIN

The measurement of mature AVP has been described several decades ago; however, based on technical challenges it was never implemented into clinical routine use. More than 90% of AVP in the circulation is bound to platelets, resulting in an underestimation of actually released amounts of AVP.[18] Furthermore, the incomplete removal of platelets from plasma samples or prolonged storage of unprocessed blood samples can lead to falsely elevated and varying AVP levels.[18,19] Once secreted, AVP is rapidly cleared from the circulation, with an *in vivo* half-life of 24 minutes.[20] AVP is unstable in isolated plasma, even when stored at –20 °C.[21] Due to its small size, AVP cannot be measured by sandwich immunoassay, but only by competitive immunoassay. Competitive immunoassays usually tend to be less sensitive than sandwich immunoassays.

On the other side, the technical advantages of copeptin measurement are well described:[1] The variant assay systems require only 15–50 μL of serum or plasma, while AVP assays need one or more milliliters of plasma. No extraction steps or other preanalytical procedures, such as, the addition of protease inhibitors, are needed. Results are available in 0.5–3 hours, whereas many of the competitive AVP immunoassays described require more than 12–24 hours, due to extensive incubation steps. Probably, the most relevant advantage of the copeptin assay is that copeptin, unlike mature AVP, is extremely stable in plasma or serum *ex vivo*. *Ex vivo* stability of copeptin (< 20% loss of recovery) was shown for serum and plasma for at least seven days at room temperature and 14 days at 4 °C.[1]

COPEPTIN AND AVP CONCENTRATION IN BLOOD

Copeptin is very robust for measurement *ex vivo*, but it behaves in a similar way to AVP in the circulation, and both markers are well correlated (Figure 15-4).[1] Copeptin concentrations in healthy volunteers have been examined now in large population studies, and range between 1 and 13 pmol/L (upper 97.5 percentile) with median

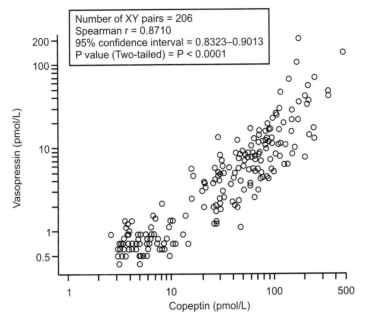

Figure 15-4 Correlation between copeptin and vasopressin.

values < 5 pmol/L.[1,22,23] Men consistently show slightly higher values compared with women, but the difference in median values is only about 1 pmol/L.[1,22] Copeptin responds to changes in plasma osmolality with a kinetic increase/decrease similar to that reported for AVP.[1,24] A recent direct comparison of AVP and copeptin showed a better correlation of copeptin to plasma osmolality, suggesting copeptin as a substitute for AVP measurements.[25] Patients with diabetes insipidus and reduced AVP have very low plasma levels of copeptin,[26,27] whilst patients with hyponatremia and the syndrome of inappropriate ADH secretion (SIADH) have elevated copeptin in their circulation.[28]

At normal concentrations, the role of AVP is to regulate the plasma osmolality by eliminating free water in the kidney. Like mature AVP, copeptin is regulated within a certain normal range, but may vary according to individual physiologic conditions. Copeptin increases to upper normal values during fasting and shows a rapid decline *in vivo* to low normal values after oral water load.[1] In two studies with healthy volunteers, copeptin showed identical changes during disordered water states or osmolality to those shown for AVP. During water deprivation, which resulted in weight loss and an increase in plasma osmolality, serum copeptin increased, which could be further pronounced by the additional infusion of hypertonic saline. This resulted in copeptin plasma values not usually seen in healthy individuals. Conversely, during hypotonic saline infusion, plasma osmolality decreased and copeptin decreased to values in the very low normal range.[24,25]

Electroloyte disturbances are common in cardiovascular and renal diseases, including the most commonly seen hyponatremia, and the pathophysiology is complex and the diagnostic approach is challenging.[29] Copeptin plasma concentrations might be valuable in the diagnostic work-up of hyponatremic conditions, which have been reported in up to 15% of hospitalized patients,[30] sometimes with a poor prognosis. In patients with SIADH, determination of copeptin together with urine sodium helped in the differential diagnosis.[28]

Whilst the normal range of copeptin mirrors the physiological AVP secretion needed to maintain plasma osmolality, in severe diseases or states, such as shock, sepsis, stroke, or cardiovascular diseases, the nonosmotic release of AVP is seen by a strong increase in plasma copeptin. This increase of copeptin has diagnostic and prognostic values.

COPEPTIN IN CARDIOVASCULAR SHOCK

The effect of experimental hemorrhagic shock on copeptin was studied in a small number of baboons.[31] After induction of hemorrhagic shock, copeptin increased more than thirtyfold after the second hour and reached a peak > 250 pmol/L after three hours of bleeding. Copeptin levels dropped again within one hour of reperfusion, and continued to decline until they reached a plateau of slightly elevated normal values at the end of the experiment. The mean arterial blood pressure followed inverse kinetics in all animals, decreasing during bleeding and increasing slowly after reperfusion.[31] This behavior of copeptin was described for mature AVP in a similar experimental setting more than 30 years ago.[32]

COPEPTIN TO RULE OUT ACUTE MYOCARDIAL INFARCTION

A particularly interesting observation on the response of circulating copeptin levels after an acute myocardial infarction (AMI) was first reported by Khan and Ng.[33] In 980 post-acute MI patients of the LAMP (Leicester Acute Myocardial Infarction Peptide) study, copeptin values were highest on day 1 after AMI. During the next 2–5 days, they declined to a stable, but still elevated, plateau.[33] Furthermore, copeptin levels were higher in patients who died or were readmitted with heart failure compared with event-free survivors. Patients with copeptin levels in the highest quartile showed a > 40% event rate during the follow-up period.[33]

Based on this observation, Reichlin and Müller examined the potential role of copeptin in the diagnosis of AMI. They studied the contribution of copeptin in the management of 487 consecutive patients with chest pain presenting to the emergency room (ER).[34] In those patients with the final gold standard diagnosis of AMI (17%), copeptin levels were already elevated 0–4 hours after the onset of symptoms, at a time when troponin T was still undetectable in many patients. As copeptin levels declined, whilst troponin levels increased, these distinct kinetics

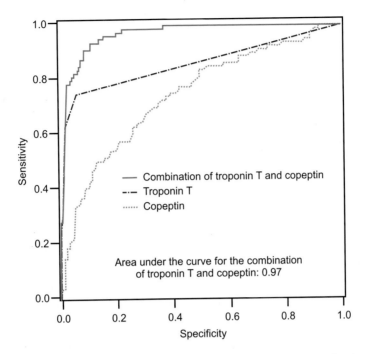

Figure 15-5 Receiver-operator characteristic (ROC) curves at presentation for the diagnosis of acute MI. Area under the ROC curves for troponin T and copeptin at presentation, and the combination of both markers in the diagnosis of acute myocardial infarction (MI). *Modified from* Reichlin T, Hochholzer W, Stelzig C, et al. Incremental value of copeptin for rapid rule out of acute myocardial infarction. *J Am Coll Cardiol.* 2009;54:60-8, with permission.

resulted in an additive diagnostic value of both markers for the diagnosis of acute MI. The area under the curve (AUC) of troponin alone in the first blood sample taken in the ER was 0.86, which was increased to 0.97 by adding copeptin (Figure 15-5). Using this double marker approach, a negative troponin and copeptin at presentation of the patient in the ER < 14 pmol/L allowed acute MI to be ruled out, with a negative predictive value of > 99%.[34]

A multicenter trial in 1293 consecutive patients with suspected acute coronary syndrome (ACS) confirmed this initial report. Combined measurement of copeptin and troponin T in the first blood sample taken at ER admission improved the c-statistic from 0.85 for troponin T alone to 0.94 for a combination of copeptin and troponin T. The effect was particularly prominent in patients presenting within three hours after chest pain onset to the ER. In this group, the combination increased the c-statistic from 0.77 to 0.91.[23]

It is important to consider that a large part of the negative predictive value is contributed by troponin. Thus, using a very sensitive troponin assay in combination with copeptin will lead to a higher NPV than a less sensitive troponin assay. An extension of the study by Reichlin and Müller shows additional value of copeptin on top of a contemporary sensitive troponin assay (unpublished). However, it is yet unclear, how the combination of copeptin and troponin may perform in a world of highly sensitive troponin assays. The present confusion on the nomenclature and clinical use of those assays[35] must be sorted out before the benefit of additional biomarkers can be fairly evaluated. The results of the ongoing CHOPIN trial (Copeptin Helps in the early detection Of Patients with acute myocardial INfarction), a multicentre trial with 2000 patients with chest pain in the ER, should help to address this issue (ClinicalTrials.gov Identifier: NCT00952744).

Release Mechanism of Copeptin and AVP in Acute MI

Why is copeptin elevated in AMI? This question is presently heavily under debate. It helps to look back a few years on what is known about AVP in this condition. In fact, the observed elevation of copeptin after acute MI has long been described for AVP, but based on the complexity of AVP measurement, this observation has never become of diagnostic relevance. However, despite insufficient assays being available, several studies tried to elucidate the AVP response in AMI.[36-38] In a sheep model of AMI, AVP was increased within two hours after inducing microembolization in the animals. In a subset of more frequently sampled animals, the peak response of AVP occurred at 40 min after embolization, and AVP was elevated for more than 12 hours.[39] But despite the very early rise of AVP (and other hormones related to stress response), none of these markers were followed up as a potential candidate for the diagnosis of AMI due to severe limitations in the measurement of these hormones. Neither AVP nor ACTH or cortisol is available in rapid and sensitive assay technology, which would allow a fast enough "vein-to-brain time" to influence the early diagnosis in an ER. It needed a stable biomarker like copeptin, to follow up on this early reports, and to show value in a clinical setting.

What triggers the rapid release of AVP/copeptin after an AMI? There are several possible explanations, but two hypotheses seem to be most likely. First, as described above, AVP is a substantial part of the endocrine stress response, resulting in ACTH and cortisol release. Therefore, it is not surprising that the body responds to acute and life-threatening diseases, such as AMI or stroke, by a rapid AVP/copeptin release. Endocrinologists discuss copeptin to be a rapid and immediate biomarker of the individual stress response.[40] However, a second trigger that leads to AVP/copeptin secretion from the posterior pituitary could be cardiac underfilling as a result of the AMI. This may lead to baroreceptor stimulation and AVP release. Also possible is a direct damage to the cardiac baroreceptors. This is supported by the fact that the highest copeptin elevation after AMI is seen in patients with electrocardiographic signs of cardiac damage.[34]

COPEPTIN IN HEART FAILURE

The role of copeptin as a biomarker in patients with CHF has been described in several studies. Patients with chronic heart failure and high levels of copeptin had a significantly poorer long-term prognosis than patients who had low plasma copeptin concentrations.[41,42] Combined measurement of plasma copeptin together with B-natriuretic peptide concentrations could further improve outcome prediction in these patients.[41,42]

Khan et al. examined the role of copeptin in 980 consecutive patients after AMI.[33] The prognostic value of copeptin was assessed alone or in combination with N-terminal B-type natriuretic peptide (NT-proBNP). Copeptin was raised in patients who died or were readmitted with heart failure compared with survivors. Copeptin and NT-proBNP were significant independent predictors of death or heart failure at 60 days. Consideration of both markers gave added prognostic information beyond existing clinical characteristics, enabling patients to be stratified into low-, intermediate-, or high-risk groups.

The same research group subsequently reported on an association of copeptin with the degree of left ventricular (LV) remodeling after AMI.[43] Thus, the AVP system may have progressive effects on LV impairment beyond the acute phase of an MI. Several actions of AVP on the heart may account for the remodeling process, including myocyte protein synthesis via the V_1-receptor,[44] increased peripheral vasoconstriction, afterload and ventricular stress,[45] and stimulation of cardiac fibroblasts.[46] These observations were strengthened by the increased risk of elevated copeptin levels and clinical heart failure in those patients. This risk stratification at an early stage after acute MI remains important and may be useful to select treatment regimes in the future, such as the use of AVP receptor antagonists (the vaptan class of drugs). Reports on those drugs exist for CHF,[47,48] but no study has yet examined the use of vaptans in the human post-acute MI patient. Only animal data is available on the improved cardiac hemodynamics after administration of conivaptan.[49]

In a subset of patients of the OPTIMAAL (Optimal Trial in Myocardial Infarction with Angiotensin II Antagonist Losartan) study, the prognostic role of copeptin in patients after AMI was further examined.[50] This multicenter setting confirmed the report by Khan,[33] and showed that copeptin is a strong marker for mortality and morbidity in patients with heart failure after AMI. The predictive value was even stronger than BNP and NT-proBNP. As described before, patients in the highest quartile (> 25.9 pmol/L) had significantly increased mortality compared with the other groups. The study also demonstrated the value of serial measurements of copeptin during the follow-up, which added predictive value over a single determination at baseline.[50]

Another heart failure follow-up study examined the role of copeptin in 786 patients across the whole spectrum of heart failure based on systolic dysfunction and BNP values.[51] The authors showed a strong and independent correlation between plasma copeptin levels and all-cause mortality. This was seen in the entire cohort of symptomatic patients with NYHA class II, III, and IV, but was most compelling in the functional classes II and III. Patients with copeptin values below the lowest quartile of 5.75 pmol/L (which is similar to the median of a healthy population) had the lowest mortality rate (< 12%) in the 24-month follow-up period, whilst patients in the highest quartile (> 21.7 pmol/L, which is above the 99th percentile of a normal population) had mortality rates > 50%.[51]

THE POTENTIAL ROLE OF COPEPTIN AND AVP RECEPTOR ANTAGONIST DRUG THERAPIES

As copeptin is a reliable biomarker of AVP release, and the new class of vaptan drugs are AVP receptor antagonists, it seems to be an obvious idea to use copeptin as a diagnostic biomarker to fine-tune vaptan therapy. The measurement of blood glucose before the administration of insulin may serve as conceptual comparison. Whilst this was and is not done for difficult to measure hormones (like angiotensin or angiotensin converting enzyme before the administration of an ACE inhibitor), the advent of copeptin as a simple way to measure AVP release may lead to a paradigm shift in the way that drug companies look at companion diagnostics. To disregard the knowledge of a circulating substance you want to block with a drug was not successful for the vaptan trials. Whilst AVP receptor antagonists have been successfully applied in experimental congestive heart failure[52,53] and hyponatremia,[54] the large clinical trials report mixed results in heart failure therapy, with no effect on mortality.[47,48] Future studies should evaluate whether treatment with AVP receptor antagonists is most effective if the vasopressinergic system is activated, as can now easily be assessed by copeptin plasma concentrations. Secondary analysis of the Biomarkers in Acute Heart Failure (BACH) trial[55] supports this reasoning. In the BACH trial, patients with low serum sodium had a worse outcome than patients with normal sodium. This is well-described for heart failure patients. Of interest, those patients with low sodium and high copeptin had a higher risk than patients with low sodium and low copeptin.[56] So the combination of serum sodium and serum copeptin could identify heart failure patients who might benefit most from vaptan treatment. Future trials need to address this issue.

Furthermore, measurement of copeptin levels may be useful in determining whether AVP receptor antagonist therapy is not only appropriate in patients with chronic heart failure and hyponatremia, but also in patients with other diseases, such as cirrhosis[57] or renal failure,[58-60] in which AVP has been shown to play a pathophysiologic role.

Also the reported ineffectiveness to AVP receptor antagonists in up to 30% of patients needs to be examined in the context of their respective copeptin levels. One could speculate if a copeptin guided adjustment of the dosage of the drug would be of help.

SUMMARY

Copeptin is the stable C-terminal fragment of the AVP precursor (CT-proAVP). Physiologically, it contributes to the correct structural formation of AVP prior to release into the circulation. The measurement of copeptin appears to be a clinically relevant method for reliably assessing AVP plasma concentrations, which cannot be determined in routine practice. This would be particularly helpful in diseases where disturbances of the vasopressinergic system contribute to or are the immediate result of the pathogenesis. Future studies should evaluate the clinical relevance of copeptin as a diagnostic and prognostic laboratory parameter in AMI, heart failure, hyponatremia, and a variety of other diseases not discussed here (like sepsis, pneumonia, or stroke).[2,61] Also, we need to understand its role in therapy monitoring of AVP receptor antagonists in heart failure, hyponatremia, and renal failure.

REFERENCES

1. Morgenthaler NG, Struck J, Alonso C, Bergmann A. Assay for the measurement of copeptin, a stable peptide derived from the precursor of vasopressin. *Clin Chem.* 2006;52:112-9.
2. Morgenthaler NG, Struck J, Jochberger S, Dunser MW. Copeptin: clinical use of a new biomarker. *Trends Endocrinol Metab.* 2008;19:43-9.
3. Morgenthaler NG. Copeptin: a biomarker of cardiovascular and renal function. *Congest Heart Fail.* 16:S37-44.
4. Holwerda DA. A glycopeptide from the posterior lobe of pig pituitaries. I. Isolation and characterization. *Eur J Biochem.* 1972;28:334-9.
5. Land H, Schutz G, Schmale H, Richter D. Nucleotide sequence of cloned cDNA encoding bovine arginine vasopressin-neurophysin II precursor. *Nature.* 1982;295:299-303.
6. Struck J, Morgenthaler NG, Bergmann A. Copeptin, a stable peptide derived from the vasopressin precursor, is elevated in serum of sepsis patients. *Peptides.* 2005;26:2500-4.
7. Acher R, Chauvet J, Rouille Y. Dynamic processing of neuropeptides: sequential conformation shaping of neurohypophysial preprohormones during intraneuronal secretory transport. *J Mol Neurosci.* 2002;18:223-8.
8. Repaske DR, Medlej R, Gultekin EK, Krishnamani MR, Halaby G, Findling JW, et al. Heterogeneity in clinical manifestation of autosomal dominant neurohypophyseal diabetes insipidus caused by a mutation encoding Ala-1→Val in the signal peptide of the arginine vasopressin/neurophysin II/copeptin precursor. *J Clin Endocrinol Metab.* 1997;82:51-6.
9. Gillies GE, Linton EA, Lowry PJ. Corticotropin releasing activity of the new CRF is potentiated several times by vasopressin. *Nature.* 1982;299:355-7.
10. Rivier C, Vale W. Modulation of stress-induced ACTH release by corticotropin-releasing factor, catecholamines and vasopressin. *Nature.* 1983;305:325-7.

11. Rivier C, Vale W. Interaction of corticotropin-releasing factor and arginine vasopressin on adrenocorticotropin secretion *in vivo. Endocrinology.* 1983;113:939-42.

12. Milsom SR, Conaglen JV, Donald RA, Espiner EA, Nicholls MG, Livesey JH. Augmentation of the response to CRF in man: relative contributions of endogenous angiotensin and vasopressin. *Clin Endocrinol (Oxf).* 1985;22:623-9.

13. Birnbaumer M. Vasopressin receptors. *Trends Endocrinol Metab.* 2000;11:406-10.

14. Holmes CL, Landry DW, Granton JT. Science review: vasopressin and the cardiovascular system part 1—receptor physiology. *Crit Care.* 2003;7:427-34.

15. Holmes CL, Landry DW, Granton JT. Science Review: vasopressin and the cardiovascular system part 2—clinical physiology. *Crit Care.* 2004;8:15-23.

16. Thibonnier M, Preston JA, Dulin N, Wilkins PL, Berti-Mattera LN, Mattera R. The human V3 pituitary vasopressin receptor: ligand binding profile and density-dependent signaling pathways. *Endocrinology.* 1997; 138:4109-22.

17. Peter J, Burbach H, Adan RA, et al. Molecular neurobiology and pharmacology of the vasopressin/oxytocin receptor family. *Cell Mol Neurobiol.* 1995;15:573-95.

18. Preibisz JJ, Sealey JE, Laragh JH, Cody RJ, Weksler BB. Plasma and platelet vasopressin in essential hypertension and congestive heart failure. *Hypertension.* 1983;5:I129-38.

19. Kluge M, Riedl S, Erhart-Hofmann B, Hartmann J, Waldhauser F. Improved extraction procedure and RIA for determination of arginine 8-vasopressin in plasma: role of premeasurement sample treatment and reference values in children. *Clin Chem.* 1999; 45:98-103.

20. Baumann G, Dingman JF. Distribution, blood transport, and degradation of antidiuretic hormone in man. *J Clin Invest.* 1976;57:1109-16.

21. Robertson GL, Mahr EA, Athar S, Sinha T. Development and clinical application of a new method for the radioimmunoassay of arginine vasopressin in human plasma. *J Clin Invest.* 1973;52:2340-52.

22. Bhandari SS, Loke I, Davies JE, Squire IB, Struck J, Ng LL. Gender and renal function influence plasma levels of copeptin in healthy individuals. *Clin Sci (Lond).* 2009;116: 257-63.

23. Keller T, Tzikas S, Zeller T, Czyz E, Lillpopp L, Ojeda FM, et al. Copeptin improves early diagnosis of acute myocardial infarction. *J Am Coll Cardiol.* 2010;55:2096-106.

24. Szinnai G, Morgenthaler NG, Berneis K, Struck J, Muller B, Keller U, et al. Changes in plasma copeptin, the c-terminal portion of arginine vasopressin during water deprivation and excess in healthy subjects. *J Clin Endocrinol Metab.* 2007;92:3973-78.

25. Balanescu S, Kopp P, Gaskill MB, Morgenthaler NG, Schindler C, Rutishauser J. Correlation of plasma copeptin and vasopressin concentrations in hypo-, iso-, and hyperosmolar states. *J Clin Endocrinol Metab.* 2011;epub.

26. Katan M, Morgenthaler NG, Dixit KC, Rutishauser J, Brabant GE, Muller B, et al. Anterior and posterior pituitary function testing with simultaneous insulin tolerance test and a novel copeptin assay. *J Clin Endocrinol Metab.* 2007;92:2640-3.

27. Fenske W, Quinkler M, Lorenz D, Zopf K, Haagen U, Papassotiriou J, et al. Copeptin in the differential diagnosis of the polydipsia-polyuria syndrome—revisiting the direct and indirect water deprivation tests. *J Clin Endocrinol Metab.* 2011;epub.

28. Fenske W, Stork S, Blechschmidt A, Maier SG, Morgenthaler NG, Allolio B. Copeptin in the differential diagnosis of hyponatremia. *J Clin Endocrinol Metab.* 2009;94:123-9.

29. Vachharajani TJ, Zaman F, Abreo KD. Hyponatremia in critically ill patients. *J Intensive Care Med.* 2003;18:3-8.

30. Hoorn EJ, Halperin ML, Zietse R. Diagnostic approach to a patient with hyponatraemia: traditional versus physiology-based options. *QJM*. 2005;98:529-40.

31. Morgenthaler NG, Muller B, Struck J, Bergmann A, Redl H, Christ-Crain M. Copeptin, a stable peptide of the arginine vasopressin precursor, is elevated in hemorrhagic and septic shock. *Shock*. 2007;28:219-26.

32. Arnauld E, Czernichow P, Fumoux F, Vincent JD. The effects of hypotension and hypovolemia on the liberation of vasopressin during hemorrhage in the unanesthetized monkey (Macaca mulatta). *Pflugers Arch*. 1977;371:193-200.

33. Khan SQ, Dhillon OS, O'Brien RJ, Struck J, Quinn PA, Morgenthaler NG, et al. C-terminal provasopressin (copeptin) as a novel and prognostic marker in acute myocardial infarction: Leicester Acute Myocardial Infarction Peptide (LAMP) study. *Circulation*. 2007;115:2103-10.

34. Reichlin T, Hochholzer W, Stelzig C, Laule K, Freidank H, Morgenthaler NG, et al. Incremental value of copeptin for rapid rule out of acute myocardial infarction. *J Am Coll Cardiol*. 2009;54:60-8.

35. Jaffe AS, Apple FS. High-sensitivity cardiac troponin: hype, help, and reality. *Clin Chem*. 2010;56:342-4.

36. Schaller MD, Nicod P, Nussberger J, Feihl F, Waeber B, Brunner HR, et al. Vasopressin in acute myocardial infarct: clinical implications. *Schweiz Med Wochenschr*. 1986;116: 1727-9.

37. McAlpine HM, Morton JJ, Leckie B, Rumley A, Gillen G, Dargie HJ. Neuroendocrine activation after acute myocardial infarction. *Br Heart J*. 1988;60:117-24.

38. Donald RA, Crozier IG, Foy SG, Richards AM, Livesey JH, Ellis MJ, et al. Plasma corticotrophin releasing hormone, vasopressin, ACTH and cortisol responses to acute myocardial infarction. *Clin Endocrinol (Oxf)*. 1994;40:499-504.

39. Charles CJ, Rogers SJ, Donald RA, Ikram H, Prickett T, Richards AM. Hypothalamo-pituitary-adrenal axis response to coronary artery embolization: an ovine model of acute myocardial infarction. *J Endocrinol*. 1997;152:489-93.

40. Katan M, Morgenthaler N, Widmer I, Puder JJ, Konig C, Muller B, et al. Copeptin, a stable peptide derived from the vasopressin precursor, correlates with the individual stress level. *Neuro Endocrinol Lett*. 2008;29:341-6.

41. Stoiser B, Mortl D, Hulsmann M, Berger R, Struck J, Morgenthaler NG, et al. Copeptin, a fragment of the vasopressin precursor, as a novel predictor of outcome in heart failure. *Eur J Clin Invest*. 2006;36:771-8.

42. Gegenhuber A, Struck J, Dieplinger B, Poelz W, Pacher R, Morgenthaler NG, et al. Comparative evaluation of B-type natriuretic peptide, mid-regional pro-A-type natriuretic peptide, mid-regional pro-adrenomedullin, and copeptin to predict 1-year mortality in patients with acute destabilized heart failure. *J Card Fail*. 2007;13:42-9.

43. Kelly D, Squire IB, Khan SQ, Quinn P, Struck J, Morgenthaler NG, et al. C-terminal provasopressin (copeptin) is associated with left ventricular dysfunction, remodeling, and clinical heart failure in survivors of myocardial infarction. *J Card Fail*. 2008;14: 739-45.

44. Fukuzawa J, Haneda T, Kikuchi K. Arginine vasopressin increases the rate of protein synthesis in isolated perfused adult rat heart via the V1 receptor. *Mol Cell Biochem*. 1999;195:93-8.

45. Goldsmith SR. Vasopressin as vasopressor. *Am J Med*. 1987;82:1213-9.

46. Fan YH, Zhao LY, Zheng QS, Dong H, Wang HC, Yang XD. Arginine vasopressin increases iNOS-NO system activity in cardiac fibroblasts through NF-kappa B activation and its relation with myocardial fibrosis. *Life Sci*. 2007;81:327-35.

47. Konstam MA, Gheorghiade M, Burnett JC Jr, Grinfeld L, Maggioni AP, Swedberg K, et al. Effects of oral tolvaptan in patients hospitalized for worsening heart failure: the EVEREST Outcome Trial. *JAMA*. 2007;297:1319-31.

48. Gheorghiade M, Konstam MA, Burnett JC Jr, Grinfeld L, Maggioni AP, Swedberg K, et al. Short-term clinical effects of tolvaptan, an oral vasopressin antagonist, in patients hospitalized for heart failure: the EVEREST Clinical Status Trials. *JAMA*. 2007;297:1332-43.

49. Wada K, Fujimori A, Matsukawa U, Arai Y, Sudoh K, Yatsu T, et al. Intravenous administration of conivaptan hydrochloride improves cardiac hemodynamics in rats with myocardial infarction-induced congestive heart failure. *Eur J Pharmacol*. 2005; 507:145-51.

50. Voors AA, von Haehling S, Anker SD, Hillege HL, Struck J, Hartmann O, et al. C-terminal provasopressin (copeptin) is a strong prognostic marker in patients with heart failure after an acute myocardial infarction: results from the OPTIMAAL study. *Eur Heart J*. 2009;30:1187-94.

51. Neuhold S, Huelsmann M, Strunk G, Stoiser B, Struck J, Morgenthaler NG, et al. Comparison of copeptin, B-type natriuretic peptide, and amino-terminal pro-B-type natriuretic peptide in patients with chronic heart failure: prediction of death at different stages of the disease. *J Am Coll Cardiol*. 2008;52:266-72.

52. Serradeil-Le Gal C, Wagnon J, Valette G, Garcia G, Pascal M, Maffrand JP, et al. Nonpeptide vasopressin receptor antagonists: development of selective and orally active V1a, V2, and V1b receptor ligands. *Prog Brain Res*. 2002;139:197-210.

53. Golestaneh L, Talreja A, Le Jemtel TH. Vasopressin antagonists in heart failure. *Curr Heart Fail Rep*. 2004;1:190-6.

54. Schrier RW, Gross P, Gheorghiade M, Berl T, Verbalis JG, Czerwiec FS, et al. Tolvaptan, a selective oral vasopressin V2-receptor antagonist, for hyponatremia. *N Engl J Med*. 2006;355:2099-112.

55. Maisel A, Mueller C, Nowak R, Peacock WF, Landsberg JW, Ponikowski P, et al. Mid-region pro-hormone markers for diagnosis and prognosis in acute dyspnea: results from the BACH (Biomarkers in Acute Heart Failure) trial. *J Am Coll Cardiol*. 2010;55:2062-76.

56. Maisel A, Xue Y, Shah K, Mueller C, Nowak R, Peacock WF, et al. Increased 90-day mortality in acute heart failure patients with elevated copeptin: secondary results from the biomarkers in acute heart failure (BACH) study. *Cric Heart Fail*. 2011. Epub ahead of print.

57. Gerbes AL, Gulberg V, Gines P, Decaux G, Gross P, Gandjini H, et al. Therapy of hyponatremia in cirrhosis with a vasopressin receptor antagonist: a randomized double-blind multicenter trial. *Gastroenterology*. 2003;124:933-9.

58. Bouby N, Bachmann S, Bichet D, Bankir L. Effect of water intake on the progression of chronic renal failure in the 5/6 nephrectomized rat. *Am J Physiol*. 1990;258:F973-9.

59. Sugiura T, Yamauchi A, Kitamura H, Matsuoka Y, Horio M, Imai E, et al. High water intake ameliorates tubulointerstitial injury in rats with subtotal nephrectomy: possible role of TGF-beta. *Kidney Int*. 1999; 55:1800-10.

60. Bardoux P, Bruneval P, Heudes D, Bouby N, Bankir L. Diabetes-induced albuminuria: role of antidiuretic hormone as revealed by chronic V2 receptor antagonism in rats. *Nephrol Dial Transplant*. 2003;18:1755-63.

61. Katan M, Fluri F, Morgenthaler NG, Schuetz P, Zweifel C, Bingisser R, et al. Copeptin: a novel, independent prognostic marker in patients with ischemic stroke. *Ann Neurol*. 2009;66:799-808.

Index

Page numbers with *t* and *f* indicate table and figure, respectively; page numbers in bold refer to formal discussion.